PRINCIPLES OF INTERNAL MEDICINE

Prof. (Dr.) Sujata K. Das and
Dr Ankush Chandra

ALLIED
HEALTH
PRESS

Principles of Internal Medicine

***Authors:* Prof. (Dr.) Sujata K. Das and Dr Ankush Chandra**

Allied Health Press
4164 Lakeshore Road
Burlington ON L7L 1A4
Canada
www.alliedhealthpress.com
Email: orders@arclereducation.com

ISBN: 978-1-77956-224-1

ABOUT THE AUTHORS

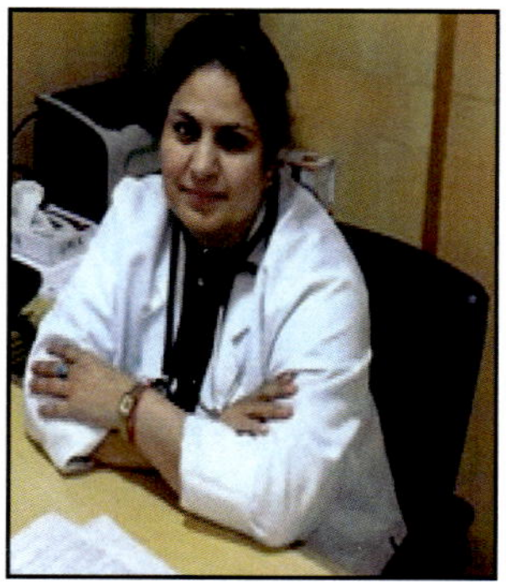

Prof (Dr) Sujata K. Dass, M.B.B.S, D.N.B, Ph.D. (Medicine) is a distinguished neuro-physician and academician, currently serving as an Attending Consultant in the Department of Neurology, B.L. Kapur Hospital, a renowned super-specialty medical institution in the New Delhi. Her illustrious career in medicine and research spans over three decades, characterized by her profound contributions to neurology and her unwavering commitment to medical education.

Dr. Dass began her educational journey at Flushing High School in New York, USA, and completed her High School Diploma thereafter she joined Queens College of the City University of New York as an undergrad student. With a passion for medicine, she pursued her MBBS degree at King George Medical College, Lucknow, U.P., India. Her academic prowess and dedication to medicine were evident early on, setting the stage for a remarkable career. Dr Dass worked under the supervision of Dr M.S. Bains, M.D. as a Visiting Fellow in cardio-thoracic surgery at Memorial Sloan Kettering Cancer Research Center, New York, USA. Dr. Dass furthered her medical training by obtaining a D.N.B. (Family Medicine) and conducted significant research on hematological changes in malaria. Her quest for knowledge and excellence led her back to New York, where she completed her Ph.D. (Medicine) at the Department of Obstetrics & Gynecology, The New York Hospital-Cornell University Medical Center under the mentorship of Prof. Brij B. Saxena. Her groundbreaking work on Sn-Proto and Sn-Mesoporphyrin and the chemoprevention of neonatal jaundice culminated in the award of her D.Sc. (Medicine).

Dr. Sujata Dass joined as the BR Ambedkar Chair Professor in July 2002 in the Institute of Biomedical Sciences, Faculty of Medicine, Bundelkhand University, Jhansi. Her tenure was marked by her dedication to advancing medical research and education. She also served as UGC National Research Award (Professor) at V.P. Chest Institute, University of Delhi. Throughout her career, Dr. Dass has received numerous awards and accolades on a global level. Notable among these are the UGC Research Award, the Fast Track Young Scientist Award from the Department of Science and Technology (DST), and the Women's Award of Highest Honour from Soka University, Japan. She has also received numerous research grants from DST, DBT and ICMR, UGC etc. These awards and grants underscore her exceptional contributions to medical science and research.

Dr. Dass is a respected member of various scientific and administrative bodies like Planning Board (IGNOU), Executive Council - Bhagat Phool Singh Mahila Vishwavidhlaya, Haryana (2008-2011) where she continues to influence the medical community with her insights and expertise. Her commitment to guiding and mentoring students in their master's and doctoral thesis highlights her dedication to nurturing the next generation of medical professionals. Dr. Dass remains a beacon of excellence and a role model for aspiring medical professionals worldwide.

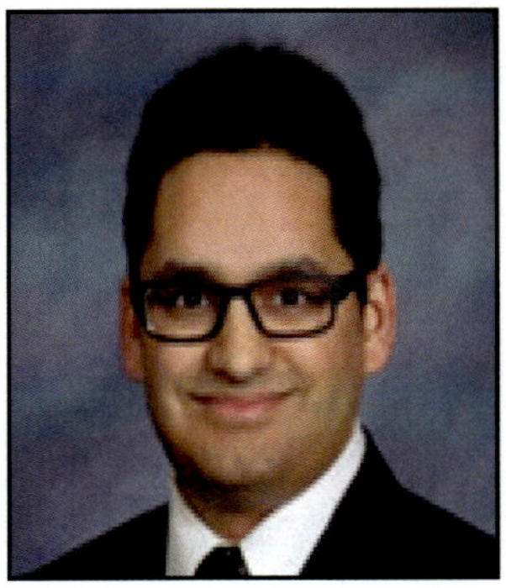

Dr Ankush Chandra, M.D., M.S. born in New York on 19th August 1989, grew up in Boston, Massachusetts, a distinguished neurological surgeon. He has made significant contributions to the field of neuroscience and neurosurgery. Ankush received his Doctor of Medicine (M.D.) degree in Neurological Surgery from Wayne State University School of Medicine, Detroit, Michigan and graduated with honors in Biomedical Research. This accolade was conferred upon him during a special convocation. Dr Chandra also holds a Master of Science (MS) degree in Medical Sciences from Boston University School of Medicine, Boston, MA, and a Bachelor's degree (BA) in Neuroscience and Biology from Boston University. His academic journey is marked by excellence and dedication, reflected in numerous awards and honors.

Ankush's research career began as a Research Fellow at Massachusetts General Hospital (MGH) Harvard University School of Medicine, Boston where he made significant contributions to neuroscience research. He also served as a Research Fellow at Merrimack Pharmaceuticals, Inc. in Cambridge, MA. One of the most notable achievements of Dr Chandra is being awarded the prestigious Howard Hughes Medical Institute (HHMI) Medical Research Fellowship in Neurosurgery at the University of California, San Francisco (UCSF) School of Medicine, spanning from 2016 to 2023. This fellowship is one of the highest honors for a young investigator in the United States.

Dr Chandra has received numerous accolades throughout his career, including the Comprehensive Academic Honors, Howard Hughes Medical Institute Medical Research Fellowship (HHMI), AOA Carolyn Kuckein Research Award, AANS Medical Student Research Fellowship, BCBS Michigan Research Award, Ralph Wadley MD Scholarship, BMA Endowed Scholarship, Wayne State Board of Governors Scholarship, Sarah and John Tait Endowed Scholarship for Cancer Research, Robert F. Troxley Award in Biochemistry, Boston University Scarlet Key Award, Commitment to Residence Life Award, Distinction in Neuroscience, and the Summer Undergraduate Research Grant. He is also a member of the prestigious Alpha Omega Alpha (AOA) Medical Honor Society. He has published more than 100 original research papers in prestigious journals, such as- JAMA Oncology, Lancet Neurology, Proceedings of the National Academy of Sciences (PNAS), Cancer Research, Journal of Neuro-Oncology, Journal of Clinical Investigation (JCI), Journal of Neuroscience, and Journal of Neurosurgery. Additionally, he has edited two volumes of the book titled "Makers of Indian History".

Dr Chandra's early interest in medicine and research was evident during his summer internship in 2007 at the New York-Presbyterian Hospital of Weill Cornell Medical College, where he was trained under the guidance of Prof. Brij B. Saxena in the laboratory of Reproductive Endocrinology, Department of Obstetrics & Gynecology. This experience provided him with a solid foundation in understanding the immunological and molecular mechanisms involved in hypothalamic-pituitary-gonadal regulation and function, after completing his High School with distinction from Springdale's School, New Delhi, India in 2007. Currently, Dr Ankush Chandra is pursuing a challenging career in Neurological Surgery at McGovern Medical School, University of Texas Health Sciences Center, Houston, Texas. He specializes in glioblastoma and brain surgery, continuing his dedication to advancing medical science and improving patient outcomes.

Dr Ankush Chandra has also served as the President and Captain of the Boston University Cricket Club, Chief Curriculum Officer-Innoworks United Academy at Boston University

Word Roots, Prefixes, and Suffixes by Chapter

Chapter 1 Infectious Diseases

hyper-: excessive (e.g., hyperthermia)
hypo-: below normal (e.g., hypothermia)
-itis: inflammation (e.g., tonsillitis)
-emia: blood condition (e.g., bacteremia)
-osis: abnormal condition (e.g., tuberculosis)
-phobia: fear of (e.g., germophobia)

Chapter 2 Respiratory System Disorders

brady-: slow (e.g., bradypnea)
a-/ an-: without (e.g., apnea)
dys-: abnormal, difficult (e.g., dyspnea)
-oxia: oxygen (e.g., hypoxia)
-ectasis: dilation (e.g., bronchiectasis)
-otomy: cutting (e.g., tracheotomy)

Chapter 3 Diseases of the Cardiovascular System

endo-: within (e.g., endocarditis)
hyper-: high (e.g., hypertension)
hypo-: low (e.g., hypotension)
-oma: tumor, mass (e.g., angioma)
-sclerosis: hardening (e.g., arteriosclerosis)
-pathy: disease (e.g., cardiomyopathy)

Chapter 4 Chronic Kidney Diseases

poly-: many, excessive (e.g., polyuria)
hyper-: high (e.g., hyperkalemia)
hypo-: low (e.g., hypokalemia)
-uria: urine (e.g., proteinuria)
-emia: blood condition (e.g., azotemia)
-lithiasis: presence of stones (e.g., nephrolithiasis)
-lysis: breakdown (e.g., dialysis)

Chapter 5 Diseases of the Gastrointestinal System

hyper-: above normal (e.g., hyperbilirubinemia)
peri-: surrounding (e.g., peritonitis)
sub-: under, below (e.g., subhepatic)
-itis: inflammation (e.g., appendicitis)
-stomy: surgical opening (e.g., colostomy)
-ectomy: removal (e.g., gastrectomy)
-algia: pain (e.g., gastralgia)

Chapter 6 Hematological Disorders

hypo-: low (e.g., hypochromic)
hyper-: high (e.g., hyperchromic)
auto-: self (e.g., autoimmune)
-emia: blood condition (e.g., anemia)
-penia: deficiency (e.g., neutropenia)
-cytosis: increase in cells (e.g., leukocytosis)
-philia: attraction to (e.g., eosinophilia)

Chapter 7 Metabolic Syndrome

hyper-: excessive (e.g., hyperglycemia)
hypo-: low (e.g., hypoglycemia)
dys-: abnormal (e.g., dyslipidemia)
poly-: many, excessive (e.g., polyphagia)
-emia: blood condition (e.g., hyperlipidemia)
-osis: condition, often abnormal (e.g., ketoacidosis)
-lysis: breakdown (e.g., lipolysis)
-oma: tumor (e.g., insulinoma)

Chapter 8 Aging and Neurological Disorders

a-/ an-: without (e.g., aphasia)
dys-: abnormal, difficult (e.g., dysphagia)
poly-: many (e.g., polyneuropathy)
neuro-: nerve (e.g., neuropathy)
-pathy: disease (e.g., neuropathy)
-plegia: paralysis (e.g., hemiplegia)
-trophy: nourishment, development (e.g., atrophy)
-algesia: pain (e.g., analgesia)

Table of Contents

LIST OF FIGURES

Figure 8.6. Neurological diseases may be linked to alterations that occur during the senescence process. The molecular-level pathological changes impact the cells of the aging organism, resulting in systemic deterioration and the development of age-related neurological diseases. Reactive oxygen species, white matter (WM), and gray matter (GM) are three distinct components of the brain

LIST OF TABLES

PREFACE

Internists are uniquely positioned to detect underlying diseases that might have been missed in early evaluations due to their extensive knowledge, ensuring timely and appropriate patient care. These specialists are at the forefront of managing chronic conditions such as diabetes, hypertension, and asthma, thanks to their comprehensive training, which provides a holistic view of the body's functioning. All physicians specializing in internal medicine undergo foundational training specific to internal medicine, which prepares them for various subspecialties within the field. Their special training equips them to tackle diagnostic challenges, manage severe chronic illnesses, and care for patients with complex, multiple health issues.

Internal medicine physicians are adept critical thinkers who thrive in challenging and dynamic environments. Their deep understanding of the body's internal and external connections allows them to integrate diverse data sets—including lifestyle, symptoms, existing conditions, and medications—in clinical and non-clinical settings. They excel in making sense of the healthcare landscape, interpreting information from colleagues, and identifying patient outcomes to deliver optimal care.

Their expertise naturally positions them as leaders within team-based care, often sought after by other medical professionals for their problem-solving abilities and capacity to identify solutions. The versatility of internal medicine opens doors to various career paths across multiple settings and disciplines, including healthcare leadership roles. Internal medicine training fosters leadership and collaboration skills, applicable across a wide spectrum of professions throughout one's career.

Internal medicine physicians are pivotal in shaping healthcare policy, advocating for meaningful change, and influencing decision-makers within the healthcare system. They are found in various roles, including hospitalists, subspecialists, CEOs, educators, and policymakers, contributing significantly both nationally and locally. This specialty provides a platform for enacting significant change in healthcare settings, leveraging their comprehensive knowledge, analytical skills, and leadership capabilities.

For patients, physicians specializing in internal medicine are invaluable, offering thorough, knowledgeable guidance through adult life and ensuring access to high-quality care. They navigate patients through the complexities of the healthcare system, connecting them with necessary resources and optimizing patient care processes at the organizational level. Their advocacy extends to healthcare policy, where they utilize their knowledge and skills to advance public health initiatives globally. As the healthcare landscape evolves, the broad perspective and in-depth understanding of physicians specializing in internal medicine become increasingly crucial. They lead in designing solutions that enhance access, reduce costs, improve quality, and eliminate disparities in care. Internal medicine's adaptability as a specialty underscores its significant role in shaping the future of healthcare, influencing policy, educating the next generation, and solving complex health issues.

The aim of this book "Internal Medicine" is to provide an exhaustive overview of the field, equipping readers with the knowledge and skills necessary to diagnose, manage, and treat a wide range of complex adult diseases. This comprehensive resource is designed to cover the breadth of internal medicine, including the latest advancements in medical science, evidence-based treatment strategies, and innovative approaches to patient care. It aims to bridge the gap between theoretical knowledge and practical application, enabling healthcare professionals to apply learned concepts in real-world clinical settings.

The readership for this book primarily includes internal medicine physicians, both practicing and in training, such as residents and fellows who seek to deepen their understanding of internal medicine. Additionally, it serves as a valuable resource for medical students pursuing a career in internal medicine, offering a solid foundation in the specialty. The book is also relevant for healthcare professionals in related fields, such as nurse practitioners, physician assistants, and specialists who collaborate closely with internists, providing them with insights into the holistic and patient-centered approach characteristic of internal medicine. Through this book, readers are expected to enhance their clinical acumen, improve patient outcomes, and contribute to the advancement of healthcare in the field of internal medicine.

Chapter

INFECTIOUS DISEASES 1

Contents

Introduction

Infectious diseases are a broad category of illnesses caused by various microorganisms, including bacteria, viruses, fungi, and parasites. Despite remarkable strides in the prevention and treatment of these diseases over the past decades, they continue to be a leading cause of morbidity and mortality globally, particularly in less developed regions. These diseases significantly impair quality of life, exacerbating poverty and deteriorating living conditions for countless individuals. Clinicians often face challenges in diagnosing infectious diseases, as they can mimic a wide array of conditions affecting numerous organ systems. The infectious diseases can be transmitted through various means, including contaminated water supplies (e.g., cholera) or person-to-person contact (e.g., tuberculosis). The risk of acquiring an infectious disease is influenced by a complex interplay of host, environmental, and microbial factors.

Orientation and Directional Terms

Term	Definition	Illustration
Infectious Diseases	Diseases caused by pathogenic microorganisms, such as bacteria, viruses, parasites, or fungi, that can spread, directly or indirectly, from one person to another.	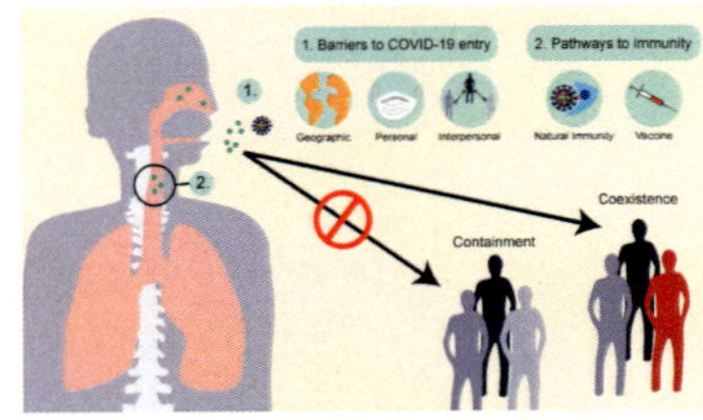
Malaria	A mosquito-borne infectious disease caused by Plasmodium parasites, leading to fever, chills, and flu-like symptoms.	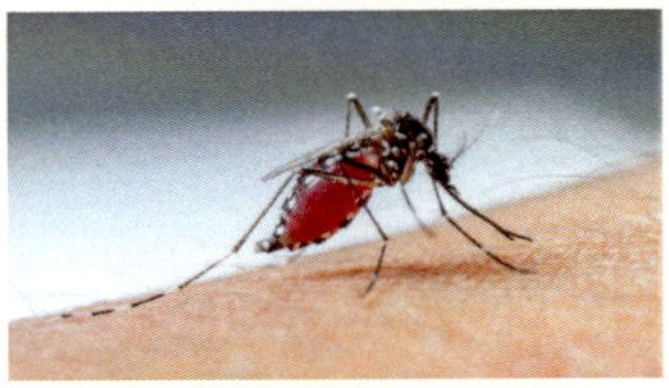
Typhoid (Enteric) Fever	A bacterial infection caused by *Salmonella typhi*, characterized by high fever, weakness, stomach pain, and headache, typically transmitted through contaminated food and water.	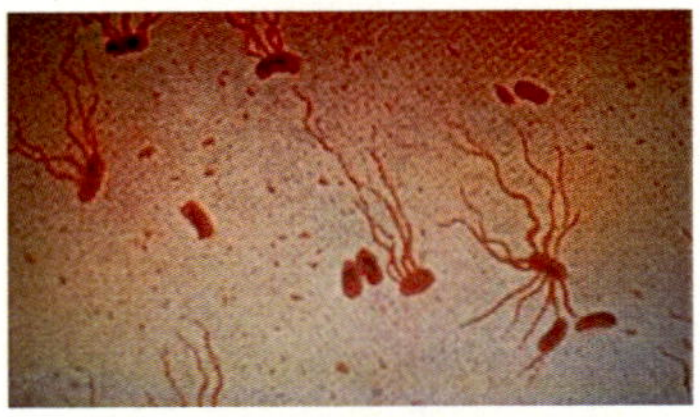
Relapsing Fever	A bacterial infection caused by *Borrelia* species, characterized by recurring episodes of fever, often spread by lice or ticks.	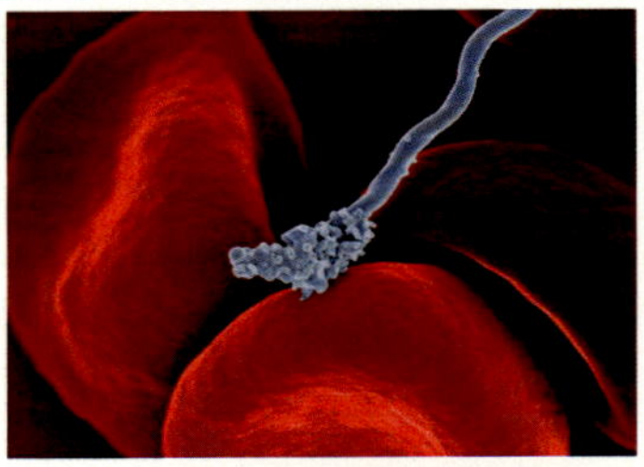
Rickettsial Diseases	A group of infectious diseases caused by *Rickettsia* bacteria, transmitted through the bite of infected ticks, mites, or lice, leading to fever, headache, and rash.	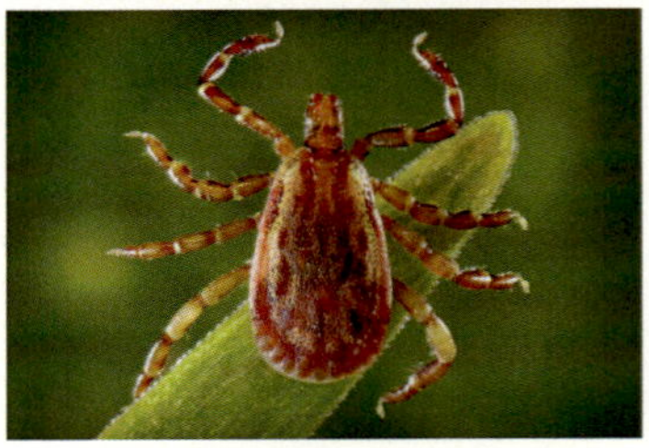

1.1. Host and Environmental Factors Influencing Infectious Diseases

For an infection to manifest, the pathogen must come into contact with the host. This interaction is heavily influenced by various factors, such as geographic location (e.g., the prevalence of malaria in high-altitude regions), environmental conditions (e.g., the existence of breeding grounds for malaria-carrying mosquitoes), disease vectors, and individual behaviors (e.g., practices leading to sexually transmitted infections). Host-specific factors, including age, immunization history, previous illnesses, nutritional status, pregnancy, coexisting conditions, and emotional well-being, can also significantly impact the susceptibility to infections (Figure 1.1).

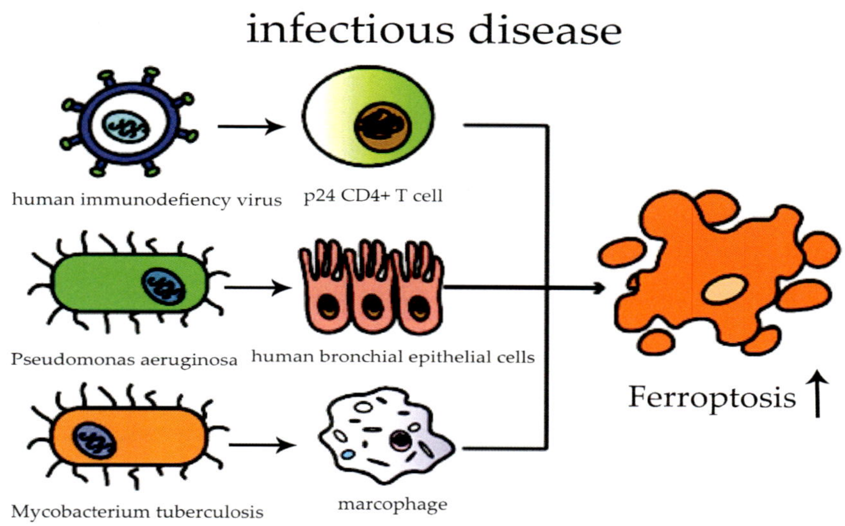

Figure 1.1. *Various pathogenic microorganisms engage in the pathogenesis of infectious diseases by inducing ferroptosis in different cells.*

Source: https://www.researchgate.net/.

Medical interventions themselves may elevate a patient's risk of infection through exposure to pathogens in healthcare settings, procedures involving injections and surgical incisions, the use of medical devices like endotracheal tubes and bladder catheters, the introduction of foreign objects into the body, alterations to the body's natural microbial flora due to antibiotic use, and the administration of immunosuppressive medications such as steroids.

1.1.1. Microbial Factors and the Dynamics of Infection

The pathogenesis of infectious diseases involves a sophisticated interplay between the pathogen and the host, impacting both entities. Pathogens typically undergo a series of steps to establish an infection, with each step requiring specific strategies to overcome the host's defense mechanisms. These strategies vary across different classes of microorganisms and even among species within a class.

1. **Invasion:** Microorganisms often initiate infection by adhering to and penetrating mucosal surfaces, employing mechanisms such as transcytosis, as observed with meningococci and gonococci.
2. **Tropism:** Successful pathogens exhibit tropism, targeting specific sites or cell types within the host. For instance, malaria parasites specifically invade liver cells before infecting red blood cells.
3. **Microbial Virulence Strategies:** Pathogens deploy various tactics to evade the host's immune response, including the production of toxins and enzymes that facilitate invasion and disease progression. Many bacteria also possess protective capsules that enable them to evade immune detection in the absence of specific antibodies.

1.1.2. The Host's Immune Response to Infection

The immune system employs two primary strategies to combat infectious agents: innate (or natural) immunity and acquired (or adaptive) immunity. Innate immunity provides immediate, nonspecific defense without prior exposure to the pathogen, involving barriers like skin and mucous membranes, phagocytosis by immune cells, and the complement system. Acquired immunity develops specific responses to particular pathogens over time, creating a memory that enhances the body's ability to respond to future exposures. It includes cellular immunity, mediated by T-lymphocytes and NK cells, and humoral immunity, involving B-lymphocytes and antibodies (Figure 1.2).

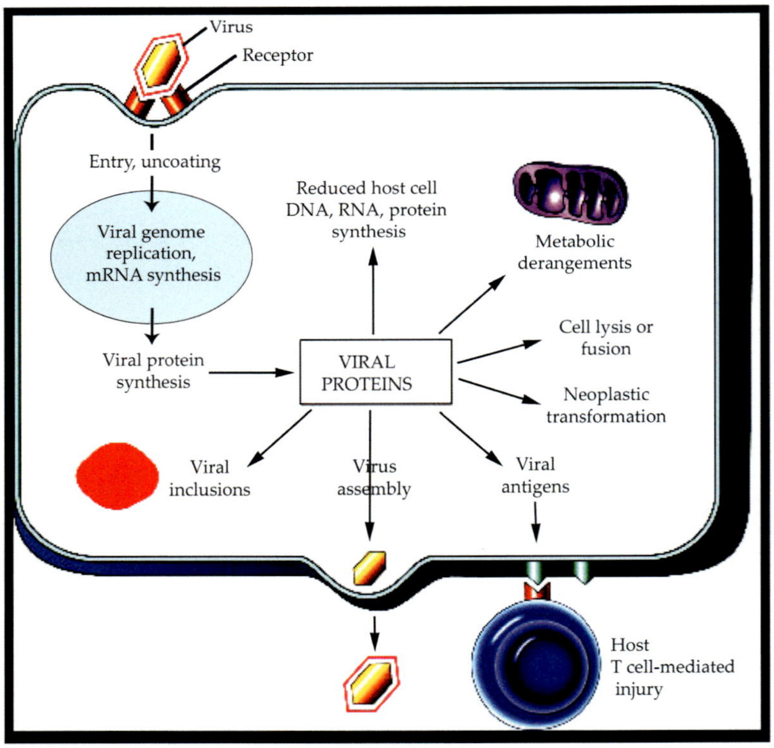

Figure 1.2. *Infection and host response.*

Source: https://ars.els-cdn.com/.

1.1.3. Laboratory Diagnosis and Treatment of Infectious Diseases

Diagnosing infections typically involves direct methods, such as microscopic examination of clinical specimens (e.g., blood films for malaria) or culture techniques, and indirect methods, such as serological tests for detecting antibodies against specific pathogens. Effective treatment requires comprehensive medical knowledge and astute clinical judgment. While some life-threatening infections necessitate immediate treatment, sometimes even before identifying the particular pathogen, other situations may call for a more cautious approach, delaying antimicrobial therapy until a precise diagnosis is confirmed. Additionally, some infections, like peritonitis and abscesses, may require surgical intervention, with antibiotics serving an adjunct role in treatment.

1.2. Acute Febrile Illnesses

1.2.1. Malaria

1.2.1.1. Etiology of Malaria

Malaria, a protozoal disease of significant global health concern, is caused by genus *Plasmodium*, with four species predominantly responsible for human infection: *Plasmodium falciparum* (known for causing malignant or severe malaria), *P. vivax* and *P. ovale* (both leading to tertian malaria), and *P. malariae* (resulting in quartan malaria). It is noteworthy that *P. falciparum* is the most lethal, accounting for the majority of malaria-related deaths worldwide (Figure 1.3).

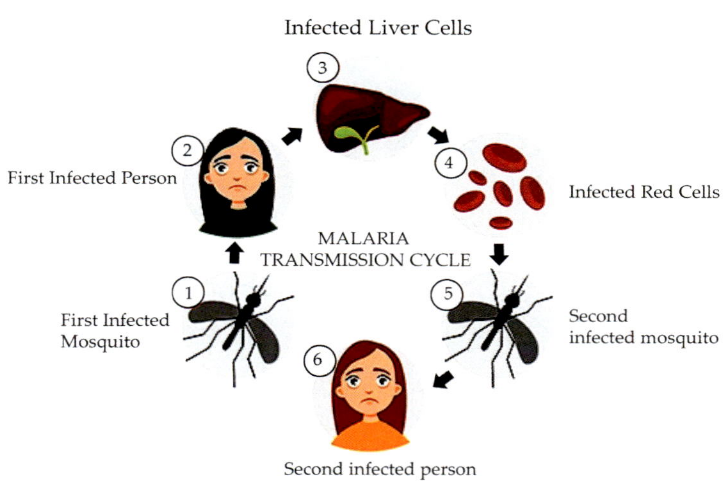

Figure 1.3. *Etiology of malaria.*

Source: https://www.medicoverhospitals.in/.

1.2.1.2. Epidemiology of Malaria

Malaria stands as one of the most prevalent infectious diseases, affecting approximately 500 million individuals annually and resulting in around 2 million fatalities. Approximately 40% of the global population, particularly those in tropical and subtropical regions, are at risk of malaria. The disease's incidence is on an upward trend, fueled by the emergence of DDT-resistant Anopheles mosquitoes, Plasmodium strains resistant to anti-malarial drugs, and alterations in global weather patterns, which may exacerbate the conditions conducive to mosquito breeding and survival.

Epidemic outbreaks of malaria are frequent in highland areas, with significant seasonal peaks observed. In countries like Ethiopia, malaria's presence is widespread, affecting a substantial portion of the population across various regions. The epidemiological distribution of malaria is determined by factors such as splenic rates in children, leading to the categorization of regions into hypo-endemic, meso-endemic, hyper-endemic, and holo-endemic based on the percentage of children with palpable spleens. These classifications reflect the intensity of malaria transmission and the population's immunity level, which varies from high in holo- and hyper-endemic areas (characterized by stable transmission) to low in hypo- and meso-endemic areas (where transmission is unstable).

1.2.1.3. Transmission of Malaria

The primary mode of malaria transmission is through the bite of infected female Anopheles mosquitoes. These mosquitoes serve as vectors, transferring the Plasmodium parasites from their salivary glands into the human bloodstream during a blood meal. Environmental conditions such as high temperatures and the availability of stagnant water bodies are crucial for mosquito breeding and, consequently, malaria transmission. Transmission patterns are highly influenced by seasonal variations, with increased incidence during rainy seasons and among populations that lack immunity to the disease.

1.2.1.4. Life Cycle and Pathogenesis of Malaria

The Plasmodium parasite's life cycle is complex, comprising both asexual and sexual phases that occur in humans and mosquitoes, respectively. The human phase of the infection begins when sporozoites are introduced into the bloodstream by a mosquito bite, subsequently migrating to the liver, where they replicate within hepatocytes, producing thousands of merozoites. These merozoites then enter the bloodstream, infecting red blood cells and leading to the symptomatic phase of malaria. *P. vivax* and *P. ovale* are unique in that they can form dormant stages (hypnozoites) in the liver, causing relapses of the disease months or even years after the initial infection (Figure 1.4).

Within red blood cells, the merozoites undergo further development, eventually rupturing the cells and releasing new merozoites into the bloodstream, which perpetuates the infection cycle. This process not only results in anemia due to the destruction of red blood cells but also contributes to the enlargement of the spleen due to its role in clearing infected and damaged cells from circulation. *P. falciparum* is particularly notorious for causing severe disease due to its ability to induce infected red blood cells to adhere to the endothelial lining of blood vessels and form clumps with uninfected cells, disrupting microcirculation and leading to severe complications.

Some Plasmodium parasites develop into gametocytes, the sexual stage capable of infecting mosquitoes and perpetuating the transmission cycle. When a mosquito feeds on an infected individual, it ingests these gametocytes, which then undergo sexual reproduction in the mosquito's gut, eventually leading to the production of new sporozoites that migrate to the mosquito's salivary glands, ready to infect another human host.

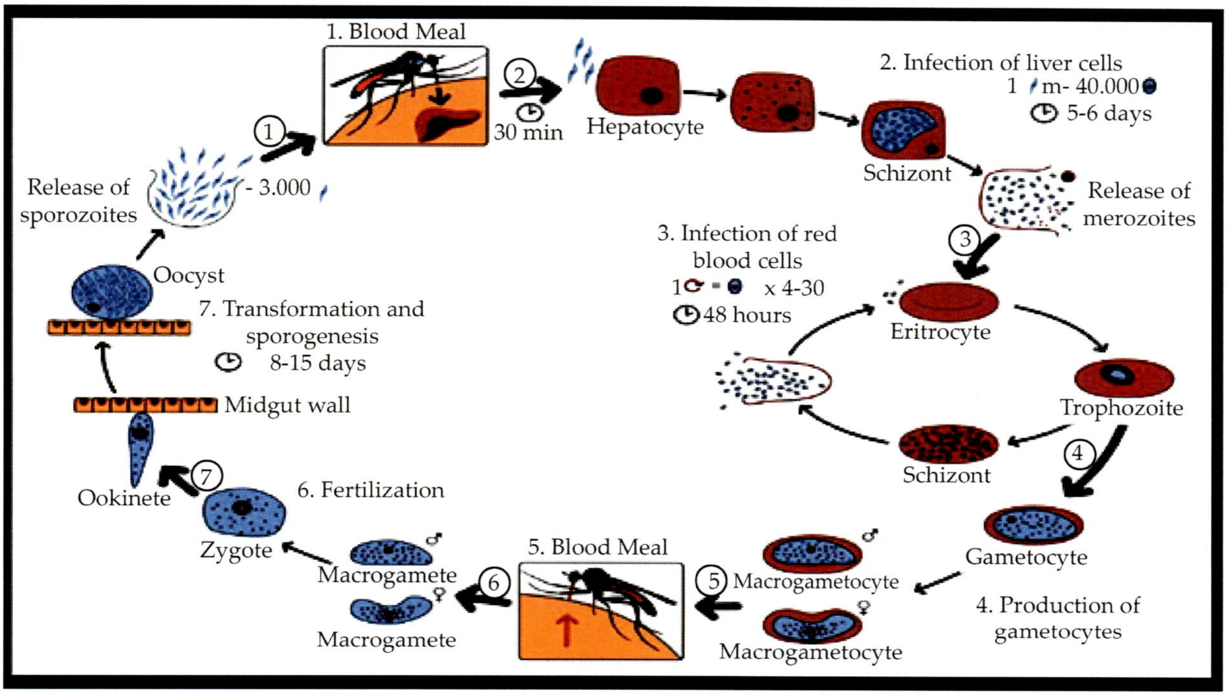

Figure 1.4. *Life cycle and pathogenesis of malaria.*

Source: https://akm-img-a-in.tosshub.com/.

1.2.1.5. Clinical Features and Incubation Period

Malaria's clinical manifestations are highly variable and deeply influenced by the species of Plasmodium parasite responsible for the infection. The incubation period, or the interval from the infecting mosquito bite to the appearance of symptoms, is a critical phase that varies significantly among the different malaria-causing Plasmodium species. For infections caused by *P. vivax*, *P. ovale*, and *P. falciparum*, symptoms typically emerge within 10 to 14 days post-bite. In contrast, *P. malariae* has a longer incubation period, with symptoms appearing anywhere from 18 days to six weeks after the mosquito bite. This variance in incubation periods is indicative of the distinct biological and pathological characteristics of each Plasmodium species, which in turn influence the clinical presentation and progression of the disease.

1.2.1.6. Diverse Clinical Presentations of Malaria

Upon the culmination of the incubation period, the clinical manifestations of malaria begin to surface. Common symptoms across all forms of malaria include fever, chills, sweats, headaches, nausea and vomiting, body aches, and general malaise. These symptoms are often cyclic in nature, corresponding to the life cycle of the parasites within the red blood cells. The severity and specific features of the disease, however, can vary dramatically depending on the infecting species:

1. ***P. falciparum***: Known for causing the most severe form of malaria, *P. falciparum* infections can lead to life-threatening complications such as cerebral malaria, severe anemia,

and respiratory distress. Symptoms can rapidly progress to severe illness without timely treatment.

2. ***P. vivax* and *P. ovale***: Infections with these species are typically characterized by tertian fever patterns, with fevers spiking every 48 hours. These forms of malaria are generally less severe than those caused by *P. falciparum* but can be complicated by relapses due to dormant liver stages known as hypnozoites.
3. ***P. malariae***: This species causes quartan malaria, with fever patterns occurring every 72 hours. *P. malariae* infections are typically milder than those caused by *P. falciparum* but can persist for extended periods, sometimes leading to chronic complications such as nephrotic syndrome.

1.2.1.7. Complications and Severity

The severity of malaria and its complications can vary widely among individuals and is influenced by a variety of factors, including the Plasmodium species, the patient's immune status, and the presence of any coexisting conditions. Complications can range from mild anemia and jaundice to severe malaria characterized by organ failure, cerebral involvement, and death.

1.2.1.8. Diagnosis and Management

Given the variability in clinical presentations and the potential for severe outcomes, timely and accurate diagnosis of malaria is crucial. Diagnosis typically involves laboratory testing to identify the presence of Plasmodium parasites in the blood. Management strategies vary according to the species of Plasmodium involved and the severity of the disease, encompassing a range of antimalarial medications and supportive care measures. In *P. vivax* and *P. ovale* infections, treatment may also include agents targeting the dormant liver stages to prevent relapses.

1. **Treatment of Uncomplicated Falciparum Malaria:** Due to widespread resistance to chloroquine and sulfadoxine-pyrimethamine, alternative oral drugs are recommended for the treatment of uncomplicated falciparum malaria in tropical countries.

The following treatments are suggested:

i. Artemisinin-based Therapies:

- Artemisinin and its derivatives originate from China and are highly effective in treating falciparum malaria in both adults and children. Common formulations include Artesunate (available for oral or intravenous administration) and Artemether (available for oral or intramuscular administration).
- **Artemether-Lumefantrine (Coartem 20/120):** A widely used option in Ethiopia, combining 20 mg of Artemether with 120 mg of Lumefantrine in a single dose. The recommended dosage is 3 tablets twice daily for 3 days for individuals weighing less than 35 kg, and 4 tablets twice daily for 3 days for those weighing more than 35 kg.
- **Side Effects:** May include dizziness, fatigue, anorexia, nausea, vomiting, abdominal pain, palpitations, myalgia, sleep disorders, arthralgia, headache, and rash.
- **Contraindications:** Not recommended for malaria prophylaxis, individuals with a history of adverse reactions, pregnant women, mothers with infants under three months, and infants under 5 kg.

ii. Quinine:

- For adults, the dose is 600 mg orally

three times a day for 5 to 7 days, either alone or in combination with tetracycline (500 mg four times a day) or doxycycline (100 mg per day) for the same duration.

- **Side Effects:** Includes cinchonism (tinnitus, hearing loss, dizziness, tremor, nausea), restlessness, blurred vision, and hypoglycemia.

iii. Mefloquine:

- Effective against all malaria species, including drug-resistant *P. falciparum*. Initial dose of 15 mg/kg followed by a second dose of 10 mg/kg after 8–12 hours.
- **Side Effects:** Nausea, abdominal cramps, vertigo, insomnia, and in rare cases, acute psychosis, and convulsions.

iv. Sulfadoxine-Pyrimethamine (Fansidar):

- A single dose of 3 tablets (each tablet containing 500 mg sulfadoxine and 25 mg pyrimethamine) is used. Not recommended for children under one year or for treating *P. falciparum* malaria due to high resistance levels.

2. **Treatment of Severe and Complicated Falciparum Malaria:** Severe cases require hospital admission and include:

i. Drug Treatment:

  - **Quinine**: The preferred treatment, administered intravenously where possible. A loading dose of 20 mg/kg over 4 hours, followed by a maintenance dose of 10 mg/kg every 8 hours until oral administration is feasible. For intramuscular administration, a 20 mg/kg loading dose is divided between two sites, followed by 10 mg/kg every 8 hours.
  - **Artesunate Injection:** 2.4 mg/kg IV or IM initially, followed by 1.2 mg/kg at 12 and 24 hours, then daily.

ii. Supportive Treatment:

- Fever reduction strategies and administration of paracetamol.
- IV or oral glucose to prevent hypoglycemia and support early resumption of oral food intake.
- Adequate hydration while monitoring fluid balance to prevent pulmonary edema.
- Consideration for blood transfusion in cases of severe parasitemia.
- Regular monitoring of renal function and blood glucose levels.
- Proper nursing care for unconscious patients, including regular repositioning, bladder catheterization, fluid management, glucose monitoring, and nutritional support.

1.2.1.9. Chronic Complications of Malaria

Tropical Splenomegaly Syndrome (Hyperreactive Malarial Splenomegaly): A condition arising from an abnormal immune response to recurrent malaria infections, commonly observed in individuals from malaria-endemic regions in tropical Africa and Asia. Characteristics include:

1. **Splenomegaly**: Significantly enlarged spleen (greater than 10 cm below the left costal margin), possibly accompanied by hepatomegaly.
2. **Hypersplenism:** Manifestations include anemia and pancytopenia, leading to increased susceptibility to infections.

3. **Immunological Indicators:** Notably high levels of serum IgM and anti-malarial antibodies, hepatic sinusoidal lymphocytes, and peripheral B-cell lymphocytosis.
4. **Clinical Presentation**: Symptoms may include an abdominal mass or sensation of dragging in the left upper quadrant, abdominal pain, and the potential for anemia and pancytopenia. Parasites may not be detectable in peripheral blood films.

Treatment:

1. **Long-Term Antimalarial Prophylaxis:** Utilizing drugs like chloroquine or mefloquine for the duration of exposure to malaria.
2. **Outcomes:** Effective prophylaxis can lead to spleen regression and liver enlargement over months.
3. **Splenectomy:** Considered only when antimalarial prophylaxis fails after at least 6 months of treatment.

Prevention of Malaria:

1. General Measures:

i. Mechanical Barriers/Methods:

- Draining standing water and modifying swampy areas.
- Use of insecticide-treated mosquito nets.
- Installing wire mesh on windows.
- Remaining indoors during peak mosquito activity times.
- Wearing long-sleeved shirts and trousers.

ii. Insecticides or Chemicals:

- Indoor spraying with insecticides such as permethrin, deltamethrin, and chlorinated hydrocarbons.
- Applying insect repellents (e.g., diethyltoluamide) to exposed skin.
  - Spraying DDT inside homes for prolonged mosquito control.

2. **Drug Prophylaxis:** Recommended for specific groups at increased risk, including pregnant women in endemic areas due to their heightened vulnerability to severe malaria, children aged three months to four years from non-immune mothers, and travelers to malaria-endemic regions.

In areas with chloroquine-resistant *P. falciparum*:

- Mefloquine (250 mg weekly), suitable during pregnancy.
- Doxycycline (100 mg daily), not for children under eight years or during pregnancy.
- Maloprim (pyrimethamine + dapsone), once weekly.
- Chloroquine + proguanil as alternatives to mefloquine and doxycycline.

In areas with chloroquine-sensitive *P. falciparum*:

- Chloroquine (2 tabs of 150 mg weekly).
- Chloroquine + proguanil combination as an alternative.

1.3. Typhoid (Enteric) Fever

Definition: Typhoid Fever: It is a systemic infection marked by fever and abdominal pain, caused by the dissemination of *Salmonella typhi*, and occasionally by *S. paratyphi* A, B, and *S. typhimurium*. These agents are non-capsulated, gram-negative, motile bacteria.

Epidemiology:

1. **Hosts:** Only human beings serve as hosts for *S. typhi* and *S. paratyphi*, making enteric fever transmissible exclusively through close contact

with acutely infected individuals or chronic carriers, via the ingestion of contaminated food or water.

2. **Carriers:** Chronic carriers, often with the bacteria harbored in their gallbladder (especially if gallstones are present), act as a source of infection, potentially affecting individuals of all ages and sexes. Enteric fever is endemic in many developing countries.
3. **Risk Groups:** The incidence of typhoid fever is notably higher in AIDS patients compared to the general population.

Pathogenesis: Following the ingestion of contaminated food or drink, *S. typhi* overcomes the gastric barrier, reaching the upper small intestine. Here, the bacteria invade the intestinal epithelium, are engulfed by phagosomes in Peyer's patches, multiply, and then disseminate through the bloodstream, causing transient bacteremia. This leads to colonization of reticuloendothelial tissues (liver, spleen, lymph nodes, bone marrow) by the bacteria. Initial signs and symptoms are minimal or absent. Symptoms like fever and abdominal pain emerge once a significant bacterial load has been achieved. Complications can include inflammation of Peyer's patches, potentially leading to intestinal hemorrhage and perforation, and gallbladder invasion.

Clinical Manifestation:

1. **Incubation Period**: Ranges from 3 to 60 days, with severity depending on the size of the inoculum, the state of the host's defense mechanisms, and disease duration.
2. First Week:

- High-grade fever with a stepladder pattern, becoming persistent.
- Symptoms include headache, malaise, abdominal pain, initially diarrhea or loose stools followed by constipation in adults (diarrhea predominates in children), relative bradycardia, splenomegaly, hepatomegaly, and epistaxis. Rose spots may appear in lighter-skinned individuals.

3. **Second Week**: Continuous fever, with patients appearing severely ill, possibly exhibiting withdrawal, confusion, delirium, or coma.
4. **Third Week:** The "typhoidal state" is characterized by extreme toxemia, disorientation, "pea-soup" diarrhea, and potentially intestinal perforation and hemorrhage.
5. **Fourth Week:** Fever diminishes, leading to resolution of symptoms and significant weight loss. Relapses may occur in approximately 10% of cases.

Complications of Typhoid Fever:

1. Gastrointestinal Complications:

- **Gastrointestinal Perforation and Hemorrhage:** These severe complications can arise during the 3rd or 4th week of illness, potentially developing even as clinical symptoms seem to improve. They pose significant life-threatening risks, requiring prompt medical and surgical intervention.

2. Less Common Complications:

- **Hepatitis:** Inflammation of the liver, affecting its function.
- **Meningitis:** Infection and inflammation of the membranes covering the brain and spinal cord.
- **Arthritis and Osteomyelitis:** Infection-induced inflammation of joints and bones.
- **Parotitis and Orchitis:** Inflammation of the parotid glands and testicles, respectively.
- **Nephritis:** Kidney inflammation, potentially affecting kidney function.
- **Myocarditis:** Inflammation of the

heart muscle, possibly leading to cardiac complications.

- **Bronchitis and Pneumonia:** Respiratory complications due to infection of the bronchi and lungs.

Note: Early diagnosis and treatment can prevent these complications.

3. Chronic Carriers:

- **Incidence:** About 1–5% of patients with enteric fever become asymptomatic chronic carriers, shedding *S. typhi* through urine or stool for more than a year.
- **Risk Factors:** Higher incidence in women and individuals with biliary abnormalities (e.g., gallstones, gallbladder cancer) and other gastrointestinal malignancies.

4. Diagnosis:

- **Indicators:** Persistent fever, relative bradycardia (found in 86% of Ethiopians), and rose spots (observed in 70% of whites and 20% of Ethiopians), alongside leucopenia.
- **Laboratory Tests**:
  - **Blood, Stool, or Urine Culture:** Culturing these specimens can diagnose the disease, with the recovery rate depending on the specimen and the disease's duration. Blood cultures are most effective in the first week.
  - **Widal Test:** Tests for O and H antigens, indicating active infection or past exposure. Its limitations include non-specificity and the requirement of a fourfold rise in titer for a definitive diagnosis.

5. Treatment:

- **Antibiotic Therapy:** Curative, with administration depending on the patient's condition and disease severity. Note that fever may persist for 4–6 days despite effective treatment.
- **First-Line Oral Drugs:** Include 4-amino quinolones (e.g., Ciprofloxacin, Ceftriaxone) for their efficacy against multi-drug resistant typhoid. Restrictions apply to children and pregnant women.
- **Alternatives:** Azithromycin, Chloramphenicol, and Norfloxacin are effective alternatives.
- **Intravenous Drugs:** For critically ill patients or those unable to take oral medications, such as Ceftriaxone.

Antibiotic Treatment Challenges:

- **Multidrug Resistance:** Increasingly reported, necessitating the use of quinolones, azithromycin, or third generation cephalosporins in affected areas.
- **Relapse:** Early antibiotic use is associated with a higher relapse rate due to inhibited immune response development.

1. Chronic Carriers:

- **Treatment:** Extended treatment with Ciprofloxacin or a combination of Ampicillin/Amoxicillin with Probenecid, and possibly Co-trimoxazole with Rifampicin, is recommended.
- **Surgical Intervention:** In some cases, gallbladder resection may be necessary.

2. Prevention and Control:

- **Sanitation Improvement:** Crucial for reducing transmission.
- **Carrier Management:** Identifying and treating chronic carriers and

preventing them from handling food.

- **Vaccination:** Recommended for travelers to endemic areas. The options including the live oral TY21a vaccine and the purified Vi polysaccharide vaccine.

1.4. Relapsing Fever

Relapsing fever is an acute, febrile illness caused by the Borrelia species, characterized by the recurrence of feverish episodes lasting several days, interspersed with symptom-free intervals. This condition encompasses two distinct types:

- **Louse-Borne Relapsing Fever (LBRF)**: Transmitted through the body louse, *Pediculus humanus* var *corporis*.
- **Tick-Borne Relapsing Fever (TBRF)**: Spread by the tick genus *Ornithodoros*.

Etiology: The disease is triggered by *Borrelia* species, spiral-shaped gram-negative bacteria. Each type of relapsing fever is caused by different Borrelia species:

- *B. recurrentis* is responsible for LBRF.
- *B. duttonii* is predominantly associated with TBRF in sub-Saharan Africa. These bacteria can vary their surface antigens, enabling them to evade the host's immune response and cause repeated febrile episodes.

Transmission:

- **LBRF**: Humans contract the disease from infected body lice. The lice become carriers after feeding on the blood of an infected person. Infection occurs when crushed lice contaminate cuts or mucous membranes.
- **TBRF**: Primarily spread through tick bites, with rodents acting as the main reservoir for Borrelia. Infected ticks can pass the bacteria to their offspring, perpetuating the cycle of infection.

Pathophysiology: After entering the human body, Borrelia multiply in the bloodstream, leading to high spirochetal densities during feverish periods and potentially invading organs like the spleen, liver, and central nervous system. The disease's severity is correlated with the density of spirochetes in the blood, while systemic symptoms are due to the release of cytokines. Organ damage, including spleen and liver enlargement and potential complications in the brain, heart, and kidneys, is common.

Clinical Features: Both LBRF and TBRF share similar symptoms, including:

- An incubation period of approximately 7 days.
- Sudden onset of high fever, headache, chills, muscle and joint pain, and insomnia.
- Signs of severe illness such as delirium, tachycardia, dry mouth, and photophobia.
- Physical findings may include hepatosplenomegaly, petechiae, and signs of meningitis.
- Jaundice in later stages of the disease.

Complications: If untreated, the disease can lead to severe complications, especially in individuals with delayed diagnosis. These may include:

- Hemorrhagic manifestations like epistaxis and blood-streaked sputum.
- Neurological complications, including meningitis, coma, and cranial nerve palsies.
- Additional risks include pneumonitis, myocarditis, and splenic rupture.

Treatment within the early stages of the disease can prevent most life-threatening complications. Untreated cases experience intensifying symptoms over 2–7 days, followed by spontaneous resolution. However, without intervention, febrile episodes can recur multiple times.

Diagnosis: The diagnosis of relapsing fever hinges on the visualization of *Borrelia* in blood, bone marrow, or cerebrospinal fluid (CSF) samples.

1. Blood Film Examination:

- **Transmission Mechanism**:
  - **LBRF**: Infection occurs through contamination of mucous membranes or skin abrasions by body fluids from crushed lice. LBRF is not transmitted by lice bites or feces.
  - **TBRF**: Transmission is via the bite of an infected tick, with Borrelia present in the tick's saliva and coxal fluid.
- **Vertical Transmission**:
  - **LBRF**: No vertical transmission.
  - **TBRF**: Yes, ticks can transmit the bacteria to their offspring.
- **Distribution**:
  - **LBRF**: Mainly in East Africa, especially Ethiopia.
  - **TBRF**: Widespread across Sub-Saharan Africa, the Mediterranean, the Middle East, and parts of Russia, India, China, and the USA.
- **Occurrence:**
  - **LBRF**: Epidemics common among the homeless and in crowded, unhygienic conditions.
  - **TBRF**: Occurs sporadically or in small, often familial clusters.
- **Vector Longevity:**
  - **LBRF**: Body lice have a short lifespan.
  - **TBRF**: Ticks can live for over 10 years.
- **Jarisch-Herxheimer Reaction:** More severe in LBRF cases.
- **Eradication:**
  - **LBRF**: Relatively easier due to the vector's characteristics.
  - **TBRF**: More challenging due to ticks' habits, vertical transmission, and longevity.

2. Laboratory Tests:

- Peripheral blood smears, stained with Giemsa or Wright stain, are commonly used, especially in resource-limited settings.
- Borrelia can be observed in blood samples taken during febrile periods before a crisis, with a higher detection rate in LBRF than TBRF.
- Other diagnostic methods include dark field microscopy of unstained blood/ CSF and serologic tests.

Treatment: Antibiotics are effective in treating relapsing fever. LBRF responds well to a single dose, whereas TBRF may require a longer course.

1. Adult Dosage:

- **Oral:** Erythromycin, Tetracycline, Doxycycline, and Chloramphenicol are used for both LBRF and TBRF, with specific dosing schedules.
- **Parenteral:** Penicillin G (procaine) is an option, particularly for patients who cannot tolerate oral medications.

  Delousing is crucial for preventing LBRF transmission and recurrence.

2. Jarisch-Herxheimer Reaction (JHR):

- Occurs within 1–4 hours of the first antibiotic dose, with more severe reactions noted in LBRF.
- It involves three phases: Chill, Flush, and Recovery, with symptoms ranging

from fever and hyperventilation to a potential drop in blood pressure.

Prevention and Control: Key strategies include reducing overcrowding, practicing good hygiene to control lice populations, eliminating tick habitats, health education, and early treatment of cases and their contacts. For TBRF, rodent control measures are also important.

1.5. Rickettsial Diseases

Rickettsiae are diminutive intracellular bacteria transmitted to humans via arthropod vectors including human body lice, fleas, ticks, and larval mites. These organisms inhabit the gastrointestinal tract of their arthropod hosts and are transmitted to humans either through the direct bite of the vector or through the inoculation of organisms contained in the vector's feces, which enters the skin via scratching at the bite site. Rickettsial infections are known for their persistence within the host body, widespread vasculitis due to the invasion of endothelial cells of small blood vessels, and the potential to affect multiple body systems. Notably, except for louse-borne typhus, humans are generally incidental hosts in the life cycle of most Rickettsia species (Figure 1.5).

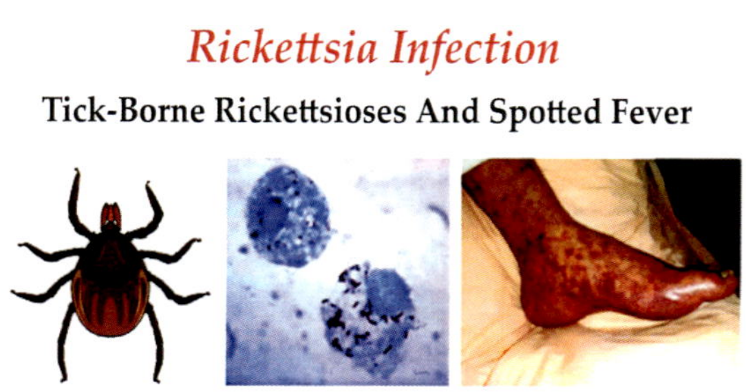

Figure 1.5. *Rickettsial diseases.*

Source: https://microbenotes.com/.

- **Classification:** Rickettsial diseases are categorized into several groups, reflecting their diverse modes of transmission and clinical manifestations:
- Tick and mite-borne spotted fever group;
- Flea and louse-borne typhus group;
- Chigger-borne scrub typhus;
- Ehrlichiosis;
- Q-fever.
- **Etiology and Epidemiology of Typhus:**
- **Epidemic Typhus (Louse-Borne):** Caused by *Rickettsia prowazekii* and transmitted through the human body louse, *Pediculus humanus corporis*. Lice become infected while feeding on the blood of an infected individual, with the bacteria proliferating within the louse's midgut and being excreted in feces. The disease often emerges under conditions of poverty, cold climates, during wars, or after natural disasters, with notable prevalence in the mountainous regions of Africa, South America, and Asia.
- **Endemic Typhus (Flea-Borne) / Murine Typhus:** This form is caused by *Rickettsia typhi*, transmitted by fleas. The disease circulates among mammalian hosts (primarily rats) and fleas, with humans becoming incidental hosts upon being bitten by infected fleas. The disease's cycle involves rickettsemic rats and lifelong carriage of the bacteria by the fleas.

Pathophysiology: Within the human body, Rickettsia species target endothelial cells of capillaries, leading to lesions in various organs including the skin, brain, lungs, heart, kidneys, and skeletal muscles. The resultant endothelial proliferation and perivascular inflammation can cause thromboses and minor hemorrhages. The primary pathology stems from increased vascular permeability, which can induce edema, hypovolemia, and subsequent organ ischemia, thus precipitating multi-system involvement and a range of complications such as pulmonary edema, cardiac dysrhythmias, encephalitis, and renal and hepatic failure.

- **Clinical Features:**
- **Incubation Period:** Typically, one week.
- **Onset:** Characterized by abrupt prostration, severe headache, and a high fever.
- **Symptoms:** Cough, severe myalgia, and a rash that begins on the upper trunk and spreads, excluding the face, palms, and soles. The rash transitions from macular to maculopapular and can become petechial if untreated.
- **Additional Signs**: Include photophobia, conjunctival injection, a dry and furred tongue, and signs of central nervous system (CNS) involvement such as meningoencephalitis.
- **Brill-Zinsser Disease:** A recrudescence of epidemic typhus, occurring years after the initial infection due to *R. prowazekii* reactivation. This form is milder but can still facilitate transmission if vectors are present.
- **Endemic Typhus Features:**
  - Considered milder than epidemic typhus.
  - Sudden onset after a 1–3-week incubation, featuring fever, headache, and cough, with a rash that appears on the fifth day and progresses to become purpuric, sparing the face and neck.
- **Complications of Typhus:** Both endemic and epidemic forms of typhus can lead to serious complications, including skin necrosis, gangrene of the digits, venous thrombosis, interstitial pneumonia, myocarditis, and oliguric renal failure.
- **Diagnosis:** The diagnosis of rickettsial diseases primarily relies on a combination of clinical symptoms, the course of the disease, and epidemiologic factors pointing to possible exposure.

1.6. Summary

Infectious diseases are disorders caused by organisms such as bacteria, viruses, fungi, or parasites. Many of these organisms are normally harmless and even beneficial, but they can cause disease under certain conditions. These diseases are a leading cause of death worldwide, particularly in low-income countries where access to clean water and healthcare is often limited. They can spread directly from person to person, through insects or animals, or by ingesting contaminated food or water.

Viruses like the flu, human immunodeficiency virus (HIV), and coronavirus are among the most known causes of infectious diseases. Bacteria, which can be responsible for illnesses such as strep throat and urinary tract infections, are another major category. Fungal infections, though less common, can affect the skin, nails, and lungs, while parasitic diseases include malaria and tapeworm infections.

The impact of infectious diseases has been profound throughout history, shaping societal structures, economies, and health systems. Modern medicine, through the development of vaccines and antibiotics, has made significant strides in controlling many infectious diseases. However, challenges such as antibiotic resistance and the emergence of new pathogens continue to pose threats to public health.

Preventative measures such as vaccination, maintaining good hygiene, using insect repellent, and practicing safe food and water habits are key in reducing the spread of these diseases. Public health strategies, including surveillance, reporting, and response systems, are crucial in managing outbreaks and epidemics.

Infectious diseases also have a significant economic impact, causing loss of productivity, healthcare costs, and hindering economic development. Research and investment in healthcare infrastructure, particularly in vulnerable populations, are essential for managing and preventing these diseases.

In summary, infectious diseases remain a major global health challenge despite advancements in medical science. Continued vigilance, research, and adherence to public health guidelines are crucial to combat the spread of these diseases and safeguard public health.

A Closer Look

Rickettsial Disease

Rickettsial diseases are a group of infectious illnesses caused by bacteria belonging to the genus Rickettsia, which primarily spread through vectors like ticks, fleas, and lice. Known for their zoonotic nature, these bacteria infect both animals and humans, making certain occupations (such as farming and veterinary work) more susceptible to outbreaks. Common types of Rickettsial diseases include Rocky Mountain spotted fever, epidemic typhus, and scrub typhus, each presenting specific characteristics based on the bacterium involved and the geographic region.

Rickettsial diseases generally affect endothelial cells lining blood vessels, causing vascular inflammation and increased permeability. Symptoms vary but often begin with fever, headache, and a distinctive rash, often mistaken for other febrile illnesses like dengue. Due to this symptom overlap, early diagnosis is challenging. The severity ranges from mild to life-threatening, particularly if left untreated, as the bacteria can cause complications such as neurological impairments, respiratory issues, and renal failure.

Diagnosis relies on clinical evaluation and laboratory tests, although these tests may not detect the bacteria until the disease has progressed, making clinical suspicion crucial. Serologic testing, polymerase chain reaction (PCR), and culture methods aid in confirming diagnosis, though availability and accuracy can vary depending on the region.

Treatment typically involves antibiotics such as doxycycline, especially for severe cases, as it is highly effective against most Rickettsial infections. Preventive measures emphasize avoiding exposure to vectors through proper clothing, insect repellents, and hygiene practices. Vaccination is still under research, as Rickettsial diseases continue to pose a public health challenge globally, particularly in rural and underdeveloped regions with limited healthcare infrastructure.

References

1. Afrizal, S. H., Handayani, P. W., Hidayanto, A. N., Eryando, T., et al., (2019). Barriers and challenges to Primary Health Care Information System (PHCIS) adoption from health management perspective: A qualitative study. *Inform. Med. Unlocked 17,* 10098.

2. Arsenault, C., Yakob, B., Tilahun, T., Nigatu, T. G., et al., (2021). Patient volume and quality of primary care in Ethiopia: Findings from the routine health information system and the 2014 Service Provision Assessment survey. *BMC Health Serv. Res. 21,* 485.

3. Cardoso, G., Neto, C., Neto, G. C. C., Andreazza, R., & Chioro, A., (2021). Integration among national health information systems in Brazil: The case of e-SUS Primary Care. *Rev. Saúde Pública 55,* S1518–S8787.

4. Chang, Y., Yao, Y., Cui, Z., Yang, G., et al., (2022). Changing antibiotic prescribing practices in outpatient primary care settings in China: Study protocol for a health information system-based cluster-randomized crossover controlled trial. *PLoS ONE 17,* e0259065.

5. Cullen, T., Flowers, J., Sequist, T. D., Hays, H., et al., (2019). Envisioning health equity for American Indian/Alaska Natives: A unique HIT opportunity. *J. Am. Med. Inform. Assoc. 26,* 891–894.

6. Dagnew, E., Woreta, S. A., & Shiferaw, A. M., (2018). Routine health information utilization and associated factors among health care professionals working at public health institution in North Gondar, Northwest Ethiopia. *BMC Health Serv. Res. 18,* 685.

7. Daneshkohan, A., Alimoradi, M., Ahmadi, M., & Alipour, J., (2022). Data quality and data use in primary health care: A case study from Iran. *Inform. Med. Unlocked 28,* 100855.

8. Eslami Andargoli, A., Scheepers, H., Rajendran, D., & Sohal, A., (2017). Health information systems evaluation frameworks: A systematic review. *Int. J. Med. Inform. 97,* 195–209.

9. Faridah, L., Rinawan, F. R., Fauziah, N., Mayasari, W., et al., (2020). Evaluation of Health Information System (HIS) in The Surveillance of Dengue in Indonesia: Lessons from Case in Bandung, West Java. *Int. J. Environ. Res. Public Health, 17,* (1795).

10. Han, D., Wang, S., Jiang, C., Jiang, X., et al., (2015). Trends in biomedical informatics:automated topic analysis of JAMA articles. *J. Am. Med. Inform. Assoc. 22,* 1153–1163.

11. Harahap, N. C., Handayani, P. W., & Hidayanto, A. N., (2021). Barriers in Health Information Systems and Technologies to Support Maternal and Neonatal Referrals at Primary Health Centers. *Healthc Inform. Res. 27,* 153–161.

12. Health, T. L. D., (2021). Digital technologies: A new determinant of health. *Lancet Digit. Health 3,* e684.

13. Higman, S., Dwivedi, V., Nsaghurwe, A., Busiga, M., Sotter Rulagirwa, H., Smith, D., Wright, C., Nyinondi, S., Nyella, E., Nsaghurwe, A., Dwivedi, V., Nsaghurwe, A., Busiga, M., et al., (2019). Designing interoperable health information systems using enterprise architecture approach in resource-limited countries: A literature review. *Int. J. Health Plan. Manag. 34,* e85–e99.

14. Hosseinpoor, A. R., Bergen, N., Schlotheuber, A., & Boerma, T., (2018). National health inequality monitoring: Current challenges and opportunities. *Glob. Health Action 11,* 1392216.

15. Iyamu, I., Xu, A. X. T., Gómez-Ramírez, O., Ablona, A., et al., (2021). Defining digital public health and the role of digitization, digitalization, and digital transformation: Scoping review. *JMIR Public Health Surveill. 7,* e30399.

16. Jacobson, R. P., Kang, D., & Houck, J., (2020). Can Patient-Reported Outcomes Measurement Information System® (PROMIS) measures accurately enhance understanding of acceptable symptoms and functioning in primary care? *J. Patient Rep. Outcomes, 9,* 39.

17. Koumamba, A. P., Bisvigou, U. J., Ngoungou, E. B., & Diallo, G., (2021). Health information systems in developing countries: Case of African countries. *BMC Med. Inform. Decis. Mak. 21,* 232.

18. Liaw, S. T., Georgiou, A., & Marin, H., (2020). Evaluation of Digital Health & Information Technology in Primary Care. *Int. J. Med. Inform. 144,* 104285.

19. Mulyanto, J., Kunst, A. E., & Kringos, D. S., (2019). Geographical inequalities in healthcare utilisation and the contribution of compositional factors: A multilevel analysis of 497 districts in Indonesia. *Health Place, 60,* 102236.

20. Nguyen, L., Bellucci, E., & Nguyen, L. T., (2014). Electronic health records implementation: An evaluation of information system impact and contingency factors. *Int. J. Med. Inform. 83,* 779–796.

21. Nsaghurwe, A., Dwivedi, V., Ndesanjo, W., Bamsi, H., et al., (2021). One country's journey to interoperability: Tanzania's experience developing and implementing a national health information exchange. *BMC Med. Inform. Decis. Mak. 21,* 139.

22. Puente, D., López-Jiménez, T., Cos-Claramunt, X., Ortega, Y., et al., (2019). Metabolic syndrome and risk of cancer: A study protocol of case-control study using data from the Information System for the Development of Research in Primary Care (SIDIAP) in Catalonia. *BMJ Open 9,* e025365.

23. Qomariyah, S. N., Sethi, R., Izati, Y. N., Rianty, T., et al., (2020). No one data source captures all: A nested case-control study of the completeness of maternal death reporting in Banten Province, Indonesia. *PLoS ONE 15,* e0232080.

24. Sheikh, A., Anderson, M., Albala, S., Casadei, B., et al., (2021). Health information technology and digital innovation for national learning health and care systems. *Lancet Digit. Health 3,* e383–e396.

25. Shiferaw, A. M., Zegeye, D. T., Assefa, S., & Yenit, M. K., (2017). Routine health information system utilization and factors associated thereof among health workers at government health institutions in East Gojjam Zone, Northwest Ethiopia. *BMC Med. Inform. Decis. Mak. 17,* 116.

26. Tamrat, T., Chandir, S., Alland, K., Pedrana, A., et al., (2022). Digitalization of routine health information systems: Bangladesh, Indonesia, Pakistan. *Bull. World Health Organ. 100,* 590–600.

27. Thomas, J. C., (2017). Contextual factors affecting health information system strengthening. *Glob. Public Health 12,* 1568–1578.

28. Wardhani, V., Mathew, S., Seo, J.-W.; Wiryawan, K. G., et al., (2018). Why and how do we keep editing local medical journals in an era of information overload? *Sci. Ed. 5,* 150–154.

29. Watsiq, A., Madjido, M., Espressivo, A., Watsiq Maula, A., et al., (2019). Health Information System Research Situation in Indonesia: A Bibliometric Analysis ScienceDirect Health Information System Research Situation in Indonesia: A Bibliometric Analysis. *Procedia Comput. Sci. 161,* 781–787.

30. Zhang, L. Z., (2005). Numerical study of heat and mass transfer in an enthalpy exchanger with a hydrophobic-hydrophilic composite membrane core. *Numer. Heat Transf. Part A Appl. 51,* 697–714.

31. Zhang, X., Hailu, B., Tabor, D. C., Gold, R., et al., (2019). Role of Health Information Technology in Addressing Health Disparities: Patient, Clinician, and System Perspectives. *Med. Care 57,* S115–S120.

Chapter

RESPIRATORY SYSTEM DISORDERS

2

Contents

Introduction

The respiratory system, essential for sustaining life, facilitates the vital process of gas exchange, ensuring the intake of oxygen from the surrounding atmosphere into the bloodstream and eliminating carbon dioxide (CO_2) from the body. The significance of this interaction cannot be overstated in terms of maintaining cellular metabolism and overall physiological functioning. In addition to its primary function, the respiratory system has a significant impact on various other physiological areas, emphasizing its intricate complexity and essential nature.

The respiratory system plays a crucial role in thermoregulation across various species, facilitating the accurate regulation of body temperature. This function has been emphasized by West's research in 2005. The central role of this system in maintaining physiological equilibrium is further exemplified by its involvement in regulating the body's acid-base balance, in conjunction with the kidneys, as described by Semenza in 2011.

Furthermore, it is worth noting that the respiratory system plays a crucial role in the regulation of blood pressure by producing substances such as the angiotensin-converting enzyme. This significant finding was first reported by Skeggs et al. in 1956. The role of this entity encompasses the metabolism of various compounds, including eicosanoids and nitric oxide, which play a crucial role in regulating physiological responses such as vasodilation and inflammation. This investigation was conducted by Moncada, Palmer, and Higgs in 1991.

The respiratory system's immune defense mechanism, specifically its ability to repel inhaled pathogens and process antigens via intravascular macrophages in specific animal species, highlights its crucial contribution to overall health and resilience against diseases. The studies conducted by Fogarty and Perri in 2007 shed light on this aspect, highlighting the system's role that goes beyond simple gas exchange.

The manifestation of dysfunction in these diverse roles can have a profound impact during periods of illness. The most severe consequence of respiratory system failure is the impairment of gas exchange, which results in hypoxemia and hypercapnia. These conditions play a significant role in the illness seen in respiratory diseases and, if not addressed, can lead to respiratory failure, which can be a potentially life-threatening result as explained by Nunn and Hill in 1960.

An extensive understanding of the physiological foundations and pathological consequences of hypoxia, hypercapnia, and respiratory failure is crucial for effectively treating respiratory conditions in a clinical setting. The terminal nature of respiratory failure, primarily caused by impaired gas exchange, emphasizes the importance of preserving the integrity of the respiratory system for survival. In 1984, Weibel conducted further investigation into these concepts, emphasizing the multifunctional roles of the respiratory system.

Orientation and Directional Terms

Term	Definition	Illustration
Lungs	The primary organs of the respiratory system responsible for the exchange of oxygen and carbon dioxide in the body.	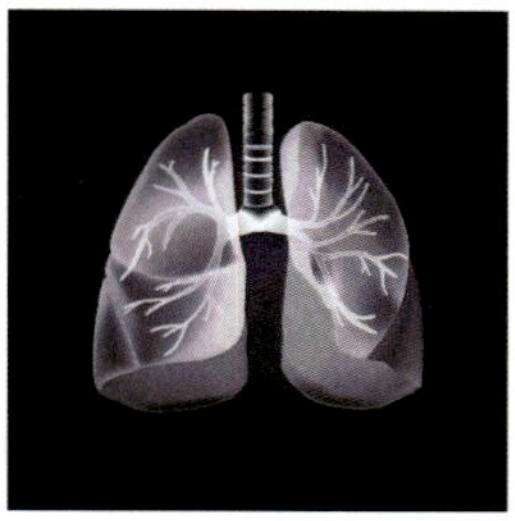
Asthma	A chronic respiratory condition marked by inflammation and narrowing of the airways, causing wheezing, shortness of breath, and coughing.	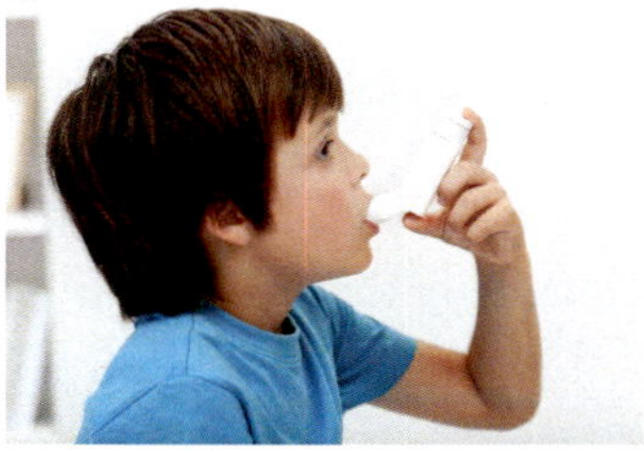
Pulmonary Disease	A group of disorders affecting the lungs and respiratory system, including conditions like COPD and bronchitis.	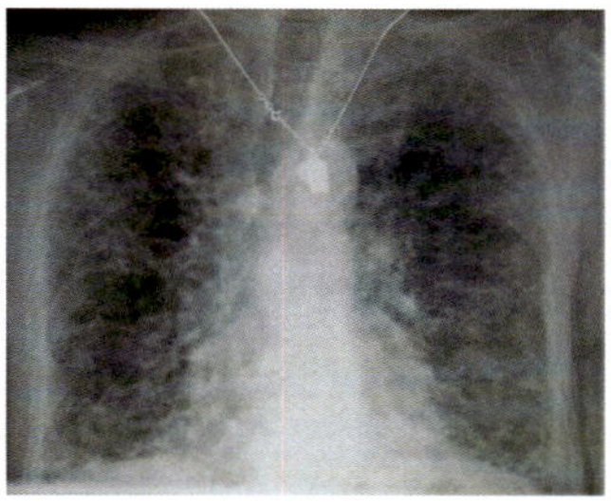
Cystic Fibrosis	A genetic disorder affecting the respiratory and digestive systems, leading to the production of thick, sticky mucus that clogs airways and glands.	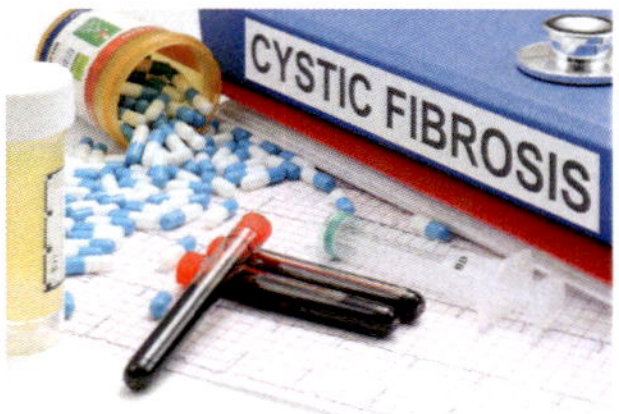
Lung Cancer	A type of cancer originating in the lungs, often associated with smoking and environmental factors, characterized by uncontrolled cell growth in lung tissue.	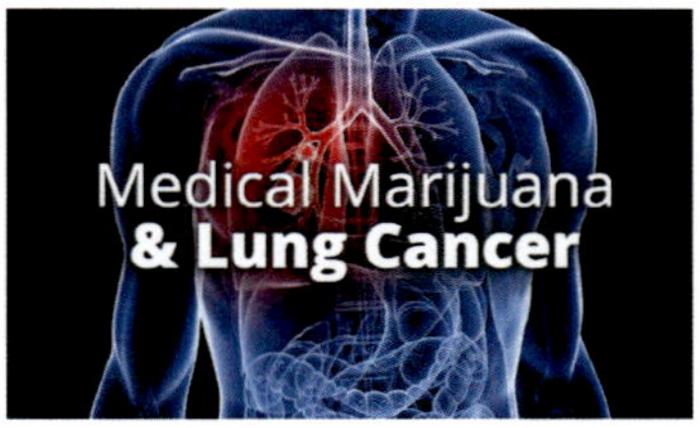

2.1. An Overview of Chronic Respiratory Diseases (CRDs)

The prevalence of CRDs that impact individuals of all age groups, including both adults and children, is steadily rising on a global scale. The precise cause of mortality and morbidity associated with respiratory diseases remains uncertain. Nevertheless, recent data released by the World Health Organization (WHO) and other organizations indicates that approximately 400 million individuals worldwide are afflicted with mild to moderate forms of Asthma and COPD exclusively. Furthermore, the annual mortality rate associated with lower respiratory tract (LRT) infection caused by Hemophilus influenzae ranges from 250,000 to 500,000 deaths. In 2015, *Mycobacterium tuberculosis* caused an LRT infection in 10.4 million individuals globally, resulting in a mortality rate of 14%. An alarming upward trend has been observed in the mortality rate of 1.6 million individuals annually due to noninfectious conditions such as lung cancer, which can be attributed to tobacco smoking or the inhalation of environmental carcinogens. Respiratory disorders contribute to 10% of the overall disability-adjusted life years (DALYs) in the human workforce, in addition to the associated mortality rate.

Respiratory diseases can be classified into two main categories based on disease pathology and mode of transmission. The first category is communicable diseases, which include infectious diseases such as tuberculosis (TB) and pneumonia. The second category is noncommunicable diseases, which do not have an infectious cause. Examples of noncommunicable diseases include asthma, chronic obstructive pulmonary disease (COPD), cystic fibrosis (CF), interstitial pulmonary fibrosis, and lung cancer. Respiratory diseases exhibit a diverse range of etiologies and are characterized by distinct diagnostic approaches. However, particularly noncommunicable CRDs are managed in a similar manner. Specifically, the treatment for these conditions typically involves the use of a bronchodilator, corticosteroids, and antibiotics. Furthermore, the investigation into the pathology of COPD has only begun in the past 20 years, and the areas with a significant prevalence of the disease lack a reliable method for diagnosing and preventing/managing the condition. This issue raises significant concerns, especially in low- and middle-income nations like India, China, as well as countries across various regions, including Asia Pacific, Latin America, and Africa.

Although the burden of CRDs is steadily increasing, the available treatment options are limited. The primary reason for this is a limited comprehension of the fundamental mechanisms that could potentially facilitate the identification of promising targets, whether they are characteristically molecular or immunological. Furthermore, the variability in the mode of drug delivery necessitates additional research to improve the deposition and effectiveness of currently prescribed medications.

We will provide a concise overview of respiratory diseases, encompassing the impact, pathology, and pathophysiology of CRDs. In addition, an examination of the presently accessible therapeutic alternatives for significant respiratory ailments will be undertaken.

2.2. The Morphology and Physiology of the Lungs

The human respiratory system is comprised of two primary components, namely the upper respiratory tract (URT) and the LRT. The URT consists of the nose/nostrils, mouth, and the initial segment of the trachea. The LRT encompasses the trachea, which gradually divides into the bronchi, bronchioles, and ultimately the functional units referred to as alveoli. The lung parenchyma provides support to the airways, while the pulmonary vasculature facilitates gas exchange. The primary role of the respiratory system is the facilitation of gas exchange, specifically the process of oxygen (O_2) absorption and CO_2 release. Gas exchange occurs within the pulmonary capillaries via the individual membranes of the pulmonary alveolus. Breathing involves two main processes: inhalation and exhalation. Inhalation involves the intake of air into the lungs, primarily through the expansion of the chest volume. The inhaled air then moves through the smaller "conductive" airways. Exhalation, on the other hand, is the expulsion of air from the lungs, which occurs when the chest volume contracts. Inhalation and exhalation are primarily facilitated by two types of muscles: the diaphragm and the intercostal muscles. The internal surface area of the lungs is estimated to be around 50–75 m^2. The mean weight of a typical human lung is estimated to be around 1 kg, with approximately 40% to 50% of this weight being ascribed to the blood present in the pulmonary vasculature. The quantification of air volume and the assessment of inhalation and exhalation are crucial in determining the existence of restrictive and/or obstructive pulmonary conditions, such as asthma and COPD.

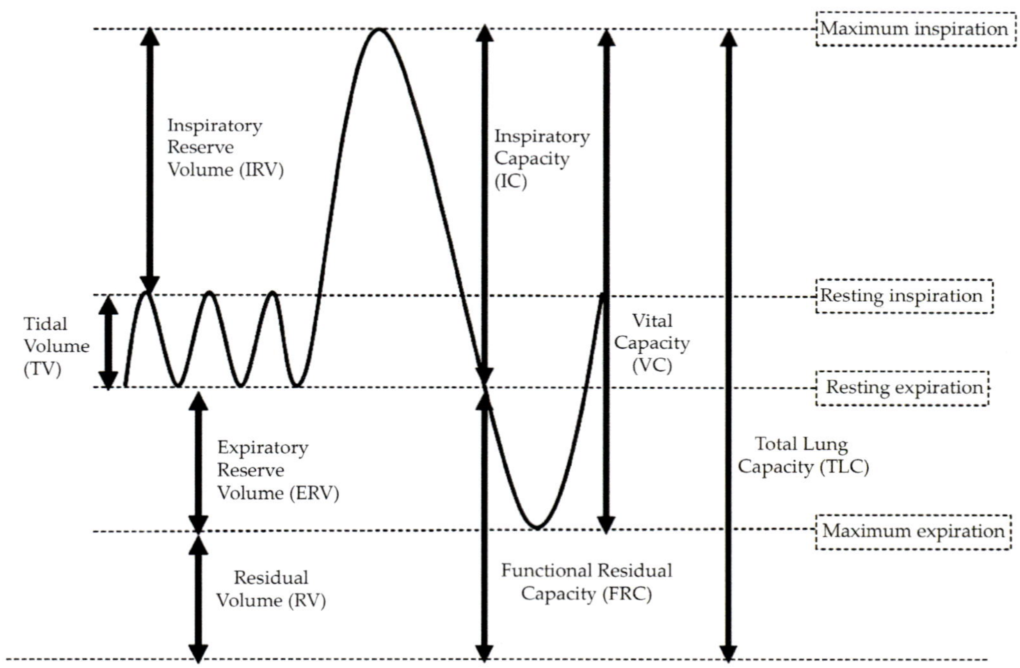

Figure 2.1. *The spirometer trace provides information on standard lung volumes and capacities. The lung volumes and capacities are indicated by the solid black and gray arrows, respectively.*

Pulmonary mechanics encompasses the effective process of gas exchange, which necessitates the involvement of multiple components. Various measurements are commonly employed to monitor the regular operation of the lungs. Spirometry is a widely employed method in clinical laboratories for assessing lung functionality. It is a reliable and consistent maximum breathing test that is widely utilized to evaluate the ventilatory capacity of the lungs. Spirometers in contemporary times offer the supplementary benefits of providing prompt computer-generated feedback to the operator regarding the test's quality and repeatability, along with a real-time graphical representation of the flow-volume curve. The commonly assessed lung volumes encompass tidal volume (TV), inspiratory reserve volume (IRV), expiratory reserve volume (ERV), and residual volume (RV). In addition to ventilatory capacity (IC), other commonly assessed lung capacities include inspiratory capacity (FRC), vital capacity (VC), and total lung capacity (TLC). Figure 2.1 presents a concise overview of the lung volumes and capacities.

In a typical human lung, there exist multiple cell types that possess distinct and specialized functions. The primary cell types encompassed within the airway are airway epithelial cells, goblet cells, ciliated cells, Clara cells, neuroendocrine cells, basal cells, as well as type I and type II alveolar cells. Furthermore, the lungs contain immune cells, stem cells, and adipose cells. Various respiratory diseases are also associated with one or more cell types. For example, the presence of risk factors is associated with the induction of lung adenocarcinomas in glandular cells located in the lungs. Disease is also associated with the functionality of particular cell types. The pathology of respiratory diseases, including neonatal respiratory failure, ILD, alveolar proteinosis, and other rare lung diseases, has been associated with the secretion of surfactant proteins and lipids. Furthermore, apart from its role as the initial barrier that separates the host-environment axis, the airway epithelia also play a significant role in modulating pulmonary inflammation and immune cell activation. Additionally, it is a vital component in pulmonary remodeling and repair. Furthermore, the pulmonary vasculature undergoes alterations such as intimal hyperplasia and smooth muscle hypertrophy/hyperplasia, which are likely caused by the chronic constriction of the small pulmonary arteries due to hypoxia. Furthermore, there is a growing recognition of the significant role played by basal cells in the airway epithelium in the process of airway remodeling. An important issue that continues to be worrisome is the absence of efficient treatment and/or management approaches for CRDs, particularly noncommunicable diseases such as asthma, COPD, CF, and IPF. This phenomenon can be ascribed to various factors, one of which is the absence of a comprehensive comprehension regarding the fundamental mechanisms that may be involved in the onset and advancement of CRDs. Therefore, the existing treatments are limited to addressing the primary symptoms of the disease and do not provide lasting relief, either in terms of prevention or cure. Furthermore, the existing drugs are inadequate in their ability to fully target biological entities, necessitating the development of more efficient drug delivery methods to alleviate symptoms of CRDs.

2.3. Overview of Respiratory Disease

The increasing population, coupled with the evolving lifestyle of the 21st century, has created an opportunity for a diverse array of diseases that pose a significant risk to human life worldwide. Respiratory disorders were identified as the most prevalent health issues impacting the extensive populations of middle- and lower-income countries globally. Respiratory diseases, despite their considerable prevalence, frequently go unnoticed or receive insufficient attention. The human lungs are the sole internal organ that is consistently subjected to a diverse array of environmental pollutants, encompassing organic, inorganic, and biological agents originating from both natural and anthropogenic sources. Consequently, these lungs face an ongoing risk of developing a spectrum of pulmonary disorders, ranging from simple to complex. These disorders have the potential to negatively impact an individual's quality of life and ultimately result in mortality. The following text provides a concise overview of several respiratory diseases that pose a significant threat to millions of lives worldwide.

2.3.1. Asthma

Asthma is a diverse and intricate lung condition that is distinguished by fluctuating airflow blockage, heightened sensitivity of the airways (bronchial), and, significantly, elevated airway inflammation. Asthma has a prevalence rate of approximately 10% among the adult population in nearly all nations, resulting in a global population of approximately 300 million individuals. Furthermore, asthma is projected to be a primary factor in 383,000 fatalities globally, with more than 80% of asthma-related deaths occurring in low- and middle-income nations. Asthma also imposes a significant economic burden, amounting to up to $USD 3100 per individual annually.

Asthma is a prevalent but inadequately comprehended respiratory condition that can occur at any stage of life. Asthma risk factors encompass various elements, such as indoor pollutants (including house dust mites and pollution), exposure to outdoor allergens (including pollen, molds, and pollution), tobacco smoke, occupational exposure to chemical fumes, and air pollution. Asthma is a multifaceted condition that can present as a "episodic" disease, characterized by periods of symptom onset and resolution following treatment. Additionally, it is worth noting that the disease may exhibit a "persistent" nature in certain individuals, as evidenced by the presence of distinct clinical symptoms associated with asthma. The primary manifestations of asthma encompass wheezing, dyspnea, dyspnea, and cough. The manifestation of symptoms can be heightened by a range of factors, including exposure to both known and unknown allergens, irritants, respiratory tract infections caused by viruses or bacteria, bacterial sinusitis, physical exertion, thunderstorms, and cold weather.

The latest knowledge in the pathophysiology of asthma has resulted in the classification of asthma into different phenotypes and/or endotypes. The identification of "treatable traits" in patients with asthma and the subsequent targeting of these traits for disease management have been recommended by the recent Lancet commission as crucial for the effective treatment of this condition. Moreover, asthma can be classified into allergic asthma, which is triggered by allergens such as pollen, house dust mites, mold, and exposure to biological/organic environmental substances. Nonallergic asthma, on the other hand, is linked to risk factors such as tobacco smoke, viral/bacterial infections, exposure to cold air, physical activity, and dietary choices. Research indicates that in most instances, asthma is primarily caused by Th2 responses, in which type 2 T-helper cells are attracted to the airways in reaction to external or internal stimuli and generate cytokines such as IL-4, IL-5, IL-9, and IL-13 at high levels. IL-4 is a crucial factor in the IgE switch process in B cells, leading to an upregulation in the production of immunoglobulin E. This, in turn, triggers the synthesis of inflammatory mediators such as histamine and cysteinyl leukotrienes. On the other hand, IL-5 is solely responsible for the recruitment of eosinophils, which contributes to the onset of allergic rhinitis in the URT. Interleukin-13 (IL-13) and IL-4, in conjunction with inflammatory mediators, induce the contraction of smooth muscles, thereby inducing bronchospasm, excessive mucus production, and heightened immune cell infiltration. Consequently, this leads to a decrease in airway diameter and an increase in airway hyperresponsiveness in the lower airways, ultimately resulting in a reduction in airflow (FEV1). The airway epithelium has been identified as a significant contributor to the regulation of Th2 responses through the production of master regulators such as thymic stromal lymphopoietin, IL-25, and IL33. These master regulators play a crucial role in controlling the expression of Th2 cytokines, which in turn contribute to the early development of asthma in childhood.

The early phase of asthma is distinguished by the presence of wheezing and heightened sensitivity of the airways to nonspecific stimuli. However, in later stages, particularly in severe forms, there is an escalation in inflammation accompanied by additional local (viral/bacterial infections) or systemic factors. This leads to the remodeling of the airways, resulting in subsequent exacerbations. The initial findings derived from animal models have led to the misconception that asthma is an allergic, eosinophilic, Th2-mediated inflammatory condition. Nevertheless, human clinical trials have demonstrated that certain types of asthma are associated with reduced or absent Th2 responses, thereby confirming the existence of distinct phenotypes in this extensively researched respiratory condition. Research conducted on individuals with severe asthma revealed increased levels of neutrophilic populations, while eosinophilic populations remained stable or showed no significant changes. Furthermore, the presence of neutrophilia, characterized by an excessive neutrophilic population, has been frequently observed in individuals with severe asthma who are currently undergoing treatment or have previously received treatment with inhaled corticosteroids (ICS). This observation prompts the consideration that ICS may potentially be accountable for this distinctive phenotype. Asthmatic individuals with neutrophilia exhibited minimal or negligible response to ICS treatment. Currently, clinicians are utilizing negative skin tests as a means of distinguishing between nonallergic asthmatics and allergic asthmatics. This involves subjecting skin cells to aeroallergens to assess their capacity to generate IgE. Furthermore, genome-wide association studies conducted on asthma in both adult and pediatric populations have revealed significant polymorphisms in IL33, ILRL1, IL18R1, IL2RB, and SMAD3 genes located on chromosome 17q21. Additionally, these polymorphisms have been found to be associated with gene expressions of ZPBP2, GSDMB, and ORMDL3. These genes are responsible for preserving the integrity and functionality of the epithelial barrier. Nevertheless, the precise genetic markers responsible for the onset of asthma in both early stages and adulthood remain poorly comprehended. Recent research has established a connection between inherent factors such as obesity and the heightened development of asthma. It has been observed that white adipose tissues release IL-1, IL-6, and TNF, which contribute to oxidative stress through inflammatory macrophages. Moreover, the process of epithelial to mesenchymal transition, the increase in thickness of the basement membrane, and the deposition of collagen contribute to the remodeling of the airways and the exacerbation of asthmatic exacerbations. These findings emphasize the significant diversity of asthma and the urgent requirement for novel therapies and strategies to address the issue.

2.3.1.1. Therapies

Clinicians consider multiple factors when providing treatment for individuals afflicted with asthma. Prior to treatment, the lung function analysis, along with sputum analysis, takes into consideration preexisting respiratory conditions and ongoing treatments. Originally, glucocorticoids were the preferred medication for treating most asthmatics due to their ability to suppress Th2 responses. However, this steroid treatment had its drawbacks. The administration of steroids for an extended period has been associated with various local and systemic adverse effects, such as dysphonia, candidiasis, osteoporosis, and adrenal suppression. Nevertheless, patients exhibiting neutrophilic asthma, or low Th2 response phenotypes demonstrated resistance. Research has demonstrated that allergic asthma, specifically pollen allergies, exhibits a positive response to β2-agonist in ICS. However, individuals who do not have allergies to viruses or bacteria are typically treated with systemic corticosteroids (SCS). In accordance with EPR-3 regulations, high concentrations of short-acting beta-agonists, such as albuterol and levalbuterol are administered. O_2 is the primary treatment for acute asthmatics. However, in later stages (chronic), these medications are substituted with epinephrine, magnesium sulfate, noninvasive positive pressure ventilation, and hospitalization.

Azithromycin has gained popularity as a long-term treatment option for patients with severe asthma in recent years. However, its use is still a subject of controversy. Gibson and his team demonstrated that the addition of azithromycin to ICS effectively decreased the number of annual exacerbations by 50% in individuals with severe asthma. Nevertheless, the epidemiological data presented by Tian et al. indicate that azithromycin does not demonstrate a substantial effectiveness in managing severe asthmatic exacerbations. To draw definitive conclusions and validate the potential of azithromycin as a viable treatment for asthma, further human cohorts are required. A recent study has brought attention to the fact that the prolonged utilization of azithromycin, an antibiotic and macrolide, has resulted in a decrease in H. The presence of influenzae in individuals with severe asthma has been observed. However, it has been noted that there is an escalation in antibiotic resistance towards azithromycin over time. This finding underscores a significant constraint in utilizing the well-known antibiotic for the treatment and management of asthma.

The application of monoclonal antibodies in disease treatment has garnered significant interest from scientific communities worldwide in the past decade. The efficacy of biological inhibitors, such as mepolizumab (anti-IL-5) and omalizumab (anti-IgE mAb), in managing exacerbations in individuals with severe asthma has been demonstrated. Omalizumab, in particular, forms an irreversible complex with immunoglobulin IgE, thereby inhibiting the synthesis of inflammatory mediators and immune cells (specifically mast cells and basophils). Consequently, it effectively regulates the pathogenesis of the disease. Busse et al. demonstrated that the administration of omalizumab has substantially decreased the frequency of exacerbations in individuals with severe asthma, in comparison to the placebo and ICS groups. Moreover, the effectiveness and safety of utilizing omalizumab or other monoclonal antibodies (mAB) were verified and documented. While the utilization of biological inhibitors (mAB) is efficient and alleviates the financial strain on medication, the expenses associated with the manufacturing, transportation, and storage of mAB continue to pose difficulties.

2.3.2. Chronic Obstructive Pulmonary Disease

COPD is a comprehensive term employed to denote a collection of progressive, obstructive-irreversible pulmonary conditions, including emphysema, chronic bronchitis, small airway deterioration, and chronic asthma. As per the World Health Organization (WHO), the global burden of disease study documented 251 million cases of COPD worldwide, with 90% of these cases originating from low- and middle-income countries. In 2015, there were an estimated 3.17 million deaths, representing 5% of the total deaths. This represents an 11.6% increase compared to the number of deaths in 1990. The Centers for Disease Control and Prevention estimated that COPD incurred an economic burden of USD $32.1 billion in 2010 in terms of medical expenses and lost workdays. This burden is projected to increase to USD $49.0 billion by 2020 in the United States. Nevertheless, the precise global prevalence of COPD remains a subject of contention. This is primarily attributed to the misclassification of asthma cases in the elderly as COPD, as well as the lack of available data from developing or underdeveloped countries in Asia and the Middle East. Consequently, the mortality rate in these regions may be underestimated by several million individuals.

Patients afflicted with any manifestation of COPD display a diverse array of symptoms. One prominent symptom is the presence of breathlessness or shortness of breath during routine activities, which tends to deteriorate over time. Conversely, individuals afflicted with severe forms of COPD and asthma encounter frequent exacerbations and subsequent visits to the emergency room throughout the year. The observed phenomenon can be attributed to the partial destruction of alveoli, known as emphysema, or the accumulation of excessive mucus and inflammatory cells in bronchioles, referred to as chronic bronchitis. This condition is particularly prevalent among individuals who smoke or have previously smoked and are afflicted with COPD. Consequently, the reduced gas exchange capacity of the lungs leads to airflow obstruction, resulting in decreased blood O_2 levels (hypoxemia) and subsequent organ failure. Furthermore, individuals afflicted with any manifestation of COPD may display typical symptoms such as persistent cough (with or without mucus), fatigue, wheezing, and chest tightness; in the majority of instances, these symptoms are misconstrued as age-related factors. Certain patients may remain asymptomatic until the disease worsens. Despite the extensive research conducted over several decades, a cure for the regeneration of damaged tissue and the restoration of lung function has yet to be found. Furthermore, COPD is a degenerative condition that deteriorates as individuals age. The current therapies aim to decelerate the advancement of disease development and offer temporary relief to patients, but they are unable to fully restore the impaired functionality of affected areas. Based on the available data sets, tobacco smoking was identified as the primary cause of COPD. Recent studies indicate that prolonged exposure to noncigarette smoke irritants, such as airborne dust particles, geogenic dust, and metal contaminants, is a significant risk factor associated with the development (in nonsmokers) or worsening (in smokers) of COPD. However, this aspect of the disease has received limited attention in existing research. Furthermore, research has substantiated the significance of hereditary factors and genetic predisposition, such as the deficiency of alpha-1-antitrypsin, in the pathogenesis of COPD. However, the precise underlying mechanisms responsible for this phenomenon remain largely uninvestigated. Nevertheless, individuals with AAT deficiency exhibit a higher susceptibility to respiratory infections, and genetic factors account for only 1% of all cases of COPD. This underscores the significant role of tobacco smoking and air pollutants as primary causes. It is noteworthy that not all individuals who smoke or have quit smoking will develop the disease. Only 20%–30% of active smokers or former smokers may develop the disease at some point in their lives. Passive smoking was identified as a risk factor for developing COPD in 51.2% of the studies (n = 87). However, the specific underlying mechanisms are still not fully understood.

The primary mechanism underlying the development of COPD involves the disruption of airflow and the entry of inflammatory cells, particularly CD8+ T lymphocytes, neutrophils, and macrophages, into the alveolar and peripheral spaces. This inflammatory response is triggered by exposure to tobacco smoke or certain environmental particles and gases. However, variations in the immune system response have been observed among different subtypes of COPD. Chronic bronchitis is a medical condition that is distinguished by the excessive production of mucus, heightened presence of inflammatory cells, overexpression of the MUC5AC gene in response to the release of serine proteases, elevated levels of reactive oxygen species (ROS) from inhaled smoke or activated macrophages. This condition leads to the constriction of the air space and subsequent harm to neighboring cells, ultimately resulting in the remodeling (fibrosis) of the airways and subsequent loss of lung elasticity. On the other hand, emphysema, which can manifest in both centrilobular and pan lobular forms, is directly caused by exposure to cigarette smoke. Inhaling smoke increases inflammation in the bronchioles and alveolar sacs, causing gradual damage to the alveolar sacs and narrower airway walls. This results in the loss of alveolar structure, function, and recoil. The precise mechanism by which innate and adaptive immune responses are activated in patients with COPD remains uncertain. Nevertheless, the excessive production of CXC, IL8, and matrix metalloproteinase (MMP) by immune cells, as well as the generation of proinflammatory mediators such as TNF±, IL1β (Th1 responses), leukotriene B4, and transforming growth factor beta (TGF²), lead to the development of local fibrosis and an imbalance in the ratio of ROS) to reactive nitrogen species. These factors have been identified as significant contributors to the worsening of the disease.

Clinicians frequently rely on noninvasive spirometry and the Global Initiative for Chronic Obstructive Lung Disease (GOLD) staging system, developed (GOLD), for the purpose of diagnosing and assessing the severity of disease progression. The GOLD staging system employs the forced expiratory volume/forced vital capacity ratio (FEV1/FVC) as a metric to assess pulmonary function. FEV1/FVC refers to the volume of air exhaled by a patient within a one-second timeframe following a single deep breath. This system classifies individuals into one of four distinct stages:

- **Stage 1:** Indicates mild chronic obstructive pulmonary disease (COPD) when the individual's FEV1/FVC ratio is ...80% of the normal range.
- **Stage 2:** If the individual's FEV1/FVC ratio falls within the range of 50% to 80% of the normal range, they are classified as having moderate COPD.
- **Stage 3:** Severe emphysema is classified when an individual exhibits a FEV1/FVC ratio ranging from 30% to 50% of the normal range.
- **Stage 4:** In Stage 4, an individual is classified as having a very severe form of emphysema or COPD if their FEV1/FVC ratio is less than 30% of normal or if their blood O_2 levels are low, as indicated by stage 3.

Patients diagnosed with GOLD stage 1 or stage 2 COPD experience a gradual decline in the FEV1 ratio and progress towards stage 3 and 4. At these stages, patients encounter severe symptoms and a decline in their quality of life. Currently, in addition to spirometry, imaging modalities such as chest X-rays and high-resolution CT scans can be employed to assess the advancement of the disease. Furthermore, the utilization of a blood gas analyzer for the purpose of monitoring O_2 and carbon monoxide levels in blood samples can prove to be advantageous.

COPD is a disease that can be prevented, but it cannot be reversed. The current treatments aim to alleviate symptoms and decelerate the advancement of the disease, but they do not offer complete recuperation, which can only be achieved through a lung transplant, which is not a viable option. The administration of pharmaceutical agents such as bronchodilators, corticosteroids, glucocorticosteroids, phosphodiesterase-4 inhibitors, theophylline, and antibiotics has been shown to induce relaxation of the muscles in the airways, enhance airflow, and reduce inflammation in the LRT. For stages 3 and 4, clinicians frequently recommend O_2 therapy to restore blood O_2 levels to their baseline. However, this treatment is temporary, and once the O_2 supply is disrupted, the patient's condition rapidly regresses to its original state. Modifying one's lifestyle, such as ceasing smoking, evading air pollution, and limiting dietary consumption, can also decelerate the advancement.

2.3.3. Interstitial Lung Diseases

ILDs encompass a diverse array of pulmonary disorders, comprising more than 100 conditions, characterized by the development of lung scarring and fibrosis. ILDs exhibit a range of characteristic manifestations, including respiratory symptoms such as coughing and difficulty breathing, a decrease in pulmonary capacities, abnormalities observed on chest radiographs, abnormal fibrosis, and inflammation detected on biopsies. ILDs can be classified into individual disorders based on specific clinical, physiological, radiological, and histopathological features. Granulomatous inflammation, without parenchymal fibrosis, is a clear sign of sarcoidosis. On the other hand, broad pulmonary fibrosis and lung distortion are specific characteristics of idiopathic pulmonary fibrosis (IPF). The intricacy of establishing a definitive diagnosis has hindered the ability to accurately estimate the prevalence rates of ILDs. Nevertheless, it seems that IDLs are prevalent globally and primarily impact adults. The most prevalent ILD is IPF, affecting approximately 3 million individuals globally and 130,000 individuals in the United States. Furthermore, there has been a reported upward trend in the incidence rate of IPF. The epidemiology of ILDs can vary depending on the specific disorder. For example, IPF exhibits a higher prevalence among individuals aged 65 years and above, whereas sarcoidosis seems to be more commonly observed among African Americans and Northern Europeans.

The prognosis of ILDs exhibits heterogeneity, encompassing a spectrum that spans from partially reversible fibrosis to chronic progressive fibrotic ILDs, which possess the potential for fatality. In particular, IPF, which is the prevailing chronic progressive fibrotic disorder, exhibits a significantly unfavorable prognosis, as evidenced by a median survival time of merely 2–5 years subsequent to diagnosis. Patients with IPF frequently experience acute exacerbations that have the potential to be fatal. The progression of IPF exhibits significant interindividual and intraindividual heterogeneity. Certain patients experience a gradual progression of their diseases, while others encounter a rapid decline in lung function. Furthermore, within the same patient, there may be alternating periods of low changes in lung function and rapid deterioration. Sarcoidosis, a prevalent inflammatory bowel disease (ILD) characterized by significant morbidity, exhibits diverse patterns of progression and outcome among patients. These variations encompass an acute onset with spontaneous regression, as well as a chronic progressive disease. Frequently, ILDs exhibit comorbidities and/or lack distinct symptoms, which can complicate the diagnosis process. Consequently, this can lead to treatment delays and negatively impact the patient's prognosis. For instance, a study revealed a delay of approximately 2.1 years in diagnosing IPF patients. In the majority of instances, ILDs are classified as idiopathic conditions, indicating that the etiology of the pulmonary injury and subsequent fibrosis remains unidentified. Nevertheless, certain instances have established a correlation between ILDs and systemic disorders, such as autoimmune diseases like rheumatoid arthritis, infections, or exposure to environmental agents that specifically inflict harm on the lungs, such as tobacco smoke or asbestos. Furthermore, certain instances of ILDs have been correlated with genetic mutations, whereby the modification of a particular group of genes is linked to an elevation in fibrosis or serves as the underlying cause of the ILDs known as Hermansky-Pudlak syndrome. Furthermore, it has been demonstrated that individuals who have undergone lung transplantation and hematopoietic stem cell transplantation exhibit an increased susceptibility to the development of bronchiolitis obliterans, a relatively uncommon form of idiopathic pulmonary disease (ILD).

The precise mechanisms underlying the development of IDLs remain largely unidentified, although they seem to be influenced by multiple factors, such as aging and injuries to the lung epithelium. Two prominent characteristics of ILDs are the existence of atypical inflammation and fibrosis within the pulmonary system. These conditions are distinguished by an excessive proliferation of inflammatory cells, such as macrophages and lymphocytes, as well as an abnormal accumulation of collagens and other extracellular matrix constituents within the lungs. Nevertheless, the role of inflammation in IPF is a subject of debate and lacks comprehensive understanding, despite the presence of evidence indicating the infiltration of polymorphonuclear cells in the lungs or the manifestation of profibrotic characteristics in activated macrophages. The primary identified characteristic contributing to the onset of fibrosis in IPF lung is the localized proliferation of fibroblasts and myofibroblasts, resulting in the synthesis of collagen and other extracellular matrix constituents subsequent to prolonged damage to the lung alveolar epithelium. The precise mechanisms underlying the accumulation and activation of fibroblasts and myofibroblasts are still not fully understood. However, it is possible that multiple pathways are involved, each with distinct dynamics, which could account for the wide range of clinical manifestations observed in different patients.

Treatment strategies are typically determined by the particular diagnosis of ILD and the extent of the disease. To prevent the progression of ILDs with a known cause, it is recommended to avoid the triggering agent. Nevertheless, as previously stated, the majority of ILD cases are idiopathic and, consequently, cannot be prevented, except by minimizing exposure to risk factors such as cigarette smoking and environmental and microbial stimuli. The therapeutic interventions for ILDs are contingent upon the particular ailment and have undergone comprehensive evaluation by Kim et al. and Richeldi et al. The treatment regimen frequently involved the administration of corticosteroids and/or immunosuppressive agents, such as prednisone, cyclophosphamide, or azathioprine, with the aim of maintaining lung function, decreasing the occurrence of acute exacerbations, and enhancing patient survival. Nevertheless, it appears that the implementation of these therapies has not yielded sustained improvement for patients in the most severe instances of progressive fibrosis. Currently, there is no proven treatment for IPF that can effectively extend the lifespan of patients. Two antifibrotic agents that have received approval have demonstrated efficacy in mitigating the deterioration of pulmonary function and decelerating the advancement of the disease in individuals afflicted with IPF and other progressive isolated lung diseases (ILDs). Their efficiency may be attributed to their ability to target multiple pathways. Their mode of operation remains inadequately comprehended. It has been observed that Nintedanib exhibits inhibitory effects on certain intracellular tyrosine kinase receptors implicated in IPF, such as profibrotic mediators, platelet-derived growth factor receptor, fibroblasts growth factor receptor, and vascular endothelial growth factor (VEGF) receptor. Conversely, pirfenidone demonstrates a wide range of antifibrotic, anti-inflammatory, and antioxidant properties, including the reduction of TGF^2 and TNF±. Nevertheless, these two antifibrotic agents have been associated with certain unfavorable occurrences, such as gastrointestinal events like diarrhea. If patients do not receive counseling and personalized practical management for these events, they may choose to stop their treatments. Clinical trials have demonstrated that the antioxidant N-acetylcysteine, either as a standalone treatment or in combination with corticosteroids or pirfenidone, shows potential in enhancing lung function and decelerating the advancement of the disease in patients with IPF. Although candidate biological immunomodulatory drugs, such as interferon gamma-1b treatment, have shown promising preliminary results in preventing the progression of IPF, clinical trials have frequently failed to detect any improvement in patients. Nevertheless, numerous treatment alternatives are still undergoing clinical trials, providing patients with optimism. Mesenchymal stem cell-based therapies have exhibited encouraging preclinical outcomes; however, further investigation is required to validate or refute these findings. Given the absence of any existing treatments, lung transplantation is the final recourse for patients afflicted with advanced progressive cases of IDLs. This procedure has demonstrated the ability to enhance survival rates. Nevertheless, the median survival rate following transplantation continues to be relatively low. For instance, the average survival time after transplantation in patients with IPF is six years. This underscores the necessity for innovative treatment approaches.

Collectively, ILDs continue to be a significant health issue for individuals for whom treatments are frequently ineffective. Although there has been some advancement in comprehending ILDs, the identification of a remedy for the most severe chronic progressive ILDs is still quite distant. Presently, the field of medical research pertaining to ILDs encompasses both fundamental investigations, involving the integration of cell culture and animal experimentation, as well as clinical investigations, encompassing clinical trials and real-world studies. The primary objective of this research is to elucidate the underlying mechanisms and molecular pathways implicated in the pathogenesis of atypical pulmonary inflammation and fibrosis. The primary aims of these studies are twofold: (1) to identify novel biological markers that can streamline the diagnosis of ILDs and track their advancement, and (2) to devise innovative treatments for currently untreatable ILDs, with the goal of enhancing the well-being and longevity of affected individuals.

2.3.4. Cystic Fibrosis

CF is a genetic disorder characterized by mutations in the cystic fibrosis transmembrane conductance regulator (*CFTR*) gene, resulting in significant disability. The CFTR gene is responsible for encoding a protein that facilitates the translation of a transmembrane channel containing chloride ions. This channel plays a crucial role in regulating the transport of anions and the clearance mechanism of mucocilia in the airways. The majority of cases of CF (70%) are attributed to genetic risk factors. The gene accountable for the onset of CF is known as "delta Phe508." This gene is frequently found to undergo a triple-base deletion, leading to the absence of the amino acid phenylalanine at residue 508 of the anticipated 1,480 amino acid CFTR protein. Furthermore, as of the present time, over 2,000 mutations have been identified that have the potential to influence the function of CFTR in humans. The mutations can be classified into different categories: protein production mutations (Class 1), which include nonsense and splice mutations that disrupt protein production; protein processing mutations (Class 2), which involve the addition or deletion of amino acids; gating mutations (Class 3), which cause the CFTR protein to remain closed; conduction mutations (Class 4), which result in dysfunction in protein functionality; and insufficient protein mutations (Class 5). It is worth mentioning that CFTR mRNA transcripts are observed in the epithelial cells in various regions of the respiratory tract, such as the nasal, tracheal, and bronchial epithelial cells. However, it is worth mentioning that the expression of CFTR mRNA in these epithelial cells is relatively low, with only 1–2 copies per cell.

The global prevalence of CF is estimated to be around 70,000 individuals, with a higher incidence observed among children of Northern European ethnicity, estimated to be 1 in every 2,500–3,000 births. The disease exhibits a significant mortality rate, with estimated survival rates ranging from 33 to 50 years across various regions globally. Furthermore, the financial impact of CF is just starting to be understood. In Germany, the cost of managing patients with CF ranges from €17,551 per patient-year to around €48,603 in the United Kingdom.

Genetic mutations and recurrent and/or persistent bacterial infections are the primary cellular mechanisms underlying CF. Significantly, the CFTR mutation results in the misfolding or malfunctioning of a protein, which can cause dehydrated mucus. This, in turn, hampers the clearance of mucus by the mucociliary system. Despite the continuous production of mucus by goblet cells and submucosal glands, the insufficient clearance of mucus by cilia may lead to the formation of mucus plugs. The presence of these mucus plugs may lead to local tissue hypoxia, specifically on the surface of epithelial cells. The occurrence of local tissue hypoxia is additionally linked to local inflammation and an elevated susceptibility to bacterial infections. Furthermore, the most significant risk factors for the progression of CF, particularly during the initial years of life, are both recurrent and persistent bacterial infections affecting the large airways.

A fundamental requirement exists for enhanced drug delivery mechanisms that can efficiently transport therapeutic drugs to the specific location of pathology. Numerous strategies can be employed to facilitate the delivery of drugs through nasal and/or pulmonary routes. These strategies encompass the utilization of commonly employed absorption enhancers, including surfactants (such as bile salts, phospholipids, fatty acids, and derivatives), cationic polymers, enzymatic inhibitors, cyclodextrins, and tight junction modulators. Additional approaches could involve exploring the effectiveness of nanoparticles, which are employed as carriers for drugs. Notable instances encompass polystyrene-based mucopenetrating particles.

2.3.5. Tuberculosis

TB presently stands as the primary cause of global mortality resulting from a solitary infectious agent. In the year 2018, approximately 10 million individuals fell ill and 1.5 million succumbed to the disease on a global scale. The geographical distribution of TB is not uniform. Around 66% of TB cases reported to the WHO in 2018 were concentrated in South-East Asia (44%) and Africa (24%), while Europe (3%) and the Americas (3%) had significantly lower incidence rates. In 2018, India had the highest number of TB cases, with 2.69 million cases, followed by China with 866,000 cases and Indonesia with 845,000 cases.

The main causative agent of TB in humans is the acid-fast bacterial species *M. tuberculosis*, characterized by a comparatively lower incidence of zoonotic cases, specifically 143,000 cases in 2018, can be attributed to the animal-adapted species *M. bovis*. Despite the absence of several classical virulence factors commonly observed in other bacterial pathogens, such as exotoxins, *M. tuberculosis* remains highly contagious when spread through aerosols emitted by individuals with active TB through sneezing, coughing, or spitting due to their lungs. The inhalation of the pathogen into the alveoli of the lower respiratory tract occurs when a susceptible individual is exposed to droplets containing the bacterium. In this context, resident macrophages, which are typically the initial cells of the immune system to interact with *M. tuberculosis* begins in the lung and subsequently leads to the internalization of the bacterium.

The bacterium possesses a collection of virulence genes that, when deactivated, lead to a decrease in pathogenicity in an experimental model of TB. However, this deactivation does not hinder the growth of mycobacteria under ideal in vitro conditions, without the presence of stress or starvation. The pathogenic elements of *M. tuberculosis* can be classified into various categories, such as lipid metabolism enzymes, cell envelope proteins, macrophage function inhibitors, protein kinases, proteases, metal transporters, gene regulators, and proteins with undefined functions like PE and PE_PGRS proteins. Upon being engulfed by alveolar macrophages, mitochondria (*M. tuberculosis* exhibits resistance to reactive O_2 and nitrogen intermediates, as well as the ability to hinder phagosome acidification and lysosomal fusion. The aforementioned functions play a crucial role in the long-term presence of the pathogen within the host during latent TB and also aid in the replication of bacteria, leading to tissue spread and subsequent damage in active TB cases and subsequent person-to-person transmission. The pulmonary TB condition can give rise to various forms of structural lung damage, such as fibrosis, cavitation, traction bronchiectasis, bronchostenosis, and parenchymal destruction.

The standard therapeutic regimen recommended by the WHO for drug-susceptible pulmonary TB entails the administration of four drugs, namely isoniazid, rifampicin, pyrazinamide, and ethambutol, for a duration of two months. Subsequently, patients are advised to continue with isoniazid and rifampicin for an additional four months. The treatment success rate for patients diagnosed, reported, and treated with TB in 2017 was 85% worldwide. However, the success rate decreases to 56% in cases of TB that exhibit resistance to both isoniazid and rifampicin, commonly referred to as multidrug resistant (MDR) or rifampicin resistant (RR). In 2018, the global incidence of multidrug-resistant TB (MDR/RR-TB) reached 484,000 cases, accounting for 3.4% of newly diagnosed TB cases and 18% of cases that had been previously treated.

Multidrug-resistant TB (MDR-TB) necessitates an extended treatment period, as per the World Health Organization's recommended regimen. This regimen comprises an initial intensive phase lasting 8 months, during which a minimum of four efficacious second-line TB drugs, along with pyrazinamide, are administered. This is followed by a continuation phase, during which at least three potent second-line anti-TB drugs are administered. Consequently, the treatment duration is extended to a total of 20 months. A shorter treatment regimen recommended by the WHO has been developed. This regimen consists of a 4- to 6-month intensive phase involving the administration of seven drugs: moxifloxacin, kanamycin, prothionamide, clofazimine, pyrazinamide, high-dose isoniazid, and ethambutol. This is followed by a 5-month continuation phase with the same drugs.

Furthermore, the administration of MDR-TB treatment is accompanied by a lower success rate and longer duration. Additionally, it incurs higher costs, with estimated per-case expenses of USD $134,000 in the United States and €57,213 in 15 European Union (EU) countries. In comparison, drug-susceptible TB treatment incurs costs of USD $17,000 and €10,282, respectively. Hence, there is a need for techniques that can enhance the efficacy of drug delivery in patients while simultaneously reducing the cost and/or duration of anti-TB treatment.

Advancements in drug delivery systems possess the capacity to enhance the effectiveness of current TB medications. These systems provide enhanced precision in targeting TB drugs, enhanced dispersion and bioavailability, and decreased occurrence of adverse reactions. Regarding TB control, potential outcomes of novel drug delivery systems may encompass enhancements in patient compliance with TB treatment protocols, accompanied by a reduction in the occurrence of default TB cases and treatment failures. Additionally, these systems could facilitate the development of novel therapeutic regimens with reduced durations.

The primary method of administering isoniazid, rifampicin, ethambutol, and pyrazinamide for the treatment of drug-susceptible TB is through oral administration. Furthermore, several second-line medications employed in the management of multidrug-resistant TB (MDR-TB), namely amikacin, kanamycin, and capreomycin, are administered via intramuscular or intravenous injection. The pulmonary route is currently under investigation as a potential method for administering TB drugs due to its potential to more efficiently target the drugs to the lungs, which are the primary entry point for *M. tuberculosis* and the main location of TB infection. In recent times, there has been an exploration of a gastric resident delivery system, which has demonstrated the ability to administer multigram doses of TB drugs over an extended period of several weeks in a swine model.

A diverse array of novel vehicles is currently under scrutiny in relation to the transportation of TB medications. These materials consist of liposomes (usually measuring 50–450 nm) made from phosphatidylcholine and cholesterol, microparticles (ranging from 1–1,000 µm) made from polylactic acid (PLA) or polylactic-co-glycolic acid (PLGA), and nanoparticles (ranging from 1–100 nm in at least one dimension) made from alginate, PLA, PLGA, or poly-ε-caprolactone (PCL). Liposomes, microparticles, and/or nanoparticles have been effectively utilized to encapsulate various TB medications. These formulations encompass the primary drugs isoniazid, rifampicin, ethambutol, and pyrazinamide, as well as the secondary drugs levofloxacin, ofloxacin, and capreomycin. One study demonstrated that the utilization of aerosolized PLGA nanoparticles resulted in enhanced bioavailability of isoniazid, rifampicin, and pyrazinamide, while also effectively eradicating *M. tuberculosis* is more effectively eradicated from the lungs of infected guinea pigs compared to conventional orally administered medications.

Liposomes, microparticles, and nanoparticles possess the capacity to be internalized by macrophages, thereby enabling the targeted concentration of TB drugs within the primary host cell of invading *M. tuberculosis*. This approach would effectively decrease the dosage and duration necessary to achieve complete elimination of the infection, consequently mitigating the adverse effects commonly associated with existing TB treatment protocols. Additionally, it is feasible to create vehicles that release their drug cargo once they have entered macrophages. As an illustration, researchers have successfully engineered nanoparticles incorporating cyclodextrin-based pH-operated valves. These valves are designed to selectively release isoniazid exclusively in an acidic milieu, such as the acidified endosomes found within human macrophages.

The development of novel delivery systems that selectively target drugs to the primary site of TB infection and pathology in humans holds promise for substantially enhancing TB control efforts. These systems have the potential to reduce the duration and dosage necessary to achieve effective chemotherapy outcomes. Implementing this approach would not only lead to a reduction in healthcare expenses, but also, more significantly, mitigate the negative consequences of TB medications on patients and enhance treatment adherence and efficacy. Hence, it is anticipated that additional investigation and experimentation with novel drug delivery systems will result in more effective yet cost-effective therapies for both drug-susceptible and drug-resistant TB.

2.3.6. Lung Cancer

On a global scale, the primary cause of death related to lung cancer is the delayed diagnosis and insufficient treatment interventions. Approximately 70% of lung cancer patients are diagnosed at an advanced stage, typically stage III or IV. This malignancy is highly invasive, rapidly metastasizing, and widespread in both males and females. According to statistical data, the mortality rate attributed to lung cancer in the United States surpasses the cumulative mortality rate of the four primary cancer causes, namely prostate, breast, colon, and pancreas. There is a strong correlation between a smoking history of 20 years or more and the likelihood of developing and dying from the condition. The development of lung cancer caused by tobacco is believed to rely heavily on the competitive interactions between genes and enzymes, specifically in relation to procarcinogens and the resulting DNA damage. Due to this rationale, it is widely accepted that lung cancer can be effectively prevented through the implementation of smoking prevention and cessation measures. The mitigation of the escalating incidence of respiratory cancers in nations experiencing a surge in smoking necessitates the implementation of public awareness and education initiatives aimed at reducing or eliminating cigarette smoking.

Lung cancer is the primary contributor to cancer-related mortality on a global scale, affecting both males and females. Based on a study conducted by Martin et al., the estimated number of new cases of lung cancer in 2012 was around 1.8 million, which constituted 12.9% of all newly diagnosed cancer cases. The Global Burden of Disease Study 2020 revealed that lung cancer imposed a significant healthcare burden and incurred substantial expenses on a global scale. A study found no correlation between the level of economic progress and cancer fatalities in men. Remarkably, the study also demonstrated a correlation between a country's economic development status and the number of women who die from lung cancer. Breast cancer continues to be the primary cause of mortality among women in developing nations.

There is a strong correlation between the occurrence and death rate of lung cancer and the past use of cigarettes. It is noteworthy that there has been a noticeable upward trajectory in the incidence of lung cancer and mortality rates among both males and females over time. This trend suggests a rise in smoking prevalence, followed by a subsequent decrease, potentially attributable to the development and execution of comprehensive smoking cessation strategies. The available data from the United States and the United Kingdom indicate a significant decline in both the prevalence and mortality rates of lung cancer since the 1990s. On the other hand, it is noteworthy that low- and middle-income countries (LMICs), specifically the BRICS nations (Brazil, Russia, India, China, and South Africa), have observed a substantial rise in cigarette smoking rates, regardless of gender. LMICs exhibit a higher mortality rate associated with lung cancer, despite having a lower incidence of the disease in comparison to higher-income countries. The observed phenomenon can be attributed to the unequal distribution of healthcare facilities, resulting in difficulties in promptly diagnosing and treating patients. In addition to sociocultural taboos, environmental pollution and/or contamination are also significant contributing factors. It emphasizes the necessity of implementing preventive measures such as the WHO Framework Convention on Tobacco Control, which should be reinforced in these countries. This can be achieved through tax policies, smoke-free zones, surveillance, support for quitting smoking, education on the negative effects of tobacco, and restrictions on tobacco advertising.

The intricate heterogeneity of lung cancer arises from its varying origins within the bronchial tree and the diverse manifestations of symptoms and signs exhibited by patients, which are contingent upon the specific type and anatomical site of the cancer. Lung cancer is conventionally categorized into two main groups: small-cell lung cancer (SCLC), which accounts for 15% of all lung cancers, and non-small-cell lung carcinoma (NSCLC), which accounts for 85% of all lung cancers. NSCLCs are commonly classified into three main subtypes: adenocarcinoma, squamous cell carcinoma, and large cell carcinoma. The stratification of lung cancer was enhanced by the inclusion of distinct histopathologic features and dependable immunohistochemical markers, enabling a clear differentiation between invasive adenocarcinomas and preinvasive lesions. Moreover, the emergence of molecular characterization techniques for lung cancers and the continuous expansion of therapeutic options have significantly influenced the current classification of lung cancer. The available data suggest that lung cancer encompasses a collection of diseases that exhibit histological and molecular heterogeneity, even when classified within the same histological subtype.

Squamous cell lung cancers are statistically significant compared to other subtypes of lung cancer due to their higher prevalence (25%–30%) and their location in the main bronchi of the lung, as well as their ability to metastasize to the carina, which is the bifurcation site of the trachea in the bronchi. Peripherally located adenocarcinomas, which are known to cause lobar atelectasis and pneumonitis, account for 40% of all lung cancers. Bronchioloalveolar cancers have been reclassified based on their origin in alveoli and their localized dissemination into interalveolar compartments. Adenocarcinoma in situ and minimally invasive adenocarcinoma (MIA) were further reclassified as lung cancers. SCLC, which account for approximately 10% to 15% of all lung cancers, originate from neuroendocrine cells known as APUD cells in the bronchus. These cells, referred to as Feyrter cells, are highly aggressive tumors that have the ability to rapidly spread into nearby lymphatic vessels and associated regional lymph nodes.

Over 70% of patients with (NSCLC) are diagnosed at advanced stages or with metastatic disease. The selection and progression of treatments for NSCLC are determined based on the specific location and stage of the tumor, taking into consideration the patient's involvement and performance status. This section presents an overview of conventional and current therapeutic approaches for NSCLC based on their stage, metastasis, and recurrence.

1. **NSCLC Stage I and II:** Surgical intervention is the prevailing primary therapeutic approach for resectable stage I and II disease. Postoperative adjuvant platinum-based chemotherapy has been suggested and demonstrated to be beneficial for patients with stage II NSCLC.
2. **Stage III Refers to Non-Small Cell Lung Cancer:** The treatment options for stage III NSCLC are divided into resectable and nonresectable disease due to the complex heterogeneity of the disease, which is heavily influenced by the involvement of regional lymph nodes. The spectrum of tumors encompasses resectable tumors exhibiting microscopic metastases to nearby lymph nodes, as well as nonresectable stage III disease characterized by distant nodal involvement. Conventionally, the treatment for stage IIIA resectable disease involves surgical intervention followed by chemotherapy exclusively. On the other hand, the treatment for nonresectable stage IIIA disease involves the administration of chemotherapy alone or a combination of chemotherapy and post-chemoradiation therapy with chemoradiation. The conventional treatment approach for stage IIIB NSCLC involves a sequential regimen of chemotherapy or external radiation therapy.
3. **Stage IV – Neoplastic Spontaneous Cell Line:** Stage IV NSCLC is observed in 40% of newly diagnosed patients due to the intricate nature of the disease. Given this rationale, the majority of treatment modalities primarily rely on combination therapy, encompassing combination chemotherapy, combination chemotherapy and targeted therapy, and external radiation therapy in conjunction with internal endoscopic radiation therapy as deemed necessary.
4. **Recurrent Non-Small Cell Lung Cancer:** The phenomenon of NSCLC recurrence or relapse subsequent to an initial intervention involving surgical intervention, radiation therapy, and/or chemotherapy. The treatment regimen for patients with stage IV NSCLC is identical to that of stage IV NSCLC, namely chemotherapy. On the other hand, patients who experience a recurrence of cancer after undergoing chemotherapy treatment have different options available. These options include: (1) external palliative radiation therapy to alleviate pain and other symptoms associated with the tumor; (2) cytotoxic chemotherapy; (3) Epidermal growth factor receptor (EGFR) inhibitors (TKIs) for patients with or without EGFR mutations, and (4) Echinoderm microtubule associated protein-like 4 (EML4-ALK) inhibitors (crizotinib) for patients with EML-ALK translocations.

2.4. Chemotherapy Efficacy and Strategies for Non-Small Cell Lung Cancer Treatment

In addition to surgical resection, chemotherapy-based treatment for NSCLC has demonstrated significant efficacy in improving patient survival rates. Various categories of chemotherapies are presently employed and increasingly being tested for the advantage of patients with NSCLC. A number of essential treatment strategies are outlined below.

2.4.1. Anti-Angiogenic Agents

The angiogenic pathways are widely recognized as a crucial focus in the treatment of NSCLC, as tumors demonstrate the formation of new blood vessels in the desmoplastic stroma to support their growth and advancement. The inhibition of angiogenesis necessary for tumor growth is widely recognized as a crucial approach, with a particular focus on targeting proangiogenic factors including VEGF, fibroblast growth factor (FGF), and platelet-derived growth factor (PDGF). Currently, bevacizumab, an anti-VEGF monoclonal antibody, has received approval as the primary treatment for advanced NSCLC when used in conjunction with platinum-based chemotherapy. Research has also suggested that bevacizumab could be advantageous for treating patients with adenocarcinoma. Nevertheless, it has been noted that over time, all patients exhibit resistance to the administration of anti-VEGF agents. This results in the creation of a tyrosine kinase inhibitor (TKI) called sorafenib, which specifically targets VEGFR-2/3, PDGFR-β, c-Kit, Raf, and Flt-3. Sorafenib has demonstrated encouraging results in various phase I and II trials, particularly in patients with NSCLC who have the K-Ras mutation.

2.4.2. Inhibitors of Insulin-Like Growth Factor

The IGF system, also known as the insulin-like growth factor system, consists of two receptors: the insulin-like growth factor 1 receptor (IGF-IR) and the IGF-IIR receptor, along with their respective intracellular ligands.

These ligands exhibit increased expression levels in various types of cancer, including lung cancer. In a phase II trial, Figitumumab, an anti-IGF-1R monoclonal antibody, demonstrated a significant improvement compared to chemotherapy alone in patients with NSCLC who had not received treatment before and had localized or metastatic disease. Cixutumumab and dalotuzumab, two additional monoclonal antibodies targeting IGF ligands, are currently undergoing clinical trials.

2.4.3. Inhibitors of Histone Deacetylase (HDACs)

Histones represent a group of fundamental proteins that form complexes with DNA within the nucleus, facilitating its condensation into chromatin. The regulation of protein expression and activity in cancer initiation and progression is mediated by HDACs. Several HDAC inhibitors have been developed and reported to modify the acetylation of important intracellular proteins involved in cell growth and proliferation. The cellular proteins that are targeted for investigation encompass tumor suppressor protein (p53), HSP90, STAT3, subunits of NFκ-B, and α-tubulin, among others. The FDA has granted approval for two HDAC inhibitors, namely suberoylanilide hydroxamic acid and romidepsin, for the treatment of cutaneous T-cell lymphoma. Multiple HDAC inhibitors are currently undergoing clinical trials for the treatment of NSCLC. These inhibitors include entinostat, Pivanex, CI-994, panobinostat, and romidepsin.

2.4.4. Proapopototic Agents

Most cancer cells are able to evade the typical apoptotic process by either increasing the expression of antiapoptotic factors or decreasing the expression of proapoptotic mechanisms, or both. Conatumumab (anti-DR1) and YM155 (antisurvivin), which are both apoptotic promoter agents, are currently undergoing clinical trials for the treatment of NSCLC. These proapoptotic agents have been found to produce significant results when used in combination with chemotherapy, as compared to chemotherapy alone.

Despite ongoing research and the development of various targeted agents, further investigations are necessary to ascertain early detection and treatment of these cancers, which could significantly enhance patients' long-term survival. The significance of pulmonary drug delivery is growing due to its unique physiological environment and superior absorption and treatment capabilities. Over the course of a decade, there has been a notable acceleration in the pursuit of enhancing the delivery of cancer therapeutic drugs to the pulmonary system. The significant endorsement of Pfizer's Exubera, an inhalation powder, has played a crucial role in the ongoing evaluation of similar approaches for numerous other prospective pharmaceuticals. Various drug carrier systems at microscopic scales, including liposomes, polymer conjugates, polymeric micelles, microparticles, and nanoparticles, are currently undergoing extensive research to facilitate targeted delivery of diverse anticancer therapeutic molecules to specific regions of the lung exhibiting cancerous conditions.

2.5. Challenges of Current Therapeutic Strategies

While extensive research has been conducted on the disease pathology and epidemiology of various infectious and noninfectious respiratory diseases, the progress in developing more efficacious therapies is still in the experimental stages. Asthma and COPD are prevalent noninfectious ailments that have a significant impact on substantial populations in both high-income and low-income nations across the globe. The disease's pathology and progression exhibit significant variations across different demographic groups and are primarily influenced by individual lifestyle choices. In the treatment of mild to moderate symptoms of chronic respiratory disorders, commonly prescribed bronchodilators such as albuterol and ipratropium, as well as recently developed long-acting β2 agnostics and long-acting muscarinic antagonists, have demonstrated efficacy. However, the effectiveness of these medications in patients with chronic asthma and COPD has been found to be incomplete. Furthermore, the efficacy of current therapeutic interventions has been compromised by individual lifestyle behaviors such as smoking or prolonged exposure to occupational dust. Furthermore, the advanced stages of the illness are distinguished by permanent harm to the lung tissue, resulting in scarring, which cannot be remedied with the currently accessible treatments.

On the other hand, respiratory diseases resulting from infectious agents are a significant cause for concern, as they tend to occur seasonally and persist within or outside the human body. The emergence of new potent mutants with heightened drug resistance, resulting from natural selection, mutations, and excessive antibiotic usage, has given rise to various pandemics on a global scale. Recent research has also brought attention to the phenomenon of cross-transfer of diverse infectious agents between different species, specifically between animals and humans, thereby impacting global populations on a broader scope. The recent occurrence of COVID-19 serves as a notable illustration, stemming from a specific member of the coronavirus family. This outbreak is attributed to the absence of inherent immunity against newly emerged mutant strains, thereby posing a significant risk to global health.

2.6. Summary

The prevalence of CRDs is a significant global burden, primarily attributed to the aging population and the absence of effective strategies to mitigate the risk factors associated with the onset and advancement of these pulmonary ailments. Moreover, the absence of efficacious interventions that could potentially be employed for the management and/or prevention of these persistent respiratory conditions exacerbates the societal and economic ramifications linked to chronic lung diseases. Furthermore, it is imperative to conduct additional research to identify innovative therapies for CRDs. Additionally, it is crucial to prioritize the efficient administration of treatments to the specific location of the disease, namely the airway epithelium, parenchyma, and bronchioles. Furthermore, the therapies should specifically focus on particular cell types that may be playing a pivotal role in the advancement of the diseases. Various biomolecular entities can be employed to optimize the drug delivery and absorption/adsorption of prescription drugs in controlled-release drug delivery systems. Additional investigation is necessary to determine the effectiveness and safety of these drug delivery vehicles.

A Closer Look

Lung Cancer

Lung cancer is one of the most common and deadly cancers worldwide, characterized by uncontrolled cell growth in lung tissues. Two primary types of lung cancer are non-small cell lung cancer (NSCLC), accounting for approximately 85% of cases, and small cell lung cancer (SCLC), known for its aggressive nature and rapid spread. Smoking remains the leading cause of lung cancer, although non-smokers are also at risk due to factors like air pollution, exposure to radon gas, and genetic predispositions.

The symptoms of lung cancer, such as persistent cough, chest pain, and shortness of breath, often appear late in the disease, leading to diagnosis at advanced stages. The asymptomatic early progression makes regular screening, particularly for high-risk groups, crucial for early detection. Techniques like low-dose CT scans are now utilized for at-risk individuals, significantly improving the detection rates of early-stage lung cancer.

Lung cancer diagnosis involves imaging studies (CT, MRI, and PET scans) and biopsies to determine the type and stage of cancer, which guide treatment planning. Treatment approaches depend on the type and stage, with options including surgery, radiation therapy, chemotherapy, targeted therapy, and immunotherapy. Immunotherapy, particularly, has shown promise in recent years, providing hope for longer survival in advanced cases.

Preventive measures focus primarily on reducing smoking rates through public health initiatives, as well as minimizing exposure to pollutants. Recent advancements in personalized medicine, where therapies are tailored to the genetic profile of the tumor, offer improved outcomes and underscore the need for continued research and support for lung cancer patients.

References

1. Aït-Khaled, N., Enarson, D., & Bousquet, J., (2001). Chronic Respiratory Diseases in Developing Countries: The Burden and Strategies for Prevention and Management. *Bulletin of the World Health Organization. 79*(10), 971–979.
2. Akins, S. A., O'Malley, P., (2000). Should Health-Care Systems Pay for Replacement Therapy in Patients with Alpha(1)-Antitrypsin Deficiency? A Critical Review and Cost-Effectiveness Analysis. *Chest. 117*(3), 875–880.
3. Al, M. J., Koopmanschap, M. A., van Enckevort, P. J., Geertsma, A., van der Bij, W., de Boer, W. J., & TenVergert, E. M., (1998). Cost-Effectiveness of Lung Transplantation in the Netherlands. *Chest. 113,* 124–140.
4. Anon, J. M., de Lorenzo, A., Garcia, Zarazaga, A., Gomez-Tello, V., & Garrido, G., (1999). Mechanical Ventilation of Patients on Long-Term Oxygen Therapy with Acute Exacerbations of Chronic Obstructive Pulmonary Disease: Prognosis and Cost-Utility Analysis. *Intensive Care Medicine. 25*(5), 452–457.
5. Bell, D. M. (2004). "World Health Organization Working Group on Prevention of International and Community Transmission of SARS. Public Health Interventions and SARS Spread, 2003."
6. Buist, A. S., (2002). Guidelines for the Management of Chronic Obstructive Pulmonary Disease. *Respiratory Medicine. 96*(Suppl. C), S11–16.
7. Chan-Yeung, M., Aït-Khaled, N., White, N., Tsang, K. W., & Tan, W. C., (2004). Management of Chronic Pulmonary Disease in Asia and Africa. *International Journal of Tuberculosis and Lung Disease. 8*(2), 159–170.
8. Chew, F. T., Goh, D. Y., & Lee, B. W., (1999). The Economic Cost of Asthma in Singapore. *Australian and New Zealand Journal of Medicine. 29*(2), 228–233.
9. Chung, F., Barnes, N., Allen, M., Angus, R., Corris, P., Knox, A., et al., (2002). Assessing the Burden of Respiratory Disease in the U.K. *Respiratory Medicine. 96,* 963–975.
10. Crockett, A. J., Cranston, J. M., Moss, J. R., & Alpers, J. H., (2001). A Review of Long-Term Oxygen Therapy for Chronic Obstructive Pulmonary Disease. *Respiratory Medicine. 95,* 437–443.
11. Demicheli, V., Jefferson, T., Rivetti, D., & Deeks, J., (2000). Prevention and Early Treatment of Influenza in Healthy Adults. *Vaccine. 18,* 957–1030.
12. Dolin, P. J., Raviglione, M. C., & Kochi, A., (1994). Global Tuberculosis Incidence and Mortality during 1990–2000. *Bulletin of the World Health Organization. 72,* 212–220.
13. Fitzner, K. A., Shortridge, K. F., McGhee, S. M., & Hedley, A. J., (2001). Cost-Effectiveness Study on Influenza Prevention in Hong Kong. *Health Policy. 56,* 215–234.
14. Fletcher, C. M. R., Peto, C., Tinker, M., & Speizer, F. E., (1976). *The Natural History of Chronic Bronchitis: An Eight Year Follow-up Study of Working Men in London*. New York: Oxford University Press.
15. Friedmann, M., & Hilleman, D. E., (2001). Economic Burden of Chronic Obstructive Pulmonary Disease: Impact of New Treatment Options. *Pharmacoeconomics. 19*(3), 245–254.
16. Ghosh, C. S., Ravindran, P., Joshi, M., & Stearns, S. C., (1998). Reductions in Hospital Use from Self-Management Training for Chronic Asthmatics. *Social Science and Medicine. 46*(8), 1087–1093.

17. GOLD (Global Initiative for Chronic Obstructive Lung Disease). (2001). "Global Strategy for the Diagnosis, Management and Prevention of GOLD." National Heart, Lung, and Blood Institute–WHO Workshop Report, NHLBI Publication 2701, National Institutes of Health, Bethesda, MD.

18. Hay, J. W., & Robin, E. C., (1991). Cost-Effectiveness of Alpha-1 Antitrypsin Replacement Therapy in Treatment of Congenital Chronic Obstructive Pulmonary Disease. *American Journal of Public Health. 81,* 427–433.

19. Hooi, L. N., Looi, I., & Ng, A. J., (2001). A Study on Community Acquired Pneumonia in Adults Requiring Hospital Admission in Penang. *Medical Journal of Malaysia. 56,* 275–284.

20. Hui, K. P., Chin, N. K., Chow, K., Brownlee, A., Yeo, T. C., Kumarasinghe, G., et al., (1993). Prospective Study of the Etiology of Adult Community Acquired Bacterial Pneumonia Needing Hospitalization in Singapore. *Singapore Medical Journal. 34,* 329–334.

21. Kiivet, R. A., Kaur, I., Lang, A., Aaviksoo, A., & Nirk, L., (2001). Costs of Asthma Treatment in Estonia. *European Journal of Public Health. 11,* 89–92.

22. LaDou, J., (2004). The Asbestos Cancer Epidemic. *Environmental Health Perspectives. 112,* 285–290.

23. Lee, P. Y., Matchar, D. V., Clements, D. A., Huber, J., Hamilton, J. D., & Peterson, E. D., (2002). Economic Analysis of Influenza Vaccination and Antiviral Treatment for Healthy Working Adults. *Annals of Internal Medicine. 137,* 225–231.

24. Lee, T. A., & Weiss, K. B., (2002). An Update on the Health Economics of Asthma and Allergy. *Current Opinion in Allergy and Clinical Immunology. 2,*195–200.

25. Leigh, J., Macaskill, P., Kuosma, E., & Mandryk, J., (1999). Global Burden of Disease and Injury Due to Occupational Factors. *Epidemiology. 10,* 626–631.

26. Lieberman, D., Schlaeffer, F., Boldur, I., Lieberman, D., Horowitz, S., Friedman, M. G., et al., (1996). Multiple Pathogens in Adult Patients Admitted with Community-Acquired Pneumonia: A One Year Prospective Study of 346 Consecutive Patients. *Thorax. 51,* 179–184.

27. Loewenson, R., (1999). Assessment of the Health Impact of Occupational Risk in Africa: Current Situation and Methodological Issues. *Epidemiology. 10,* 632–639.

28. Low, D. E., & McGeer, A., (2004). SARS—One Year Later. *New England Journal of Medicine. 349,* 2381–2382.

29. Mölken, M. P., Ruttenvan, Van Doorslaer, E. K., & Rutten, F. F., (1992). Economic Appraisal of Asthma and COPD Care: A Literature Review 1980–1991. *Social Science and Medicine. 35*(2), 161–175.

30. MRC (Medical Research Council Working Group). Long-Term Domiciliary Oxygen Therapy in Chronic Hypoxic Cor Pulmonale Complicating Chronic Bronchitis and Emphysema. Lancet. (1981). 1(8222), 681–686.

31. Murray, C. J. L., & A. D., Lopez, eds. (1996). The Global Burden of Disease: A Comprehensive Assessment of Mortality and Disability from Diseases, Injuries and Risk Factors in 1990 and Projected to 2020. Cambridge, MA: Harvard University Press.

32. NIOSH (National Institute of Occupational Safety and Health). (1999). Work-Related Lung Disease Surveillance Report 1999. NIOSH Publication 2000, 105. http://www.cdc.gov/niosh/docs/2000-105/2000-105.html.

33. Paltiel, A. D., Fuhlbrigge, A. L., Kitch, B. T., Liljas, B., Weiss, S. T., Neumann, P. J., & Kuntz, K. M., (2001). Cost-Effectiveness of Inhaled Corticosteroids in Adults with Mild-to-Moderate Asthma: Results from the Asthma Policy Model. *Journal of Allergy and Clinical Immunology. 108*(1), 39–49.

34. Postma, M. J., Jansema, P., van Genugten, M. L., L., Heijnen, M.-L. A., Jager, J. C., de Jong-van den Berg, L. T. W., (2002). Pharmacoeconomics of Influenza Vaccination for Healthy Working Adults. *Drugs. 62*(7), 1013–24.

35. Ramsey, S. D., Patrick, D. L., Albert, R. K., Larson, E. B., Wood, D. E., & Raghu, G., (1995). The Cost-Effectiveness of Lung Transplantation: A Pilot Study. *Chest. 108,* 1594–601.

36. Ruchlin, H. S., & Dasbach, E. J., (2001). An Economic Overview of Chronic Obstructive Pulmonary Disease. *Pharmacoeconomics. 19*(6), 623–642.

37. Sant'Anna, C. A., Stelmach, R., Feltrin, M. I., Zanetti, Filho, W. J., Chiba, T., & Cukier, A., (2003). Evaluation of Health-Related Quality of Life in Low-Income Patients with COPD Receiving Long-Term Oxygen Therapy. *Chest. 123*(1), 136–141.

38. Scanlon, P. D., Connett, J. E., Waller, L. A., Altose, M. D., Bailey, W. C., Buist, A. S., & Tashkin, D. P., (2000). Smoking Cessation and Lung Function in Mild-to-Moderate Chronic Obstructive Pulmonary Disease: The Lung Health Study. *American Journal of Respiratory and Critical Care Medicine. 161,* 381–390.

39. Schmidt, C. D., Elliott, C. G., Carmelli, D., Jensen, R. L., Gengiz, M., Schmit, J. C., et al., (1983). Prolonged Mechanical Ventilation for Respiratory Failure: A Cost-Benefit Analysis. *Critical Care Medicine. 11,* 407.

40. Scott, J. A., G., Hall, A. J., Muyodi, C., Lowe, B., Ross, M., Chohan, B., et al., (2000). Aetiology, Outcome, and Risk Factors for Mortality among Adults with Acute Pneumonia in Kenya. *Lancet. 355,* 1225–30.

41. Scuffham, P. A., & West, P. A., (2002). Economic Evaluation of Strategies for the Control and Management of Influenza in Europe. *Vaccine. 20,* 2562–78.

42. Smith, K. J., & Pesce, R. R., (1994). Pulmonary Artery Catheterization in Exacerbations of COPD Requiring Mechanical Ventilation: A Cost-Effectiveness Analysis. *Respiratory Care. 39,* 961–7.

43. Smith, K. R., (2000). National Burden of Disease in India from Indoor Air Pollution. *Proceedings of the National Academy of Sciences of the United States of America. 97*(24), 13286–93. [PMC free article]

44. Speizer, F. E., Fay, M. E., Dockery, D. W., Ferris, B. G., Jr. (1989). Chronic Obstructive Pulmonary Disease Mortality in Six, U. S., Cities. *American Review of Respiratory Disease. 140,* S49–55.

45. Stoloff, S., Poinsett-Holmes, K., & Dorinsky, P. M., (2002). Combination Therapy with Inhaled Long-Acting β2-Agonists and Inhaled Corticosteroids: A Paradigm Shift in Asthma Management. *Pharmacotherapy. 22*(2), 212–226.

46. Sudre, P., Jacquemet, S., Uldry, C., & Perneger, T. V., (1999). Objectives, Methods, and Content of Patient Education Programmes for Adults with Asthma: Systematic Review of Studies Published between 1979 and 1998. *Thorax. 54,* 681–7.

47. Sullivan, S. D., & Weiss, K. B., (2001). Health Economics of Asthma and Rhinitis: II. Assessing the Value of Interventions. *Journal of Allergy and Clinical Immunology. 107,* 203–210.

48. Toevs, C. D., Kaplan, R. M., & Atkins, C. J., (1984). The Costs and Effects of Behavioral Programs in Chronic Obstructive Pulmonary Disease. *Medical Care. 22,* 1088–100.

49. Trapido, A. S., Mqoqi, N. P., Macheke, C. M., Williams, B. G., Davies, J. C., & Panter, C., (1996). Occupational Lung Disease in Ex-Mineworkers—Sound a Further Alarm! *South African Medical Journal. 86*(5), 559.

50. Van den Boom, G., Mölken, M. P., Ruttenvan, Molema, J., Tirimanna, P. R., van Weel, C., van Schayck, C. P., (2001). The Cost Effectiveness of Early Treatment with Fluticasone Propionate 250 Microg Twice a Day in Subjects with Obstructive Airway Disease. Results of the DIMCA Program. *American Journal of Respiratory and Critical Care Medicine. 164*(11), 2057–2066.

51. Weiss, K. B., & Sullivan, S. D., (2001). The Health Economics of Asthma and Rhinitis: I. Assessing the Economic Impact. *Journal of Allergy and Clinical Immunology. 107,* 3–8.

52. WHO (World Health Organization). (2000). "Global Burden of Disease 2000: Deaths by Age, Sex and Cause for the Year 2000." WHO, Geneva.

Chapter

DISEASES OF THE CARDIOVASCULAR SYSTEM

3

Contents

Introduction

Cardiovascular disease (CVD) serves as an umbrella term for a diverse range of conditions affecting the heart and the entire circulatory system, encompassing both the network of blood vessels and the heart itself. These conditions are primarily concerned with impairing the system's ability to either move or circulate blood throughout the body. This broad categorization includes a variety of both congenital (present from birth) and acquired (developing after birth) diseases that afflict the circulatory system's components. As noted by Nichols et al. (2014), CVDs are among the most significant contributors to morbidity and mortality worldwide, highlighting the critical impact of these conditions on global health.

The scope of CVDs is extensive, including conditions like atherosclerosis, which is characterized by the buildup of plaques within the arteries. Atherosclerosis can manifest in several forms, including coronary artery disease (affecting the arteries that supply the heart), cerebral artery disease (affecting the arteries that supply the brain), and peripheral artery disease (affecting arteries that supply blood to the extremities). These conditions can lead to severe complications, such as myocardial infarction (commonly known as a heart attack) and ischemic stroke, which occurs when the blood supply to part of the brain is interrupted. According to Lloyd-Jones et al. (2010), myocardial infarction and stroke are among the leading causes of death associated with CVD, underscoring the severe consequences of these complications.

Furthermore, CVDs encompass conditions such as heart failure, a condition in which the heart is unable to pump blood efficiently, leading to fluid buildup and shortness of breath. Cardiac valvulopathies, which involve dysfunction of the heart valves, and arrhythmias, or irregular heartbeats, also fall under the broad category of CVD. Rheumatic heart disease, another significant condition, results from damage to the heart muscle and valves caused by rheumatic fever, a consequence of streptococcal bacterial infection. Congenital heart diseases, present from birth, affect the structure and function of the heart and are a major concern for pediatric health. Additionally, deep vein thrombosis (DVT) and pulmonary embolism, which involve the formation of blood clots in the deep veins and the lungs, respectively, are critical conditions that fall under the CVD spectrum.

The prevalence and impact of CVDs are staggering. As highlighted by the World Health Organization (2011), CVDs are the leading noncommunicable cause of death in Europe, accounting for approximately 50% of all deaths, and about 30% of deaths worldwide. The burden of these diseases is particularly pronounced in low- and middle-income countries, where a significant proportion of premature deaths before the age of 60 are attributable to noncommunicable diseases, including CVDs. This underscores the global challenge posed by CVDs and the urgent need for effective prevention, management, and treatment strategies to mitigate their impact on public health.

Rare CVDs are organized into a systematic classification to facilitate a comprehensive understanding and targeted approach towards diagnosis, treatment, and research. This classification categorizes rare cardiovascular conditions into several distinct classes based on their characteristics and the parts of the cardiovascular system they affect.

1. **Rare Afflictions of Systemic and Pulmonary Circulation (Class I and II):** These conditions involve abnormalities in the circulation of blood either throughout the body

(systemic) or within the lungs (pulmonary). Diseases in this category can significantly impact oxygen and nutrient delivery to tissues and the removal of CO_2 and waste products.

2. **Rare Cardiomyopathies (Class III):** This group includes diseases that affect the heart muscle itself, altering its structure or function. These conditions can lead to heart failure, arrhythmias, or sudden cardiac death if not properly managed.
3. **Rare Congenital Cardiovascular Disorders (Class IV):** Congenital cardiovascular disorders are heart and circulatory system abnormalities present from birth. These can range from simple defects with no symptoms to complex problems with severe, life-threatening symptoms.
4. **Rare Cardiac Arrhythmias (Class V):** These are unusual heart rhythms that can be too fast, too slow, or irregular. Rare arrhythmias can lead to complications such as stroke or sudden cardiac death if not adequately addressed.
5. **Cardiac Tumors and Cardiovascular Affections Related to Cancer (Class VI):** This category covers rare heart tumors and cardiovascular complications related to cancer or its treatment. These conditions are complex and require specialized care.
6. **Cardiovascular Sickness in Pregnancy (Class VII):** Pregnancy can exacerbate or unveil existing cardiovascular conditions, or new CVDs can arise as a direct result of pregnancy. These conditions necessitate careful management to protect both mother and child.
7. **Other Types of Rare Cardiovascular Illness (Class VIII):** This is a catch-all category for rare CVDs that do not fit neatly into the other classes. It encompasses a wide range of conditions, each with unique features and challenges.

i. **Etiology of Cardiovascular Diseases:** The cause of CVDs is multifactorial, involving a combination of clinical (e.g., dyslipoproteinemia, hypertension) and behavioral factors (e.g., sedentary lifestyle, overnutrition, smoking, and stress). Additionally, environmental aspects like trace element concentrations in soil can also play a role. Atherosclerosis, characterized by the buildup of plaques within the arteries, stands out as a primary cause of many cardiovascular conditions.

ii. **Diagnosis and Prognosis:** The diagnosis and prognosis of CVDs are often enhanced by the use of specific biomarkers, including proteins and nucleic acids like microRNAs and non-protein coding RNAs. These markers help in understanding the disease's progress, its impact on the body, and the effectiveness of treatment strategies.

iii. **Epidemiological Studies:** These studies are critical in identifying individual, environmental (including air pollution and exposure to second-hand smoke), and societal risk factors for CVDs. By ranking these factors according to their impact on morbidity and mortality, epidemiological research aims to develop strategies to reduce the burden of CVDs. The ultimate goal is to mitigate risk factors, enhance preventive measures, and identify effective treatments within a health system that integrates research findings into clinical practice.

Orientation and Directional Terms

Term	Definition	Illustration
Vasculitis (Angiitis)	Inflammation of blood vessels, which can lead to vessel damage, restriction of blood flow, and potential organ damage.	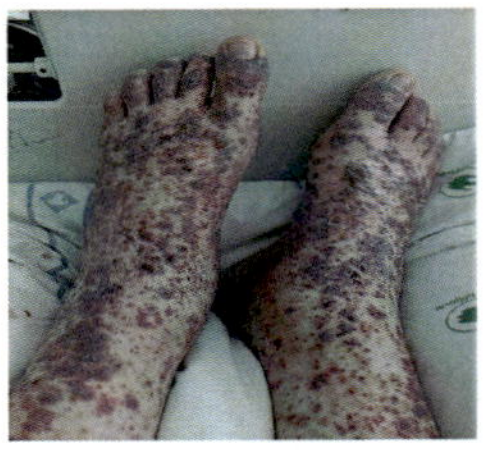
Autoimmune Disorders	Diseases in which the immune system attacks the body's own cells and tissues, mistaking them for foreign invaders.	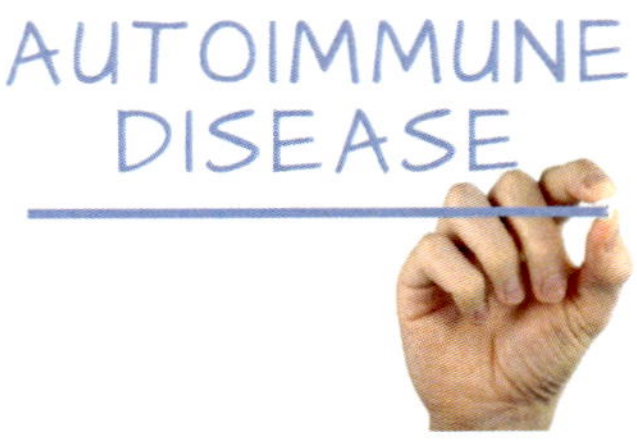
Venous Malformations (VMs)	Congenital vascular anomalies characterized by malformed, dilated veins, often leading to pain and swelling.	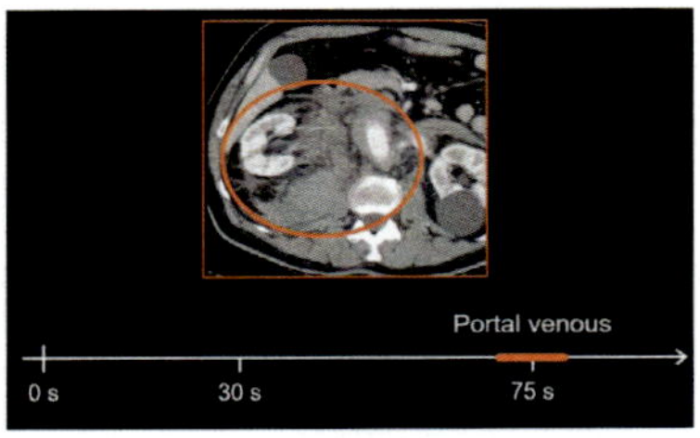
Capillary Malformations	Small, superficial vascular anomalies in capillaries, often presenting as red or pink birthmarks on the skin, such as port-wine stains.	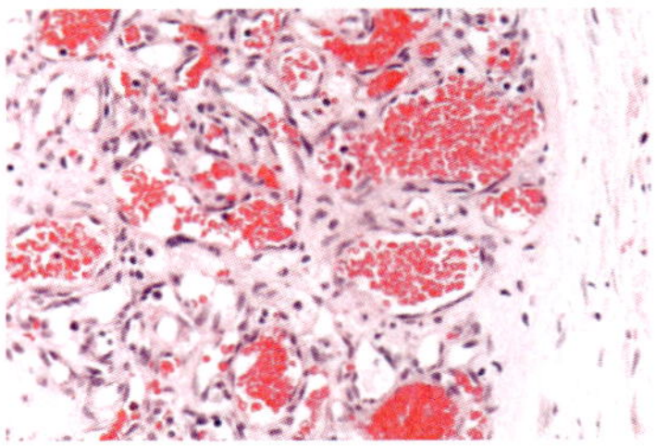
Lymphatic Malformations	Congenital malformations of the lymphatic system, leading to the formation of fluid-filled cysts or masses in the body.	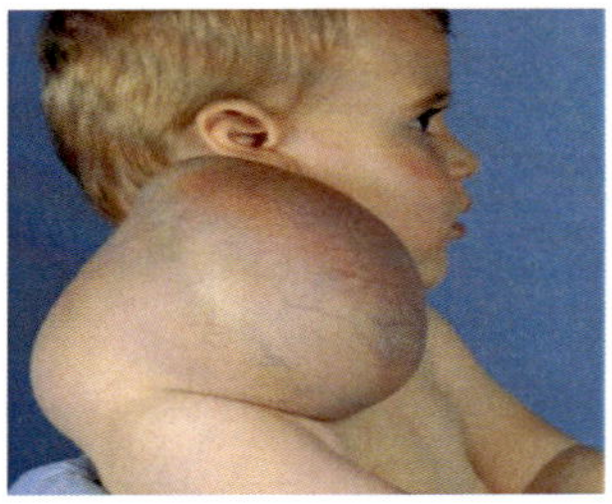

3.1. Vascular Disorders and Vascular Diseases

Vasculopathy encompasses a range of diseases that impact the blood vessels, including degenerative, metabolic processes (such as diabetic vasculopathy), inflammatory disorders, and thromboembolic conditions.

Vasculitis, also known as angiitis, is characterized by a localized or extensive inflammation of the vascular wall, regardless of the type (such as arteries, arterioles, capillaries, venules, and veins), size (big, medium, or tiny), quantity, and location of the blood vessels.

Vascular physiological and pathological pathways can be influenced by ethnicity and gender. Information collected from a large group of people, such as the relationship between a risk factor and a specific disease or complication linked to a particular gene mutation, may not accurately reflect the characteristics of a smaller, more uniform group. Sex disparities in the occurrence, frequency, illness, and death rates associated with CVD, encompassing disorders specific to each gender and symptoms that vary depending on gender, as well as the development of shared pathophysiological mechanisms between genders (such as hypertension and atherosclerosis), contribute to health inequalities. The efficacy of therapy is influenced by variations in pharmacodynamics and kinetics based on sex and race.

3.1.1. Ethnic Differences

Health inequities can be attributed to ethnicity. Individuals belonging to specific ethnic groups experience premature CVD. The occurrence rates of hypertension and diabetes are notably influenced by ethnic ancestry.

The American Heart Association and National Institute of Health have reported that the prevalence of coronary disease among African American men and women is 40%, whereas European-American men and women had rates of 30% and 24%, respectively. These disparities are primarily attributed to genetic variations among ethnic groups, rather than being influenced by living circumstances and dietary choices. In addition, African American women who have coronary disease face a risk of myocardial infarction that is twice as high as that of European American women.

- **In the United States of America:** African Americans are at a higher risk for hypertension. There is a higher prevalence of obesity and diabetes among Latinos in North America. The prevalence of coronary artery disease is higher among individuals of South Asian descent. Individuals of African-Caribbean heritage have the highest stroke rate, and the prevalence of diabetes is significantly greater in these two ethnic groups compared to the White population.
- **In the United Kingdom:** South Asians have a higher prevalence of myocardial infarction compared to non-South Asians, regardless of gender.

Stroke prevalence is higher among black individuals compared to white individuals, regardless of gender.

Indian and Pakistani men have the highest prevalence of CoAD. The White ethnic group exhibits a higher rate of revascularization compared to the black and Asian ethnic groupings.

Individuals belonging to several ethnic groups exhibit variations in fat storage patterns across different body regions.

The Black ethnic group exhibits the highest frequency of overweight and obesity among young children. Black Caribbean, Indian, Pakistani, and Bangladeshi men exhibit a significantly greater incidence of diabetes.

However, it is important to note that these disparities might be attributed not solely to genetic variations, but also to unique cultural and social customs. Differentiating the impact of ethnicity from that of socioeconomic status might provide challenges. Furthermore, racial, and ethnic groups can exhibit genetic variation.

3.1.2. The Impact of Gender

Sex differences in CVD are influenced by a combination of hormonal, genetic, and environmental variables. The hormonal secretion of an organism is influenced by its environment, which subsequently impacts brain function. These hormones exert their effects on the genome of neural cells that possess their corresponding receptors. As an illustration, the ventromedial, ventrolateral, and arcuate nuclei house neurons that are sensitive to estrogen. The ventromedial nucleus has a faster response rate compared to the arcuate nucleus.

Furthermore, the release of hormones by the adrenal gland and gonads (testis and ovary) is regulated not only by ambient temperature (heat or cold), perceived danger, and sexual stimulation, which trigger adaptive reactions, but also by circadian rhythms influenced by environmental cues (light and darkness).

The hippocampus, which is heavily influenced by the dentate gyrus mossy fiber system, can experience neuronal loss as a result of recurrent psychosocial stress. Adrenal hormones, which provide short-term protection, function in tandem with brain excitatory amino acids, resulting in long-term harm and allostatic load if the adaptive response is not effectively regulated and continues. The effects of gonadal hormones might vary depending on their concentration and duration of exposure, resulting in both protective and detrimental effects.

The determination of sex is primarily influenced by the X and Y chromosomes, which give rise to a distinct pattern of expression distinctive to each sex. Males have a solitary copy of each type (XY genotype), while females have two copies of the X chromosome (XX genotype), with one of the X chromosomes being turned off during embryogenesis (X-chromosome inactivation).

Typically, premenopausal women have a reduced risk of CVD compared to males of the same age. Males typically acquire hypertension at an earlier age compared to females. The SRY locus, located on the Y chromosome, controls the transcription of tyrosine hydroxylase (TH; or Tyr 3-monooxygenase), an enzyme that determines the rate of catecholamine synthesis, including noradrenaline. This gene is responsible for a gender-specific variation in sympathetic activity, which makes men more susceptible to hypertension compared to women.

The Y chromosome contains genes associated with inflammation and innate immunity that are connected to the activation of macrophages. Conversely, the X chromosome exerts an influence on the expression of genes linked to apoptosis, lipid oxidation, and the production of reactive oxygen species (ROS) within the mitochondrion.

Certain chromosomal loci associated with lipid metabolism in persons from European countries demonstrate sex-specific effects. Specifically, the HMGCR and NCAN genes, which encode 3-hydroxy 3-methylglutaryl coenzyme-A reductase and neurocan (or chondroitin sulfate proteoglycan CSPG3), respectively, indicate such effects.

A sex-specific single-nucleotide polymorphism in the CPS1 gene locus, responsible for producing mitochondrial carbamoyl–phosphate synthase-1, has a more pronounced impact on women compared to males. This gene is involved in hepatic nitrogen urea metabolism and the production of arginine, a precursor of nitric oxide (NO).

The androgen receptor gene is located on the X chromosome and exhibits a polymorphism associated with a significantly diverse amount of CAG repeats. Genetic variations in this gene exert a more pronounced influence on males than to females. Genetic variations also impact enzymes responsible for the production, transformation, and breakdown of sex steroids.

Multiple processes in both women and men are regulated by estrogens, such as estradiol, and androgens, such as testosterone and dihydrotestosterone.

3.1.2.1. Estrogen Signaling

The primary site of estradiol synthesis is the granulosa cells located in the ovaries, while in men, it is present in Sertoli cells. It attaches to different types of cytosolic ERα and ERβ (specifically, ligand-activated transcription factors NR3a1–NR3a2) in cardiomyocytes (CMCs) and vascular smooth muscle cells (vSMCs) as well as endothelial cells (ECs). It also binds to plasmalemmal estrogen receptor GPER1 (or GPR30) in vascular endotheliocytes and smooth myocytes, renal intercalated and tubular cells, and cells of the hypothalamic–pituitary–adrenal axis.

The initiation of fast (nonenomic) signaling by sex steroid hormones, which are synthesized by the adrenal cortex, ovary, and testis, is facilitated by estrogen receptors located in the plasma membrane. In conjunction with the membrane estrogen receptor GPER1, sex steroid receptors such as NR3a1 and NR3a2 can localize to the plasma membrane. Specifically, NR3a1 has been shown in caveolae that are connected with proteic complexes. The translocation of NR3a1 to the plasma membrane necessitates its palmitoylation at Cys447. NR3a1 and NR3a2 are essential and adequate for prompt signaling initiated by estrogen. Caveolin-1 functions as a structural framework for various signaling molecules, such as trimeric G protein, Src, PI3K, GFR, and MNAR, which are activated by the E2–NR3a1 couple within caveolae. This activation process enables the rapid generation of early signals, such as the influx of Ca^{2+} ions. Additionally, certain NR3a1 molecules are transported to the nucleus through a nuclear localization sequence or to mitochondria, facilitated by the presence of heat shock protein HSP90. In order to facilitate the development of the female reproductive tract and mammary gland, the presence of nuclear NR3a1 is essential.

NR3a2 inhibits detrimental heart pathology, such as hypertrophy and fibrosis. The interaction between E2 and NR3a2 triggers the activation of PI3K and initiates the transcription of the RCAN gene, which encodes the regulator of calcineurin (PP3). Furthermore, the E2 and NR3a2 complex initiates the production of the natriuretic peptides ANP and BNP, which inhibits the development of abnormal heart muscle growth through the action of by extracellular signal-related kinases (ERK) in the CMC. In contrast, atherogenic 27-hydroxycholesterol functions as an endogenous selective estrogen receptor modulator (SERM) that is abundant inside the pathological arterial wall. The binding of E2 to NR3a is competitively prevented, resulting in the inhibition of both the immediate vasodilation mediated by NO and the delayed transcriptional effects of E2.

Estrogens are additionally produced within the central nervous system through the synthesis of cholesterol or through the conversion of aromatizable androgens in presynaptic terminals. Estrogens have the ability to undergo diffusion. Both NR3a1 and NR3a2 are synthesized in nuclei located in the forebrain and brainstem, which play a crucial role in the regulation of cardiac frequency and blood pressure. These nuclei include the solitary tract and parabrachial nuclei, as well as the rostral ventrolateral medulla. Their production contributes to the enhancement of baroreflex mediated by the sympathetic nervous system. These brain nuclei include renin, angiotensinogen, angiotensin convertases ACE1 and ACE2, and angiotensin Agt2 receptors (such as AT1 and AT2), which are responsible for regulating the local renin-angiotensin axis (RAA). Angiotensin-2 and aldosterone induce the generation of ROS in the brain through the action of NAD(P)H oxidase, resulting in an increase in sympathetic nerve activity. Estrogens, through NR3a1 and NR3a2, inhibit the production of ROS within the subfornical organ (SFO). The administration of estradiol has been observed to decrease hypertension produced by Agt2 and aldosterone in male and ovariectomized female rodents.

Nevertheless, NR3a1 and NR3a2 have distinct regulatory effects on blood pressure. There is no observed impact on heart frequency and blood pressure in male rats when E2 is injected into the paraventricular nucleus (PVN). Actived CNSNR3a1 has been observed to provide protection against Agt2-induced hypertension in female mice, whereas PVNNR3a2 and RVLMNR3a2 have been found to provide protection against aldosterone-induced hypertension. Activated CNSNR3a2 maintains resting blood pressure in both female and male mice through RVLMCaV channels. Thus, in both female and male rodents, distinct NR3a subtypes play a role in providing E2-mediated protection in various nuclei.

The production of NO synthase NOS1 is higher in the SFO and PVN of female mice compared to male mice. Furthermore, estrogens promptly induce the synthesis of NO by nitric oxide synthase 3 (NOS3) through NR3a1 in the vascular endothelium, regardless of gender.

The kidney is influenced by estrogens in menopausal women as their salt sensitivity develops. This is likely due to the fact that estrogens promote the activity of NO and reduce the AT1/AT2 ratio, hence maintaining the kidney's ability to handle sodium ions (Na^+). Salt loading during estrogen peaks in premenopausal women reduces filtration fraction and leads to a prolonged dilatation of the renal vasculature. Salt loading has been observed to increase the filtration fraction in postmenopausal women. Furthermore, NR3a1 plays a role in the modulation of the renal ACE1/ACE2 ratio through the action of estrogens. ACE2 is responsible for the conversion of vasoconstrictive, prohypertrophic, and proproliferative angiotensin-2 into Agt (1–7).

The presence of GPER1 on arterial and venous endotheliocytes and smooth myocytes inhibits vasoconstriction induced by endothelin-1 and prostanoid, hence reducing superoxide generation and providing protection against hypertension. In addition, GPER1 induces the activation of NOS3 within the vascular endothelium. Additionally, it reduces the development of vSMCs and mitigates vascular inflammation.

In order to enhance lipidemia, estrogens exert their effects on low-density lipoproteins (LDLs) and the LDL receptor (LDLR). The synthesis of LDLR is upregulated by estradiol, leading to an increase in sterol 27-hydroxylase CyP27a1 activity, hence impeding the creation of LDL. Furthermore, estrogens increase the formation of the apolipoprotein ApoA1 in the liver, as well as the production of ApoE.

Additionally, they enhance the creation of ABCa1, thereby promoting the reverse transport of cholesterol. However, they impede the development of ScaRb1, thereby extending the duration of circulating high-density lipoproteins (HDLs).

A variety of leukocytes, including macrophages, B and T lymphocytes, and mastocytes, have been found to exhibit sex hormone receptors within atherosclerotic plaques. Consequently, estrogens have the potential to exert an influence on the inflammatory response. Estrogens induce the anti-inflammatory M2 trait in macrophages, decrease LDL oxidation, activate endothelial cells, and promote the attachment of neutrophils and monocytes to the endothelium. Additionally, they hinder NOx activity and thus inhibit the generation of ROS.

The anti-inflammatory properties of estradiol have been observed to mitigate the production of tumor-necrosis factor superfamily member TNFSF1 and inhibit its release. Furthermore, it stimulates NR3a2 and subsequently inhibits Iκ B[3], which suppresses inflammation induced by NF°B.

NOS3 is facilitated by estrogen in promoting angiogenesis in peripheral artery disease (PAD). Proangiogenic estrogens promote the movement of endothelial progenitor cells and their integration into areas where new blood vessels are formed. This is achieved through the stimulation of NOS3 and the activity of matrix metalloproteinase 9 (MMP9) in the bone marrow.

Elevated levels of circulating female sex hormones have been found to provide protection against the formation of abdominal aortic aneurysm (AAA) by mitigating inflammation and reducing matrix metallopeptidase activity inside the aortic wall. A greater abundance of the plasminogen activator inhibitor PAI1 in female animals hinders the formation of MMP2 and MMP9, hence safeguarding against the development of AAA. Estrogens decrease the levels of MMP2 and MMP9, as well as the infiltration of immune cells in AAA, resulting in a slower rate of dilation compared to animals that have undergone ovarian resection. Furthermore, the generation of NO induced by estrogens provides protection against AAA. The aortas of female mice have elevated levels of NR3a1 and reduced activity of MMP.

Conversely, people have higher levels of 3-hydroxyanthranilic acid (3HAA), indoleamine (2,3)-dioxygenase (IDO), and kynureninase in AAA samples compared to neighboring aorta segments. The enzyme in the kynurenine route of tryptophan metabolism responsible for the production of 3HAA is indoleamine dioxygenase, which serves as the initial and rate-limiting enzyme. The administration of angiotensin-2 in a short period of time promotes the formation of AAAs in APOELoΩ mice but does not have the same effect on APOE EΩ and Ido oΩ animals, where the deterioration of the elastic lamina and the expansion of the aorta decrease. Angiotensin-2 stimulates the activation of interferon-γ, leading to the upregulation of IDO and kynureninase expression. This, in turn, increases the production of IDO in medial smooth myocytes and subsequently elevates its content in the aorta wall and plasma of 3HAA. Consequently, the synthesis of MMP2 is upregulated through the activation of NFκB.

Postmenopausal women have an increased chance of developing cerebral aneurysms. However, estrogen replacement therapy helps to prevent intracranial aneurysms. This protection is achieved by the mediation of estrogens by estrogen receptor beta (NR3a2) and the synthesis of NO in the cerebral blood vessels.

3.1.2.2. Androgen Signaling

The synthesis of testosterone occurs in the Leydig cells of the testes and theca cells of the ovaries. 5α-reductase converts it into the more powerful 5α-dihydrotestosterone (5α-DHT).

Both forms of androgens are associated with a ligand-activated transcription factor known as androgen receptor (AR or NR3c4), which is found in various cell types including endotheliocytes, smooth myocytes, platelets, and macrophages. Two versions (ARa–ARb) are present in the majority of organs, exhibiting different degrees of expression depending on the type of tissue. Aromatase converts testosterone to E2 mainly in the brain.

The process of androgen signaling is associated with various biological processes, including metabolism, cell proliferation, differentiation, death, and protein production, regardless of gender. Androgens have the ability to initiate alternative fast (nonenomic) signaling pathways following their interaction with membrane-associated or cytosolic androgen receptors (ARs), which subsequently release intracellular calcium ions (Ca^{2+}) and activate various kinases such as mitogen activated protein kinase (MAPK), protein kinases A, B, and C (PKA, PKB, and PKC). Aortic endotheliocytes exhibit interactions between membrane-associated ARs and Src and caveolin-1.

Postmenopausal women exhibit a higher incidence of age-related hypertension compared to men of the same age. There is a potential association between hypoandrogenism and hypertension in older males, indicating that maintaining a normal androgen concentration may have antihypertensive effects. The activation of NOS3 in vascular endotheliocytes is facilitated by testosterone through the PI3K-PKB pathway in a prompt manner. Conversely, in a cohort of youthful, overweight, hypoandrogenic male rats, the administration of testosterone for a duration of 10 weeks yields enhancements in body weight and lipid profiles, but at the expense of elevated blood pressure. Ruptured abdominal aortic aneurysm (RAAA) constituents in the kidney have the potential to increase blood pressure through the action of androgens. Male animals can experience Agt2-induced hypertension through renal inflammation, with a higher infiltration of renal lymphocytes observed in male mice compared to female mice.

NR3a reduces the production of adhesion molecules in endotheliocytes that are exposed to atherogenic stimuli. On the other hand, NR3c4 increases the production of VCAM-1 in male-derived endotheliocytes because of a higher concentration of NR3c4 (whereas this effect is not observed in cells of female origin).

Endothelial dysfunction has been found to be associated with androgen deprivation in males. Conversely, hyperandrogenemia in women is associated with an increased propensity for atherogenesis and arterial calcification.

Androgens stimulate angiogenesis in both males and females with hypoxia resulting from occlusive peripheral artery disease. This is achieved by the activation of NR3c4, which leads to an increased production of vascular endothelial growth factor (VEGF) and its receptors in endotheliocytes. Additionally, VEGF-induced phosphorylation of PKB and NOS3 is also observed. The administration of DHT enhances the migration, proliferation, and tubulogenesis of male-derived endotheliocytes, but not in females.

In male animals, there is a notable presence of androgens, which leads to increased expression of RAAA components. This, in turn, promotes the recruitment of macrophages and the degradation of the extracellular matrix through the action of MMPs. Consequently, the formation of AAA is facilitated. However, the castration of male mice restricts the genesis and expansion of AAA induced by Agt2, resulting in levels comparable to those observed in intact female mice. Androgens can increase MMP activity in male rodents, making them more susceptible to AAA.

3.1.2.3. Steroid Hormone Metabolism Enzymes

Steroids are a class of lipophilic chemicals with low molecular weight that mostly originate from cholesterol. Fluids typically contain them in either a conjugated state, where they are connected to a hydrophilic group like sulfate or glucuronide derivatives or coupled to proteins. Unconjugated steroids in the plasma predominantly exhibit binding affinity towards carrier proteins, namely albumin (20–50%), serpin-A6 (also known as corticosteroid-binding globulin), and sex hormone-binding globulin.

The synthesis of steroid hormones is crucially carried out in the mitochondria of steroidogenic cells found in the adrenal gland, gonads, placenta during gestation, and brain. The synthesis of androgens and corticosteroids (mineralo- and glucocorticoids), ovary estrogens and progestins, and testis (mostly androgens) occurs in the adrenal gland. Adipose tissue in men contains aromatase, which is a precursor to estrogens obtained from androgens.

The endocrine messengers exert their effects on target cells, including those inside the central nervous system, subsequent to their release into the bloodstream. Neurosteroids with auto- and paracrine actions are also produced by the latter. They have a high degree of diffusion across the plasma membrane. Target cells undergo the processing of circulating steroids, resulting in the formation of active metabolites.

The process of removing a portion of the cholesterol side chain results in the production of C21-steroids belonging to the pregnane series, such as progestins and corticosteroids. Additionally, it leads to the complete removal of C19-steroids from the androstane series, including androgens. Furthermore, it causes the loss of the 19-methyl group in the estrane series, which includes estrogens.

The characterization of steroids is determined by the presence or lack of functional groups, primarily hydroxy, keto (oxo, and aldehyde, at specific places throughout the carbon skeleton. These sites are particularly notable at positions 3, 5, 11, 17, 18, 20, and 21. A multitude of stereoisomers are generated by functional groups that exhibit unique three-dimensional conformations but sharing the same chemical formula. These stereoisomers are distinguished by their kind, number, location, and orientation.

The enzymes implicated in the process of steroid production are listed in Tables 3.1 and 3.2. Mitochondrial desmolases, also known as lyases, are enzymes that selectively hydroxylate neighboring carbon atoms on the cholesterol side chain through the utilization of molecular oxygen, reduced nicotinamide adenine dinucleotide phosphate (NADPH), and cytochrome P450.

In addition to cytochrome-P450, O_2, and NADPH, membrane-bound mitochondrial or microsomal hydroxylases are also necessary.

Table 3.1. *Enzymes of Steroid Synthesis (Part 1; CyPiXj: Cytochrome-P450 Family i, Subfamily x, Polypeptide j [i, j: Integers, x: Letter])*

	Other Name
Type	**Action**
CyP11a1	Mitochondrial cholesterol side-chain cleavage enzyme.
	Converts cholesterol to pregnenolone.
CyP17a1	Steroid 17α-hydroxylase and (17,20)-lyase.

	Converts pregnenolone and progesterone into their 17α-hydroxylated products and subsequently to dehydroepiandrosterone (DHEA) and androstenedione.
CyP21a2	Steroid 21-hydroxylase.
(CyP21, CyP21b)	Catalyzes 21-hydroxylation of steroids.
	Converts 17-hydroxyprogesterone and progesterone into 11 β-deoxycortisol and deoxycorticosterone, respectively.
	Required for adrenal synthesis of mineralocorticoids and glucocorticoids.
CyP11b1	Mitochondrial steroid 11β-hydroxylase 11β-, 18-, and 19-hydroxylation of steroids, aromatization of androstenedione to estrone.
	Production of cortisol and corticosterone from 11β-deoxycortisol and deoxycorticosterone, respectively.
CyP11b2	Mitochondrial aldosterone synthase; steroid 18-hydroxylase.
	Catalyzes the conversion of corticosterone and then 18-hydroxycorticosterone into aldosterone.
CyP19a1	Aromatase, estrogen synthase.
	Converts C19 androgens to C18 estrogens.

Androstenediol and androstenedione are weak androgen and estrogen steroid hormones and intermediates in the synthesis of estrone and testosterone. Androstenedione is converted to testosterone and estrone by the 17β-hydroxysteroid dehydrogenases (HSDH17β1, HSDH17β3, and HSDH17β7) and aromatase, respectively. Androstenediol is processed by the 3β-hydroxysteroid dehydrogenases HSDH3β1 and HSDH3β2 into testosterone. The three estrogens, estrone (E_1), a weakly active E_2 precursor, which is also named the estrogen of the menopause; estradiol (E_2), the most active estrogen; and estriol (E_3), a weakly active E_2 metabolite, which is also called the estrogen of pregnancy, are produced by aromatase. Both estriol and estrone can interact with the estrogen receptor and thus antagonize estradiol action

Table 3.2. *Enzymes of Steroid Synthesis (Part 2; AKR Aldo–Keto Reductase)*

	Other Name
Type	**Action**
SRd5a1/2/3	Steroid 5α-reductases, 3-oxo 5α-steroid 4-dehydrogenases
SRd5a1/2	Convert testosterone into more potent dihydrotestosterone and progesterone or corticosterone into their corresponding 5α 3-oxosteroids.
AKR1c3	17β HSDH5, brain 3α HSDH2.
	Preferentially transforms androstenedione to testosterone.

The oxidoreductases cytosolic and microsomal hydroxysteroid dehydrogenase are reliant on either NADP(H) or NAD(H) as their substrate.

The substrate of this membrane-bound aromatase is 4-androstenedione or testosterone, which undergoes a series of hydroxylation and subsequent loss of the C19 methyl group.

In addition to its electron transfer partners, ferredoxin and ferredoxin reductase, mitochondria house the cholesterol desmolase CyP11a1, which facilitates the cleavage of cholesterol sidechains to produce pregnenolone, a C21 molecule.

Pregnenolone has the capacity to undergo conversion into either progesterone, resulting in the production of glucocorticoids, androgens, and estrogens, or 17κ-hydroxypregnenolone, which likewise gives rise to androgens and estrogens. Androgen production in the adrenal gland is restricted to dehydroepiandrosterone and androstenedione, while testosterone is produced by 17β-hydroxysteroid dehydrogenase (17HSDH) in the Leydig cells of the testis. Estrogen synthesis in granulosa cells of the ovary necessitates the presence of the aromatase complex, which utilizes the substrates androstenedione and testosterone to generate estrone and estradiol, correspondingly.

Progesterone undergoes hydroxylation at carbon 21, resulting in the formation of 11-deoxycorticosterone (DOC). Additionally, corticosterone is hydroxylated at carbon 11, and it is a significant glucocorticoid in mammalian species that do not make cortisol. Cortisol, the primary glucocorticoid produced by the adrenal glands in humans, is synthesized through the conversion of 17κ-hydroxyprogesterone into 11-deoxycortisol.

Aldosterone is formed through further hydroxylation and redox reactions at carbon 18. Mitochondria also harbor various additional steroidogenic enzymes, including 3β-hydroxysteroid dehydrogenase, 11β-hydroxylase, and aldosterone synthase.

The entry of cholesterol into the mitochondria is controlled by the steroidogenic acute regulatory protein, StAR. This process relies on the machinery of the outer mitochondrial membrane, which includes translocator protein (Tspo), voltage-dependent anion channel VDAC1, Tspo-associated acylCoA-binding domain-containing protein ACBD3, and protein kinase-A regulatory subunit PKAr1[1] [43].

The liver is the primary location for catabolism. It encompasses a range of reaction types:

- The secondary alcoholic group is formed through the reduction of a double bond at C4 and an oxo(keto) group at C3.
- The oxo group at C20 undergoes reduction to form a secondary alcoholic group.
- Oxidation of a 17β-hydroxyl group
- Further hydroxylations at various positions

The sulfate group (SO_2L4)9 and/or glucuronosyl groups (glucuronidation) are conjugated by Mg^{2+}-dependent steroid sulfokinases and glucuronyl transferase, resulting in the formation of steroid sulfates and glucuronides, respectively. This process leads to the creation of hydrophilic molecules that can be more readily eliminated by the kidney.

The conversion of cortisol into its inactive metabolite cortisone is facilitated by the enzyme corticosteroid 11β-dehydrogenase HSD11β2.

The metabolism of steroids and pharmaceuticals involves the participation of four human aldo-keto reductases (AKR1c1–AKR1c4), which are also referred to as hydroxysteroid (HSDHs) and dihydrodiol dehydrogenases (DHDHs). According to Table 3.3, the enzymes in question facilitate the transformation of aldehydes and ketones into their respective alcohols by utilizing NADH and/or NADPH as cofactors. In humans, the aldo–keto reductase superfamily also includes aldehyde (AKR1a1) and aldose reductase (AKR1b1) and aldose reductase-like proteins AKR1b10 of the small intestine and AKR1b15, δ(4-3)-ketosteroid 5β-reductase AKR1d1, aldo–keto reductase-1C-like proteins AKR1cL1 and AKR1cL2 (or testis-specific AKR1e2), and aflatoxin aldehyde reductases AKR7a2 and AKR7a3.

Table 3.3 presents the involvement of aldo-keto reductases (AKRs) in the metabolism of steroid hormones.

Table 3.3. *Aldo–Keto Reductases (AKRs) in Steroid Hormone Metabolism*

Gene Chromosomal Locus	Protein Reaction
AKR1C1 10p14–p15	AKR1c1, 20α-hydroxysteroid dehydrogenase.
	Progesterone→20α-hydroxyprogesterone; 5α-dihydrotestosterone→3β-androstanediol.
AKR1C2 10p14–p15	AKR1c2, type-3 3α-hydroxysteroid dehydrogenase.
	5α-Dihydrotestosterone→3α-androstanediol.
AKR1C3 (17β HSDH5)	AKR1c3, type-2 3α-hydroxysteroid dehydrogenase, type-5.
10p14–p15	17β-hydroxysteroid dehydrogenase, prostaglandin-F synthase.
	Δ^4-Androstenedione→testosterone; PGh_2→$PGf_{1\alpha}$;
	PGd_2→11β PGf_2.
AKR1C4 10p14–p15	AKR1c4, type-1 3α-hydroxysteroid dehydrogenase.
	3-ketosteroid→3α-hydroxysteroid.
AKR1D1 7q32–q33	AKR1d1, steroid 5β-reductase.
	Δ4-3-ketosteroid → 5β-dihydrosteroid.

AKR1c1 is responsible for the conversion of progesterone into the inactive 20κ-dihydroxyprogesterone, AKR1c2, and liver-specific AKR1c4 dihydrotestosterone into the less active 3κ-diol. On the other hand, AKR1c3 functions by catalyzing the reduction of prostaglandins PGd2 and PGh2, as well as the oxidation of (9°, 11β) PGf2 to PGd2. Additionally, AKR1c3 exhibits a preference for converting androstenedione into testosterone. AKR1c1, AKR1c2, and AKR1c3 are enzymes that facilitate the conversion of deadly aldehydes resulting from lipid peroxidation into compounds with reduced toxicity.

The liver is the main location where steroid hormones with a β-4-3 functionality, such testosterone and progesterone, are metabolized. These hormones are then transformed into tetrahydrosteroids, which are subsequently excreted. The process of conjugating steroid hormones involves two distinct phases. Firstly, the dihydrosteroids are reduced by either 5α- or 5β-steroid reductases, resulting in the formation of the corresponding dihydrosteroids. Subsequently, the 3-oxo group of the dihydrosteroids is further reduced by ketosteroid reductases, leading to the formation of tetrahydrosteroids. The AKR1C subset (AKR1c1–AKR1c4) in humans decreases the levels of 5α- and 5β-dihydrosteroids.

The involvement of AKR1C isozymes in the metabolism of testosterone and progesterone has been observed. They possess pluripotency yet exhibit a cell-specific expression pattern and a clear predilection for specific substrates. The liver is responsible for the production of all four isozymes. AKR1c1 to AKR1c3 exhibit significant expression levels in the mammary gland and prostate, while demonstrating different expression patterns in the lung, mammary gland, prostate, and testis. Conversely, AKR1c4 demonstrates specificity towards the liver.

Adenocarcinoma cells in the prostate, along with stromal, endothelial, and uroepithelial cells, have been found to express AKR1c3. The quantities of AKR1c1 to AKR1c3 are higher in prostate epitheliocytes compared to stromal cells, with the rate of synthesis increasing in prostate malignancies. AKR1c3 in the mammary gland induces a pro-estrogenic condition by converting androstenedione into testosterone. This testosterone, when turned into 17β-estradiol by aromatization by CyP19 aromatase, changes active progesterone into inactive 20°-hydroxyprogesterone. As a result, the estrogen/progesterone ratio is modified.

The AKR1C enzymes facilitate the reduction of ketosteroids at the 3-, 17-, or 20-position, with different degrees of catalytic activity depending on the specific substrate. The 5-alpha pathway is associated with the 5-alpha-steroid reductase AKR1d1. Pregnane (3,20)-dione exhibits strong binding affinity towards the pregnane X receptor (PXR or NR1i2) and constitutive androstane receptor (CAR or NR1i3). Activated hepatic NR1i3 enhances the activity of cytochrome-P450 CyP3a4, which is responsible for the metabolism of almost 50% of ingested medications.

Furthermore, 5β-reduced pregnanes are a class of neuroactive hormones that are produced within the brain and have been associated with the process of vasodilation. They play a role in both regulating steroid receptors and altering neuronal excitability by acting on gene expression through nuclear steroid hormone receptors. Additionally, they also influence ligand-gated ion channels. Allosteric modulators of the GABAA receptor are responsible for either inhibiting or stimulating neurotransmission.

The AKR enzymes can be effectively inhibited by unsaturated fatty acids (FAs) through competitive inhibition. The susceptibility of AKRs to fatty acids (FAs) exhibits variability, with docosahexaenoic, palmitoleic, and linoleic acid being identified as the most effective inhibitors for AKR1c1, AKR1c2, and AKR1c4, respectively. Fatty acids (FAs) exhibit the highest level of inhibitory efficacy against the enzyme 3β-hydroxysteroid dehydrogenase AKR1c3. In addition to detoxifying dietary and environmental xenobiotics, sulfate conjugation has a role in the conversion of steroid and thyroid hormones, catecholamines, cholesterol, and bile acids. The transfer of the sulfonate group from phosphoadenosine phosphosulfate (PAPS) to acceptor substrates is facilitated by cytosolic sulfotransferases (SulTs). There are 13 SulT isoforms in humans, which can be divided into four categories. The SULT1 subfamily consists of SulT1a1 to SulT1a3, SulT1b1, SulT1c2 to SulT1c4, and SulT1e1, while the SULT2 subfamily comprises SulT2a1, SulT2b1a, and SulT2b1b. In contrast, the remaining subfamilies consist of a single element, namely SulT4a1 and SulT6b1, respectively.

Distinct SulT1c3 isoforms (SulT1c3a, SulT1c3c, and SulT1C3d) are encoded by splice variants. While SulT1c3a exhibits a lower level of activity and demonstrates specificity towards hydroxyl-chlorinated biphenyls, SulT1c3d demonstrates a wider range of substrate specificity, encompassing the sulfation of bile acids, thyroid hormones, pyrenes, and hydroxyl biphenyls.

3.1.3. Vasculitis (Angiitis)

Vasculitides are characterized by the proliferation of inflammatory leukocytes within the walls of blood vessels, which can be attributed to a range of immunological mechanisms and potentially induced by pathogenic pathogens. Vasculitis affects the walls of arteries and veins, regardless of their size, in many organs, with a notable predilection for the skin.

Vasculitides can be categorized based on the dimensions of blood vessels or histological analysis, such as lymphocytic, leukocytoclastic, and granulomatous categories.

Large arteries are affected by Giant cell (GGA) and young women (Takayasu) arteritis, as well as autoinflammatory Behçet disease (BD). Some potential complications that may arise are inflammatory blockages and aneurysms.

Livedoid vasculitis, alternatively referred to as segmental hyalinizing vasculopathy and livedo reticularis, predominantly manifests in females, primarily characterized by the presence of thromboses and ulcerations in the lower limbs.

Eosinophilic granulomatosis with polyangiitis (EGPA), formerly known as Churg-Strauss syndrome, primarily impacts the tiny and medium-sized blood vessels of individuals aged 30 to 45, regardless of gender. In addition to the lung and skin, this condition frequently affects the heart, kidney, colon, and nerves.

Granulomatosis with polyangiitis, formerly known as Wegener's granulomatosis, primarily impacts the vascular system in the nasal cavity, sinuses, auditory system, pulmonary system, and renal system of individuals in the middle-aged or older population.

3.1.4. Vascular Wall Disorders

Wall disorders in large arteries and veins appear not only in the presence of risk factors, such as smoking, long periods without bodily motion, hypertension, diabetes, obesity, and a family history of vasculopathies, but also most often in a context that encompasses ageing, one of the most important cardiovascular event predictors, injury, ciliopathies replication stress, air pollution, and sleep disorders, among other factors.

3.1.4.1. Hemostasis and Thrombosis

The vascular endothelium, when intact and healthy, maintains a surface that inhibits blood clotting. Thrombomodulin serves as a cofactor for thrombin and is an integral membrane protein located on the wetted surface of endotheliocytes. The activation of the anticoagulant serine peptidase protein-C occurs promptly upon its binding to thrombin. The Ca^{2+} ion is essential for the activation of protein-C by the thrombin-thrombomodulin complex. Additionally, this compound inhibits the activation of clotting factor-V by thrombin. There are two unique anticoagulant activities of thrombomodulin: (1) it hinders the clotting ability of thrombin and the activation of fibrinogen, and (2) it expedites the activation of the anticoagulant protein-C. The activation of the serine peptidase inhibitor antithrombin, also known as serpin-C1, is induced by heparan sulfate proteoglycans present on the surface of endotheliocytes. This activation leads to the inactivation of thrombin and factor-Xa.

Furthermore, the endothelium is responsible for the synthesis of protease inhibitors, including prostacyclin and NO. Certain categories of active platelets have the ability to produce NO, which in turn activates the sGC-PKG axis and restricts their own adhesion and aggregation. PKG phosphorylates vasodilator-stimulated phosphoprotein (VASP), inhibiting the activation of integrin-$\alpha 2B^2 3$, which is responsible for stabilizing the initial rolling, adhesion, and recruitment of platelets to the injury site. PKG represses the activation of integrin-$\alpha 2B^2 3$ through the regulation of thromboxane receptor activation and the inhibition of IP3R-associated cyclic guanosine monophosphate (cGMP) kinase substrate (IRAG).

In the event of injury to any portion of the vasculature, the subendothelial matrix becomes susceptible to exposure to blood. The matrix components initiate the process of hemostasis, which involves the development of a blood clot largely consisting of platelets and fibrin, occurring within a matter of seconds. Hemostasis is the process of halting bleeding from a broken blood vessel, therefore preventing hemorrhage and ensuring that blood flow remains normal in other parts of the circulatory system. The initial phase of wound healing includes the process of blood coagulation, wherein blood, a mixture of cells and plasma, undergoes a transformation from a liquid to a gel state. This transformation is facilitated by the localized creation of a hemostatic plug.

The process of primary hemostasis involves the aggregation of activated platelets, which are minute pieces of a nuclear cells generated from megakaryocytes, followed by the creation of platelet plugs.

Platelets in humans exhibit subpopulations based on the presence or absence of NOS3, a protein responsible for the production of NO, an endogenous inhibitor of platelet function. Roughly 20% of platelets exhibit a deficiency in NOS3, resulting in an inability to generate NO and impaired sGC-PKG signaling. The primary function of NOS3 platelets is to initiate adhesion to collagen or von Willebrand factor. Additionally, they activate integrin-α2Bβ3, which induces aggregation between platelets. Furthermore, NOS3 platelets produce MMP2, which facilitates the recruitment of NOS3+ platelets to the forming aggregate. On the other hand, platelets that possess intact NOS3–sGC–PKG signaling constitute the majority of the aggregate (thrombus) due to their elevated PGhS1 (COx1) concentration and increased production of thromboxane-A2. This amplification of platelet aggregation is facilitated by the synthesis of thromboxane-A2, which eventually restricts the size of the aggregate through the action of NO.

Secondary hemostasis refers to the concurrent accumulation of insoluble fibrin produced during the proteolytic coagulation cascade, resulting in the formation of a net structure within and surrounding the platelet plug. This process serves to enhance the strength and stability of the blood clot.

The process of hemostasis is dependent on the equilibrium between procoagulant factors, such as platelets and components of the coagulation cascade, and anticoagulant factors, including protein-C and -S, fibrinolysis, and serpins.

A pathological thrombus is the result of blood coagulation in the absence of vascular contusion, but not intrinsic vascular injury, as a blood clot in hemostasis. Thrombosis may be influenced by an increased ratio of NOS3+/NOS3L platelets.

Thromboembolism occurs when a blood clot breaks and sheds, leading to the presence of an embolus in the bloodstream and causing blockage in a distant blood vessel.

The integrity of venous walls can be compromised, leading to the formation of thrombi that are subsequently sheared and generate emboli. The majority of venous thrombus is composed of fibrin, which is encapsulated within red blood capsules. Pulmonary embolism can be induced by venous thrombi. VTE is a term that encompasses both (DVT) and pulmonary embolism.

When exposed to increased flow rate and shear, arterial thrombus primarily consists of aggregated platelets. The primary cause of arterial emboli is typically the occurrence of ischemia and infarction in the heart, brain (stroke), gastrointestinal tract, kidney, or leg.

Both arterial and venous thrombosis are associated with increased risk due to obesity and dyslipidemia. Venous thrombosis is commonly associated with conventional acquired risk factors, which encompass malignancy, immobilization, surgery, fractures, and pregnancy.

Neutrophils play a crucial role in the defense of the host organism. They accomplish this by processing pathogens through phagocytosis and generating toxic substances to directly eliminate intruders. Additionally, dying neutrophils combine their DNA with toxic constituents from their cytosolic granules and subsequently release them as neutrophil extracellular traps (NETs), which effectively capture and neutralize microorganisms. Extracellular traps of neutrophils consist of structured arrangements of processed chromatin, specifically neutrophil DNA, and histones, which are connected to secretory and cytoplasmic proteins that are released by neutrophils in the context of inflammation. Nevertheless, the presence of improper NETosis can have detrimental effects, as it promotes prolonged and severe inflammation and thrombosis. The release of neutrophil extracellular traps (NETs) into the vasculature has the potential to induce platelet adhesion and initiate the extrinsic and intrinsic coagulation cascade. Additionally, they result in harm to the pulmonary epithelia and endothelium. In contrast, two deoxyribonucleases, namely Dnase1 and Dnase1L3, are responsible for the degradation of extracellular nuclear and mitochondrial DNA (mtDNA), resulting in the presence of circulating neutrophil extracellular traps (NETs) in a partially redundant fashion. Nevertheless, Dnase1 interferes with NETs, yet it does not cause their dissolution.

RIPK3, a protein kinase that interacts with the receptor tumor necrosis factor receptor superfamily (TNFRSF), has a role in inflammation, apoptosis, necroptosis, and hemostasis. It enhances platelet activation. Platelets are recruited by adenosine diphosphate (ADP), thrombin, and thromboxane-A2 following vascular injury. These molecules bind to their corresponding G-protein-coupled receptors and initiate the activation of integrin inside-out signaling. This activation is mediated ERKs and leads to the production of granules. The production of RIPK3 in platelets, when it interacts with G13, triggers the activation of PKB and facilitates platelet aggregation and spreading on fibrinogen through PKB1 or PKB2. This activation also leads to the secretion of a second wave of dense granule content in response to thrombin, thromboxane-A2, and clot retraction. The G13 subtype specifically facilitates platelet aggregation generated by thrombin and TxA2 but does not affect aggregation triggered by ADP. In the context of cell necrosis and clearance, RIPK3 functions autonomously from its substrate, which is known as mixed lineage kinase domain-like pseudokinase. Hence, RIPK3 has a preference for the development of arterial thrombi.

In contrast, heparin, a sulfated polysaccharide, exerts its anticoagulant effects by binding to antithrombin (serpin-C1) and subsequently enhancing the interaction between antithrombin and thrombin (FIIa), as well as activating clotting factors FV IIa and FIXa to FXIIa. This mechanism effectively impedes the completion of the coagulation cascade.

3.1.4.2. Inflammation and Angiogenesis

Inflammation of the vascular wall is caused by injury, infection, and lipid peroxidation. Furthermore, hypertension, and diabetes are linked to chronic inflammation. High levels of inflammatory markers predict future cardiovascular events.

Hypertension is associated with both macro- and microvascular disease. It affects endothelial integrity and thus vascular permeability, allowing inflammatory leukocyte recruitment.

In addition to vasoconstriction, angiotensin-2 induces redox stress, inflammation, endothelial dysfunction, and vascular remodeling with fibrosis. It causes PTPRc+ leukocytes to accumulate in aortic perivascular adipose tissue and increases MMP2 expression in these leukocytes, which promotes Agt2-primed vascular inflammation and injury. Agt2 increases the production of ROS in the aortic and perivascular media, as well as VCAM-1 and CCL2, leading to perivascular infiltration of monocytes, macrophages, and T lymphocytes. When MMP2 is present, it increases the density of monocytes as well as activated CD4+ helper and CD8+ cytotoxic T cells in the spleen. MMP2 is produced in greater amounts in CD4+ effector TH1 cells than in TH2 or naive TH0 cells. Furthermore, TH1 cells can promote MMP2 synthesis in macrophages. Agt2 promotes EGFR phosphorylation, as well as ERK1 and ERK2, in vascular smooth myocytes through heparin-binding epidermal growth factor (HBEGF) shedding.

Matrix metallopeptidases produced by vSMCs, and endothelial cells not only degrade matrix constituents (e.g., collagen, elastin, and fibronectin), but also shed growth factors (e.g., HBEGF and matrix-bound latent transforming growth factor-β), cytokines, and chemokines, favoring inflammation, as well as autacoids (e.g., big endothelin-1 and other vasoactive peptides). MMP2 specifically cleaves (activates) CCL7 and CXCL12 and processes S100.

Tissue inhibitors of metallopeptidases (TIMPs) bind to the catalytic site of MMPs, inhibiting their activity. TIMP2 is one of four TIMPs (TIMP1-TIMP4) that can either inhibit or activate MMPs; proMMP2 activation requires TIMP2 in conjunction with MMP14. In addition to MMP2, other MMP types may be involved in Agt2 action.

MMP2 deficiency, on the other hand, reduces Agt2-induced redox stress, inflammation, endothelial dysfunction, medial hypertrophy, and vascular stiffness without increasing SBP. MMP2 from both vascular and immune cells contributes to impaired acetylcholine-induced vascular relaxation and endothelial dysfunction. Immunocytes contribute to Agt2-induced hypertension because Mmp2 deletion in immune cells lowers blood pressure.

Atherosclerosis (Atherosclerosis—Biological Aspects) can be defined as a widespread inflammatory disease of the vasculature. Inflammation is present at all stages of atherogenesis, from initial lesions to fatty streaks, evolved plaques, and end-stage complications such as thromboembolism following unstable plaque rupture due to an excessive inflammatory episode. Atherosclerosis is caused by oxidized LDLs that carry cholesterol. Activated endotheliocytes express adhesion molecules that promote the diapedesis of circulating leukocytes, activated macrophages, lymphocytes, and smooth myocytes, resulting in the release of cytokines and chemokines. The procoagulant cytokine stimulates the synthesis and secretion of fibrinogen, the plasminogen activator inhibitor PAI1 (serpin-E1), and acute phase proteins like C-reactive protein (CRP), amplifying the inflammatory and procoagulant response. Inflammatory cytokines (such as IL1, TNFSF1, and CRP) promote the formation of adhesion molecules, resulting in a vicious cycle. C-reactive protein promotes tissue factor production by monocytes while inhibiting NO production, thereby contributing to the formation of a proinflammatory and prothrombotic milieu. Anti-inflammatory medications can lower cardiovascular risk.

Furthermore, systemic autoimmune rheumatic diseases, a group of disorders that share chronic inflammation causing connective tissue and organ damage (rheumatoid arthritis, systemic lupus erythematosus, ankylosing spondylitis, gout, psoriatic arthritis, systemic sclerosis, polymyositis, dermatomyositis, Sjögren's syndrome, mixed connective tissue disease, and systemic vasculitis), can be associated with medium- and large-vessel vasculitides.

Angiogenesis plays a role in both organogenesis and repair, as well as inflammatory diseases. Cellular (monocytes, macrophages, and endotheliocytes) and molecular mediators and inhibitors (angiostatin, endostatin, osteonectin, thrombospondin, and, under some circumstances, TGFβ; cytokines IL1, IL4, IL6, interferon alpha (Ifnα), and Ifnβ; and chemokines CXCL4, CXCL9, and CXCL10) are involved in this programmed cascade of events.

Growth factors (EGF, FGF1, FGF2, HGF, IGF1, PDGF, TGFβ, and VEGF), cytokines (TNFSF1, IL1, IL6, IL13, IL15, and IL18), chemokines (CCL2, CXCL1, CXCL5, CXCL7, CXCL8, CXCL12, and CX3CL1), cell adhesion molecules (endoglin, integrins, selectins, pecam1, and vcam1), and matrix components (collagen-1, fibronectin, laminin, and he

Endotheliocytes then produce matrix metallopeptidases and plasminogen activators, which degrade the basement membrane and perivascular extracellular matrix. These cells proliferate and migrate, forming a sprout that grows, tubulates, matures, and anchors to another vessel or creates a capillary network, with endotheliocytes producing subsequent generations of sprouts from the primary sprout.

Mastocytes play a role in both innate and acquired immunity, as well as inflammation, allergies, and autoantibodies. They produce histamine, TNFSF1, IL1β, IL6, CXCL8, and VEGF. Proinflammatory substance-P and IL33, two major disease agents, work together to stimulate TNFSF1 synthesis and secretion from mastocytes by activating the tachykinin (neurokinin/substance-P) receptors TacR1 (NK1R or SPR) and IL1RL1 (IL33R). Due to this mutual excitation, IL33 increases SP-primed TNFSF1 production in mastocytes by more than 100-fold. Mastocyte-derived tryptase can cleave extracellular IL33 into its mature active form, activating mastocytes and releasing soluble IL1RL1, which modulates the effects of IL33. Substance P also stimulates mastocytes to secrete histamine. Furthermore, IL33 and SP promote the synthesis of both TacR1 and IL1RL1 receptors. Furthermore, IL3 promotes SP-induced VEGF release by mastocytes. IL33 also increases the frequency and magnitude of mastocyte degranulation and chemokine production, exacerbating chronic inflammation even at low levels. TacR1 and IL1RL1 receptors interact; TacR1 binds to IL1RL1 and its coreceptor, IL1RAP (IL1R accessory protein); IL33 may also bind to TacR1 and IL1RL1. In mastocytes, the stem cell factor receptor (SCFR) forms a complex with IL1RL1 and IL1RAP to promote cross-activation. Tetramethoxyluteolin, a natural flavonoid, inhibits mastocytes stimulated by IL33, SP, or both, reducing chronic inflammation.

3.1.4.3. Oxidative and Nitrosative Stresses

Accumulation of ROS, which are toxic byproducts of aerobic metabolism, causes redox stress, which reduces fitness and ability to maintain balance. H coined the term oxidative stress. According to Sies, "a disturbance in the prooxidant-antioxidant balance in favor of the former." The rate of ROS production increases with age, and ROS is responsible for the accumulation of cellular and tissue deterioration over time in the postreproductive phase of life.

Injurious oxidative stress is defined by a shift in the oxidative-reductive balance towards a more oxidative state as a result of increased ROS production by prooxidant enzymes and decreased antioxidant defense mechanisms that scavenge excess ROS.

Deleterious reductive stress is defined by an abnormal increase in reducing equivalents, such as reduced glutathione and reduced NADPH, increased activation of antioxidant enzymes, and decreased prooxidant capacity, which shifts the redox balance from oxidative to reduced states.

Exercise is an oxidant stimulus used in redox biology research; free radicals produced during exercise regulate muscular and systemic adaptation to physical activity. However, exercise causes oxidative or reductive stress depending on the individual. Using redox markers (e.g., glutathione, F2-isoprostanes, and protein carbonyls) in plasma, red blood capsules, and urine samples before and 2 days after exercise, concentrations of the oxidant markers, F2-isoprostanes and protein carbonyls, increase or decrease, whereas the amount of glutathione decreases or increases, respectively [16].

Redox stress, which refers to the oxidation-reduction reaction disorder, is a combination of oxidative and reductive stress. Both contribute to the pathogenesis of CVD, so redox stress is the preferred term.

The inactivation of glutathione peroxidase (GPOx1) causes both oxidative and reductive stress. Reductive stress leads to Sglutathionylation of the cytoplasmic protein Tyr phosphatase PTPn1 (SHP2) and vascular remodeling.

3.1.4.4. Reactive Oxygen and Nitrogen Species

ROS and reactive nitrogen species (RNS) are produced by all layers of the vascular wall. These include superoxide anion radical ($O\cdot_2^-$), hydrogen peroxide (H_2O_2), hydroxyl radical (OH•), nitric oxide (NO•), and peroxynitrite (ONOO–).

SOD can convert superoxide into hydrogen peroxide. The oxidation of glutathione, ascorbic acid, NADPH, hydroquinone, catechol, and riboflavin by hydrogen peroxide and H_2O_2 catalysis produces the hydroxyl radical, which glutathione can scavenge. Oxy- and methemoglobin can produce hydroxyl radicals from hydrogen peroxide.

Superoxide rapidly reacts with anti-inflammatory, anticoagulant, and vasodilator NO to form the oxidant peroxynitrite. The latter oxidizes tetrahydrobiopterin, a NOS cofactor, which reduces NO availability and causes endothelial dysfunction. Among ROS and RNS, the hydroxyl radical and peroxynitrite are not considered signaling molecules; however, these highly reactive agents contribute to redox stress and tissue damage.

3.1.4.5. ROS and RNS Sources

The primary sources of vascular ROS include:

NAD(P)H oxidases (NOx1-NOx2, NOx4-NOx5)

Mitochondrial electron transport chain (ETC) involved in oxidative phosphorylation, primarily ETCcomplexes I and III (i.e., NADH-ubiquinone and ubiquinone-cytochrome-C reductase).

Uncoupled NO synthase and, to a lesser degree.

- **Xanthine Oxidase:** Prostaglandin-G/H synthases (cyclooxygenases)
- **Lipoxygenases:** The endothelial cytochrome-P450 epoxygenase CyP2c9 produces vasodilatory epoxyeicosatrienoic acids (11,12) EETs.

Myeloperoxidase [17].

- **Mitochondrial Electron Transport Chain:** ROS in the heart are primarily produced by mitochondrial ETC, as well as mitochondrial and extramitochondrial enzymes like NOxs. SOD2 rapidly degrades superoxide produced in the mitochondrial matrix to hydrogen peroxide, which then diffuses out of the mitochondria.
- **NAD(P)H Oxidases:** The NOX enzymes produce $O\cdot_2^-$, with the exception of NOx4, which primarily produces H_2O_2. They can be found in caveolae, membrane rafts, the endoplasmic reticulum, endosomes, and mitochondria.

Constitutively active canonical NOx1

and NOx2 function in a complex formed by their regulators and binding partners.

NOx1 = P22PhOx-NoxO1-NoxA1-Rac1/2

NOx2: P22PhOx, NOxO2, NOxA2, P40PhOx, and Rac1/2

NOx4 is constitutively active in the presence of oxygen. Calcium-dependent NOx5 is controlled by cytosolic calcium levels. Although NOx2 and NOx4 generate ROS in CMCs and fibroblasts, NOx1, NOx4, and NOx5 operate in vascular smooth myocytes.

NOx complexes produce $O\cdot_2^-$ on the extracytoplasmic face of cellular membranes, resulting in plasma membrane-bound NOxs outside the cell and intracellular NOxs within organelles.

NOx4 subtypes in the outer mitochondrial membrane, as well as mitochondrial ETC, are major ROS sources in diabetes. NOx4 regulates the migration and differentiation of vascular smooth myocytes, cardiac cells, fibroblasts, and stem cells. When exposed to TGFβ, NOx4 inhibits the phosphatase DUSP1 (MAPK phosphatase MKP1), inactivating P38MAPK. This phosphorylates SRF, which binds to MRTF and activates smooth muscle α-actin, promoting vSMC differentiation. In addition, NOx4 activates RhoA.

3.1.4.6. Xanthine Oxidoreductase (Dehydrogenase/Oxidase)

Xanthine dehydrogenase (XDH) and oxidase (XOx) are interconvertible forms encoded by the same gene, XDH (XOR). XOx uses hypoxanthine or xanthine as a substrate and O_2 as a cofactor (electron acceptor) to produce superoxide and uric acid, whereas XDH uses NAD+ as a cofactor (electron receptor) to generate NADH. Hypoxia, inflammation, apoptosis, and ROS generation from other sources all contribute to the conversion of XDH into XO. Xanthine oxidase contributes to the cellular redox status. It produces oxygen radicals in granulocytes, endothelial, epithelial, and connective tissue cells. It is involved in the detoxification of aldehydes. Rather than generating free radicals, it acts as a messenger in the activation of neutrophils and T lymphocytes, as well as the activation of defense mechanisms. However, it has been linked to cytotoxicity and tissue injury, particularly in cases of inflammation and ischemia.

3.1.4.7. Lipoxygenases

Arachidonate lipoxygenases ALOx5, ALOx12, and ALOx15 are linked to CVD development. Arachidonic acid (AA) is oxidized by ALOxs into hydroperoxides, which are then reduced to hydroxides and leukotriene. Each ALOx subtype produces different metabolites based on the target AA carbons.

Arachidonate lipoxygenases regulate Agt2-induced NOx activity in vSMCs. Redox stress stimulates ALOx5 synthesis in response to excess ROS formation by NOx or mitochondrial ETCs. It converts AA into 5HETE and LTa4, which serve as substrates for several enzymes that produce proinflammatory molecules LTb4, LTc4, LTd4, and LTe4, activating endotheliocytes, macrophages, neutrophils, mastocytes, T lymphocytes, and foam cells.

Both ALOx12 and ALOx15 play a role in inflammation and redox stress. The generated AA metabolites 12HPETE and 15HPETE, as well as their reduced counterparts 12HETE and 15HETE, are pro- and anti-inflammatory. They oxidize LDL. The metabolite 15HETE promotes ROS production through mitochondrial ETC and NOx4. Under hypoxia, 15HETE stimulates endotheliocyte migration and pulmonary arterial smooth myocyte proliferation via P38MAPK activation, promoting pulmonary vascular remodeling and hypertension. NOx4 is linked to ALOx12 and ALOx15 activity in diabetic hearts.

3.1.4.8. Myeloperoxidase

Myeloperoxidase (MPOx), encoded by the MPO gene, generates a single-chain precursor that is then cleaved into light and heavy chains that tetramerize. It is abundantly stored in neutrophils, where it forms the majority of neutrophil azurophilic granules, as well as in monocytes and macrophages to a lesser extent. This heme protein is generated during myeloid differentiation. This microbicide is a component of the host's immune defense. It also affects endothelial function.

Myeloperoxidase catalyzes H_2O_2 and halide or semihalide ion reactions to produce hypohalous acids, including hypochlorous acid ($HOCl^-$) and hypothiocyanous acid (HOSCN), which are effective microbicides. $HOCl^-$ reacts with nitrogen and sulfur atoms in cysteine residues, particularly glutathione. Cys oxidation can deactivate or activate cellular molecules.

Myeloperoxidase is involved in redox stress and inflammation, and it can be used as a marker of atherosclerosis plaque instability. Glutathione sulfonamide, produced by $HOCL^-$, can indicate MPOx damage. Smoking produces high levels of thiocyanate (SCN^-),19 a small acidic pseudohalide thiolate that reduces H_2O_2 by MPOx and increases hypothiocyanous acid. The POx-SCN-H_2O_2 axis is a component of host defense.

Thiocyanate can act as an antioxidant by interacting with peroxidases and protecting cells from redox damage caused by hypohalous acids like HOCl and HOBr. It reduces toxicity caused by the MPOx-Cl^--H_2O_2 axis at concentrations of 100–400 μmol/l in the nervous system, lungs, and other organs, including endotheliocytes. It also detoxifies H_2O_2 produced by the LPOx-SCN-GluOx axis. On the other hand, SCN can be cytotoxic. However, diseases associated with increased SCN and HOSCN levels are also linked to exposure to other toxic agents (e.g., cyanide, tobacco smoke, and cyanogenic glucosides), which can contribute to pathogenesis.

Hypothiocyanous acid reacts with thiols, oxidizing Trp and damaging protein Tyr phosphatases, resulting in hyperphosphorylation within the cell, altering MAPK signaling, and initiating apoptosis. It can also oxidize LDLs and HDLs, as well as NO.

3.1.4.9. Cytochrome-P450

CyP450 oxidoreductase (POR), also known as NADPH-CyP450 reductase (CPR),20 catalyzes the oxidative metabolism of a variety of xenobiotics by inserting an oxygen atom into a substrate. Processing by CyP450 enzymes is inefficient because substrate oxidation generates varying amounts of superoxide and/or hydrogen peroxide.

Microsomal CyP450 monooxygenases perform three types of NADPH-dependent oxidations, which include:

The cytochrome-P450 epoxygenases (HETEs) produce (5,6)-, (8,9)-, (11,12)-, and (14,15)-EETs through a regio- and stereo-selective olefin epoxidation of AA.

Allylic oxidation of AA (lipoxygenase-like reaction) yields 5-, 8-, 9-, 11-, 12-, and 15-hydroxyeicosatetraenoic acids (HETEs).

AA ω- and (ω-1)-hydroxylases CyP1a1, CyP1a2, CyP4a11, and CyP4a22 catalyze the formation of 16- (ω-4) to 20HETEs (ω) at or near the terminal carbons.

Four EET regioisomers, (5,6)-, (8,9)-, (11,12)-, and (14,15)-EETs, serve as auto- and paracrine messengers. EETs' primary vasodilation mechanism is smooth myocytic large-conductance Ca^{2+}-activated K^+ channels (big potassium) [22]. Activation of endothelial TRP channels by EETs, with subsequent Ca^{2+} influx, is another endothelial-derived hyperpolarizing factor. They also reduce inflammation in blood vessels and promote angiogenesis through the EPHb4-coupled PI3K-PKB pathway or the sphingosine kinase SphK1. They convert eicosapentaenoic acid (EPA) into vasoactive epoxy derivatives and endocannabinoids, whereas soluble epoxide hydrolase converts EETs to dihydroxyeicosatrienoic acids (DHETs), reducing many of their effects.

3.1.4.10. Heme Oxygenases

HOx1 and HOx2 are membrane-bound heme oxygenases that catalyze the rate-limiting step of heme catabolism by converting heme to CO, biliverdin, and ferrous iron using molecular oxygen and electrons supplied by CyP450 oxidoreductase. Heme is a potent hydrophobic prooxidant that intercalates in membranes and causes phospholipid peroxidation.

The HOx1 subtype is expressed constitutively in the liver, spleen, and bone marrow, but it can be induced in most organs by redox stress, heat shock, nutrient depletion, disrupted intracellular calcium homeostasis, cytotoxin exposure, and proinflammatory stimuli. It synthesizes the second messenger CO, a gaseous vasodilator that protects the hepatic microcirculation and other vascular beds from oxidative stress. The HOx2 isoform is found in the brain, liver, spleen, and testis.

Heme oxygenase HOx1 protects against redox stress by competing with CyP450 for binding to their common redox partner, CyP450 oxidoreductase, which reduces CyP450 activity and associated ROS production. Induction of HOx1 slows CyP1a2's microsomal production of hydrogen peroxide and hydroxyl radicals. Furthermore, HOx1 partially protects against CyP2e1-induced oxidative injury.

3.1.4.11. Crosstalk

Crosstalk exists between ROS sources. Hydrogen peroxide can activate NOx, causing xanthine dehydrogenase to transform into xanthine oxidase. Peroxynitrite causes superoxide production. Furthermore, mitochondrial ETC and NOx can interact to induce each other, resulting in the formation of an oxidative cycle. Hyperglycemia promotes this interference.

ROS partner production is dependent on the vessel's location. ROS-related protein expression varies among vSMCs, endothelial, immune, and other hematopoietic cells.

3.1.4.12. Redox Signaling

At low concentrations, certain ROS, such as superoxide and hydrogen peroxide, act as signaling mediators in redox signaling (or redox control).

ROS stimulates intracellular signaling effectors such as the MAPK module with ERK1, ERK2, and ERK4, protein Tyr kinases Src and Syk, and various redox-sensitive isoenzymes of the PKC set, as well as redox-sensitive transcription factors like AP1, ETS, HIF1, NFκB, and P53.

Hydrogen peroxide has a longer half-life than superoxide and, unlike superoxide, can cross lipidic membranes via diffusion or aquaporins to initiate intracellular signaling. Superoxide enters the cell through the anion chloride channel ClC_3.

Superoxide and hydrogen peroxide can stimulate cell growth and proliferation by oxidatively activating signaling molecules (such as PKB, Src, PLC, and MAPK) or inactivating protein Tyr phosphatases.

ROS, at low concentrations, regulate both vascular smooth myocyte proliferation and contraction-relaxation states.

3.1.4.13. Antioxidant Defense

Organisms use both enzymatic and non-enzymatic antioxidant defense to prevent an overload of highly reactive, short-lived free radicals. Redox-sensitive proteins are limited to signaling nanodomains in cardiovascular cells. Antioxidant protection occurs in four stages: preventive, chain-breaking, repairing, and adaptive. (1) The first line of antioxidant defense consists of enzymes such as superoxide dismutases (SOD1-SOD3), glutathione peroxidases (GPOx1-GPOx8), and catalase. Extracellular SOD is produced by vSMCs (not ECs). (2) The second line of defense, which includes vitamins C and E and most likely carotenoids, prevents the accumulation of secondary radicals produced by chain reactions such as lipid peroxidation. (3) The third level of defense involves enzymatic prevention and removal of secondary radicals.

Stress response, triggered by transcription factors NFκB and NFE2L2, involves protein cysteine reduction and oxidation. ROS promote the formation of NFE2L2, which stimulates the synthesis of numerous antioxidant enzymes.

When exposed to redox stress, MAP3K5 initiates a cellular response induced by ROS. ROS promote angiotensin-2-induced MAP3K5 activation. In unstressed cells, MAP3K5 homo-oligomerizes to form the inactive MAP3K5-TRdx signalosome. When stimulated by ROS, this signalosome releases its inhibitor TRdx, forming a fully activated complex with TRAF2 and TRAF6.

Antioxidants such as superoxide dismutases, catalase, glutathione peroxidases (GPOxs), and the thioredoxin-thioredoxin reductase couple counterbalance ROS production (Table 3.4). Glutathione peroxidase, catalase, and peroxiredoxins all catabolize hydrogen peroxide.

Catabolism of reaction oxygen species (ROS) (*Cat* catalase [encoded by the CAT gene], *GPOxi* type-*i* glutathione peroxidase [encoded by the GPX1–GPX8 genes], *GsR* glutathione reductase [encoded by the GSR gene], *PRdxi* type-*i* peroxiredoxin [encoded by the PRDX1–PRDX6 genes], *TRdxRdi* type-*i* thioredoxin reductase [encoded by the TXNRD1–TXNRD3 genes]).

Table 3.4. *Catabolism of Reaction Oxygen Species (ROS)*

Enzyme	Reactants	Products
GsR	$G^{SS}G$	G^{SH}
–	NADPH	$NADP^+$
GPOx1	G^{SH}	$G^{SS}G$
–	H_2O_2	H_2O
Cat	H_2O_2	O_2, H_2O
PRdx2	$TRdx^{SH}$	$TRdx^{SS}TRdx$
–	H_2O_2	H_2O
TRdxRd1	$TRdx^{SS}TRdx$	$TRdx^{SH}$
–	NADPH	$NADP^+$

The disulfide bridge characterizes the oxidized form (SS or S2). The removal of hydrogen peroxide prevents the formation of the highly reactive hydroxyl radical, which is produced when hydrogen peroxide reacts with Fe^{2+} (Fenton's reaction). In various intracellular antioxidant reactions, such as H_2O_2 removal, the reduced form of glutathione (GSH) is oxidized into glutathione disulfide (GSSG), which can then be excreted from cells or converted back to GSH by NADPH-dependent glutathione disulfide reductase.

3.1.4.14. Superoxide Dismutases

Superoxide dismutases (SOD3), SOD1 (cytosolic copper and zinc), and SOD2 (mitochondrial manganese) convert $O\cdot_2^-$ into hydrogen peroxide and molecular oxygen, preventing peroxynitrite formation (Table 3.5). SOD dismutates $O\cdot_2^-$ into H_2O_2 by reducing and re-oxidizing a redox active transition catalytic metallic ion, such as copper

(SOD with its oxidized and reduced metal ion: $SODCu^{2+}$ and $SODCu^{+}$, respectively) and manganese ($SODMn^{3+}$ and $SODMn^{2+}$) [23].

Table 3.5. *Superoxide Dismutases in Vascular Walls*

Isoform	Catalytic Metallic Ion	Metal Delivery	Location
SOD1 (homodimer)	Cu^{2+}	CCS, G^{SH}	Nucleus, cytosol, endosomes, lysosomes, peroxisomes, IMS
–	Zn^{2+}	–	–
SOD2 (homotetramer)	Mn^{3+}	ND	Mitochondria matrix.
SOD3 (homotetramer)	Cu^{2+}	Atox1,	Cell surface, extracellular matrix, and fluids
–	Zn^{2+}	ATP7α	–

Source: Atox copper chaperone antioxidant, ATP7α copper-transporting ATPase-7α, CCS copper carrier and chaperone for superoxide dismutase, and IMS intermembrane space of the mitochondrial envelope.

The SOD3 isozyme is anchored in the extracellular matrix via heparan sulfate proteoglycans, collagen, and fibulin 5.

3.1.4.15. Catalase

Catalase is primarily found in peroxisomes, where it produces H_2O_2 through β-oxidation of long-chain fatty acids. Except in the heart, heme-containing homotetrameric catalase is found in the mitochondrial matrix. Catalase activity is highest in red blood capsules, followed by the liver and kidney, and lowest in the brain, heart, and skeletal muscle.

It neutralizes hydrogen peroxide, which prevents the accumulation of hydroxyl radicals. Catalase degrades H_2O_2 through two distinct mechanisms. Dismutation occurs when another H_2O_2 molecule reduces the oxyferryl heme back to the ferric form, with H_2O_2 acting as both an oxidant and a reductant. Catalase can also use other electron donors (a peroxidative mechanism).

3.1.4.16. Peroxiredoxins

Ubiquitous homodimeric peroxiredoxins are nonheme peroxidases that detoxify both low- and high-molecular-mass peroxides. The majority of PRdxs use thioredoxin as a donor of reducing equivalents (hydrogen), but PRdx6 is a reduced glutathione-dependent peroxidase. Glutaredoxins and cyclophilins are additional electron donors for peroxiredoxin.

Peroxiredoxins are found in various subcellular compartments, including the mitochondrion (e.g., PRdx3 and PRdx5) and the cytosol (e.g., PRdx1, PRdx2, and PRdx6), with PRdx4 residing primarily in the endoplasmic reticulum and PRdx5 also in the cytosol and peroxisomes.

Peroxiredoxins are phosphorylated in response to extracellular signals, redox status, and oligomerization. They contain one or two active cysteines that are susceptible to oxidation by H_2O_2, which reacts with the thiolate deprotonated form of cysteine. Peroxiredoxins are classified into three types: typical (PRdx1–PRdx4), atypical 2-Cys (PRdx5), and 1-Cys forms (PRdx6). They also lower ONOO– and lipid peroxide levels.

Antioxidant sestrins can regenerate oxidized peroxiredoxins, scavenge ROS, and inhibit NOx4 expression, particularly in glomerular mesangiocytes and TORC1-induced ROS.

3.1.4.17. Glutathione Peroxidases

Glutathione peroxidase GPOx1 is one of the most abundant GPOX family members, along with epithelial GPOx2, which is highly expressed in the intestine, and secreted GPOx3, among other subtypes. GPOx1 resides in the cytosol, mitochondria, and peroxisomes.

The intracellular antioxidant enzyme GPOx1, which contains selenocysteine, converts hydrogen peroxide to water, limiting its accumulation and subsequent harmful oxidative effect on nucleic acids, proteins, and membrane lipids, as well as preventing carcinogenesis and CVD.

GPOx1 can also reduce lipid and other soluble hydroperoxides that have been released from membrane lipids. It also reduces phospholipid and monoacylglycerol hydroperoxides, including linoleoyl lysophosphatidylcholine hydroperoxide, but not tri- or diacylglycerol hydroperoxides. GPOx4 reduces the other types of membrane-associated phospholipids. GPOx1 may also function as peroxynitrite reductase.

GPOx1 expression is controlled by various mechanisms, including transcription, post-transcription, translation, and post-translation. Estradiol and ROS help regulate GPOx1 transcription. Selenium stabilizes mRNA, preventing nonsense-mediated decay. Translation requires Sec insertion sequence (SecIS)-binding proteins like SBP2. GPOx1 can be oxidatively inactivated by excess ROS or NO after translation, whereas the kinase Abl phosphorylates (activates) it.

3.1.4.18. Oxidative Stress

ROS have negative effects when present at high and sustained concentrations. The reversible and irreversible oxidation of cellular proteins, lipids, carbohydrates, RNA, and DNA affects cellular function. The mtDNA is particularly susceptible to ROS and RNS. Generalized oxidation leads to cell dysfunction, apoptosis, or necrosis.

ROS are involved in inflammation. Macrophages, in particular, release glutathionated peroxiredoxin-2, which acts as an alarmin (or damage-associated molecular pattern molecules), activating the innate immune response and producing TNFSF1.

ROS play a role in the initiation and progression of CVD. They participate in proinflammatory signaling within vascular endothelial cells (vECs) and vSMCs, which then produce cell adhesion molecules and chemokines. They also activate MMPs.

Major vascular risk factors (hypertension, dyslipidemia, diabetes, and smoking) are linked to higher vascular ROS production. A chronic metabolic disturbance promotes inflammation and redox stress, resulting from an imbalance between pro- and antioxidants, as well as their sources and sinks. Obese sedentary people have more NOx activity in their skeletal muscles and higher blood ROS levels than lean active people. An adequate diet that reduces redox stress protects against obesity-related disorders. Mitochondrial superoxide production accounts for 1–2% of the molecular oxygen consumed. However, excess mitochondrial $O\cdot_2^-$ affects the perivascular neutrophil niche. Lysophosphatidylcholine is involved in both mitochondrial ROS production and endotheliocyte activation, most likely due to electron leakage across the mitochondrial membrane. Hydrogen peroxide from mitochondrial $O\cdot_2^-$ affects the caliber of the coronary resistance artery.

Chronic production of inflammatory and vasoconstrictive prostaglandins exacerbates hypertension by inducing inflammation and vasoconstriction.

The oxidation and glycation of LDLs produce proinflammatory and proatherogenic adducts. High-density lipoproteins, on the other hand, reduce lipoprotein oxidation and thus the formation of oxidized LDLs (oxLDLs), with the antioxidant effect being mediated by HDL-associated paraoxonase.

ROS in atherosclerotic lesions stabilize HIF1α, which is produced in hypoxic regions of plaques and favors the M1 macrophage phenotype, leading to atherogenesis.

FAK, PTPN11, NOx, ROS, and ScaRb3 all play a role in oxLDL-induced macrophage migration. In contrast, ROS activation of ScaRb3 in extracellular vesicles prevents endotheliocyte migration.

Growth factors (e.g., platelet-derived growth factor and TGFβ), cytokines (e.g., TNFSF1 and IL1β), and hemodynamic stress (shear and stretch) affect the expression and activity of vascular NOxs. The autacoids angiotensin-2, endothelin-1, and thrombin activate NOx. Agt2 not only stimulates NOx, but it also increases the expression of its subunits, causing ROS to be produced by ECs, vSMCs, and adventitial fibroblasts via the AT1 receptor. Thrombin, alongside PDGF, TGFβ, and TNFSF1, activates NOx in vSMCs. Endothelin-1 stimulates NOx activity in ECs via the ETA receptor.

Angiotensin-2 disrupts mitochondrial function through endothelial NOx, PKC, and ONOO−, increasing mitochondrial H_2O_2 production and decreasing endothelial NO availability. Manganese-containing superoxide dismutase SOD2, as well as peroxiredoxins PRdx3, and/or PRdx5, reduce mitochondrial ROS levels and protect against mitochondrial oxidative damage. The mitochondrial ATP-sensitive potassium channel in vascular smooth myocytes and endotheliocytes is involved in Agt2-induced mitochondrial ROS production because it increases K^+ influx and alkalinizes the mitochondrial matrix. Mitochondrial permeability transition pore opening contributes to Agt2-mediated ROS production.

In some diseases, vascular endotheliocytes and smooth myocytes express more NOx1. The interaction between thrombospondin-1 and neurophilin (CD47) activates NOx1. Cyclic stretch on vessels induces the formation of myocyte-enhancing factor MEF2b, which initiates NOx1 production and shifts the vSMC phenotype to a proliferative state. Hyperglycemia stimulates both NOx1 and NOx4 syntheses, resulting in ROS-induced PKC-dependent downregulation of PKG production and repression of the NO-sGC-cGMP-PKG signaling pathway.

Inducible NOx2, which is more abundant in fibroblasts and immunocytes, aids in recruiting macrophages to inflammation sites to remove infectious pathogens. However, NOx2 overexpression in the endothelium promotes prolonged leukocyte infiltration of the vasculature and thrombosis.

Hydrogen peroxide (H_2O_2) produced by constitutively active brown adipocytic NOx4 protects the vasculature through PKG. In addition, adipocytic NOx4 slows obesity-related inflammation as well as T2DM progression. Endoplasmic reticular stress, on the other hand, activates NOx4, which generates superoxide and hydrogen peroxide. Intermedin-1–53, an N-terminal fragment of adrenomedullin-2, lowers NOx4 production.

Vasculopathies involve RNS, specifically NO•, an endothelial function marker, and its derivatives. In healthy vessels, NO inhibits circulating leukocyte adhesion to the wetted endothelial surface, causing vasodilation. In addition to endotheliocytes, circulating hematopoietic cells are major sources of NO in the blood. Excess NO production, which is often caused by NOS2 hyperactivity, is harmful to the vasculature. Obese mice's perivascular adipose tissue causes NOS3 uncoupling, converting it from NO producer to $O\cdot_2^-$ generator, exacerbating the underlying pathology.

In endothelial and smooth muscle cells, the oxidation state of hemoproteins (ferric versus ferrous) influences NO signaling. The redox state of hemoglobin (Hbα) at the myoendothelial junction influences NO activity. In the ferric state, Hbα has a reduced affinity for NO, allowing it to diffuse between endotheliocytes and smooth myocytes. Reduced ferrous Hbα suppresses the NO-sGC-cGMP-PKG axis and vasodilation of resistance arteries in both the systemic and pulmonary circulations. The flavoprotein methemoglobin reductase [24] also inhibits NO signaling at the myoendothelial junction. In contrast, methemoglobin reductase converts soluble guanylate cyclase (sGC) heme iron from ferric to ferrous, allowing NO sensing and subsequent arterial dilation. Furthermore, cGMP is not only degraded by the phosphodiesterases PDE3 and PDE5, but also exported from the cell.

3.1.4.19. Receptor for Advanced Glycation End Product

Receptor for advanced glycation end products (RAGE), a proinflammatory multiligand receptor for advanced glycation end products, generates ROS through NOx activation and mitochondrial production amplification, thereby operating via redox stress.

RAGE is present in a variety of cell types, including endothelial progenitor cells, cardiac endotheliocytes, vascular smooth myocytes, nervous system cells, pancreatic β cells, renal mesangiocytes, osteoblasts, and inflammatory leukocytes. Its cytoplasmic domain interacts with the formin diaphanous-1, activating Rac1 and NOx in aortic smooth myocytes exposed to the RAGE ligand S100b.

The RAGE connects to proinflammatory members of the S100-calgranulin set (S100a8, S100a9, and S100a12), which are predominantly expressed by neutrophils, monocytes, and activated macrophages. S100a8 is a potent antioxidant, in addition to high-mobility group box-containing protein HMGB1, amyloid β-peptide and β-sheet fibrils, lysophosphatidic acid, αMβ2-integrin (CR3), and complement component C1q.

AGEs are the byproducts of non-enzymatic glycation and oxidation of proteins and lipids in vascular cells, CMCs, neurons of the central and peripheral nervous systems, alveolar pneumocytes, podocytes, and inflammatory leukocytes, among others. Glyoxalase-1, a detoxifier of glycation precursors like 3-deoxyglucosone of the AGE N 1-carboxymethyl lysine, protects the heart from diabetes-induced redox damage, inflammation, fibrosis, and diabetic cardiomyopathy.

3.1.4.20. Lipid Peroxidation

Lipids, with their reactive double bonds, are susceptible to oxidation. Lipid peroxidation produces isoprostanes and malondialdehyde (Table 3.6).

Table 3.6. *Lipid Peroxidation (Source)*

Reagent	Reactant	Product
Free radical	Lipid	Lipid radical ($L^{\bullet}$)
Lipid radical	G^{SH}	Lipid hydroxide (LH)
Lipid radical	$O\cdot_2^-$	Lipid peroxyradical ($LOO^{\bullet}$)
Lipid peroxyradical	G^{SH}	Lipid hydroxyperoxide (LOOH)
Lipid hydroxyperoxide	G^{SH}	Lipid alcohol (LOH)

Isoprostanes are stable prostaglandin-like compounds formed by AA peroxidation and then released from cellular membranes into the bloodstream by phospholipases. Isoprostane levels in plasma and urine are associated with cigarette smoking, hypercholesterolemia, obesity, type 2 diabetes, and hyperhomocysteinemia.

Peroxidation of polyunsaturated fatty acids (PUFAs) yields malondialdehyde. It interacts with proteins, specifically lysine residues, to form Lys-Lys crosslinks, as seen in oxLDL ApoB.

3.1.4.21. Protein Tyrosine Nitration

Proteins are also oxidized and associated with pathophysiological processes other than ageing. Protein tyrosine nitration, which adds a nitro group ($-NO_2$), is mediated by RNS like peroxynitrite (ONOO–) and nitrogen dioxide ($NO\cdot_2$). This reaction has two steps: oxidizing the phenolic ring of tyrosine to tyrosyl radical (Tyr•) and adding $NO\cdot_2$ to the Tyr with a nitrating agent. Myeloperoxidase, with its transition metal center, can react with ONOO– to facilitate nitration. Nitrotyrosine formation on enzymes such as sarcoplasmic reticulum Ca^{2+} ATPase (serca2a), manganese-containing superoxide dismutase (MnSOD or SOD2), prostacyclin synthase, tyrosine hydroxylase, and aldolase-A reduces their activity. On the other hand, nitrotyrosine in fibrinogen increases its activity and speeds up clot formation.

3.1.4.22. Protein Glutathionation

SGlutathionation, the formation of a disulfide bridge between a reactive cysteine residue and the tripeptide glutathione, regulates the redox state of many cellular proteins (e.g., NOS3, ryanodine receptor, SERCA, and Na^+–K^+ ATPase, affecting their function and intracellular Na^+ and Ca^{2+} handling). SGlutathionation of hemoglobin can be used to detect redox stress.

3.1.4.23. Ageing

Ageing is associated with a decline in organ function and metabolism. It is associated with chronic inflammation, also known as inflammaging, redox stress, and arterial stiffening. Arterial redox stress contributes to arterial stiffening by promoting elastin degradation and collagen overproduction, as well as inflammation.

Many lipids are synthesized from precursors within the body, but some essential FAs must be obtained through food consumption. Fish contains EPA and docosahexaenoic acid (DHA), which are essential long chain ω3 fatty acids. Vegans eat no animal products, and vegetarians eat no meat or fish; semi-vegetarians eat fish, seafood, and occasionally poultry; lacto-vegetarians consume dairy products, and lacto-ovo-vegetarians eat eggs.

Lipids can be classified into eight types: FAs, glycerolipids, glycerophospholipids, sphingolipids, sterol and prenol lipids, saccharolipids, and polyketides. Their concentrations vary from attomolar to micromolar. The goal of lipidomics is to investigate lipid fate and signaling, as well as the effects of nutritional supplementation and its role in immune and inflammatory responses, cardiovascular and pulmonary disease. Oxylipins are signaling lipids that play an important role in the initiation and termination of inflammation.

Oxylipins are lipophilic messengers generated by oxygenation by cyclooxygenases (COxs; or prostaglandin-G/H synthases), cytochrome-P450 enzymes (CyPs), and lipoxygenases (LOxs), in addition to the non-enzymatic auto-oxidation of PUFAs, such as the ω6-fatty acids arachidonic (AA) and linoleic acid (LA) in addition to ω3-fatty acid α-linolenic acid (α LA), the plasmatic concentrations of which change not only with diet but also during ageing.

Oxylipins play a role in immunity, and thus inflammation, as well as vasomotor tone and blood coagulation. They can also be used as bactericides.

Eicosanoids are oxylipins made from AA, which is a component of cellular membrane phospholipids. Cyclooxygenases produce class II (2 double bonds) prostaglandins (PGs) and thromboxanes (Txs) from AA. Dihomo-γ-linolenic acid (DGLA) and EPA are the precursors to Class-I and III PGs and Txs, respectively.

Lipoxygenase products include:

- HETEs from AA mediate neutrophil chemotaxis and degranulation.
- The hydroxyoctadecadienoic acids (HODEs) from LA
- Hydroxyeicosapentaenoic acids from the EPA.

Lipoxygenase LOx5 produces leukotrienes and other metabolites from AA, including proinflammatory 5HETE, 5oxoETE, and LTb4, as well as 9HODE and trihydroxyoctadecenoic acids (triHOMEs) from LA. ALOx12 and ALOx15 generate 12HETE, 12oxoHETE, and proinflammatory 9HETE from AA.

CyP enzymes produce epoxides, including EETs from AA and epoxyoctadecamonoenic acids (EOMEs) from LA, which dilate arteries. Soluble epoxide hydrolase converts these products into dihydroxyoctadecenoic acids and DHETs.

3.1.4.24. Ageing, Inflammation, and Oxidative Stress

Inflammaging is caused in part by elevated alarmin levels, which activate pattern recognition receptors. Toll-like (TLRs) and nucleotide-binding oligomerization domain-like receptors (NLRs) are found not only in innate immune cells, but also in neurovascular units and blood-brain barriers. TLR2, TLR4, NLRP1, and NLRP3 are among the pattern recognition receptors activated during ageing in neurons, astrocytes, microgliocytes, endotheliocytes, and possibly pericytes.

CVD is linked to chronic obstructive pulmonary disorder (COPD) through chronic inflammation, ageing, reduced sirtuin activity, and cigarette smoking.

Desmosine and isodesmosine are involved in elastin crosslinking and can be used to detect elevated elastin fiber turnover and degradation, such as in COPD and atherosclerosis complications.

Sirtuins (SIRT1–SIRT7) are NAD+-dependent protein (histone) deacetylases that regulate lifespan and health. Sirtuin-1 regulates endothelial function by deacetylating NOS3. It also inhibits senescence and angiogenesis by deacetylating P53 and STK11 (LKB1), as well as FoxO1 and notch-1. It also activates the liver X receptor (NR1h2/3), which is involved in reverse cholesterol transport, thereby increasing cholesterol efflux. It has antioxidant properties. Additionally, it inhibits NFκB. Sirtuin-1, on the other hand, inhibits vascular smooth myocyte proliferation and atherothrombosis by downregulating endothelial tissue factor formation while increasing tissue inhibitor of metallopeptidase TIMP3 expression. Prolonged moderate exercise training increases FoxO3a expression, reduces redox stress, and increases SIRT1 activity in the heart and adipose tissue of elderly rats.

Sirtuin-3 inhibits cardiac hypertrophy because it regulates ROS concentrations. Sirtuin-6 protects endotheliocytes from telomere and gene damage, while Sirtuin-7 interacts with P53 to protect CMCs from apoptosis, redox, and genotoxic stress.

ROS are involved in ageing. However, dietary antioxidants like vitamins C and E do not slow ageing. Mitochondria are a major source of ROS, and thus mediate aging-related processes. MitoQ ([dimethoxy methyl dioxo-cyclohexadien decyl] triphenyl methanesulfonate), a derivative of the potent antioxidant ubiquinone conjugated to triphenylphosphonium that accumulates within mitochondria, can be taken orally to prevent mitochondrial redox damage. It thus attenuates the production of proliferative, proinflammatory, and profibrogenic mediators (e.g., tumor growth factor, connective tissue growth factor, and PDGF) by neighboring and infiltrating cells in the liver (i.e., activated hepatic stellate cells, which form a collagen-rich matrix, Kupffer cells, and cholangiocytes, in addition to injured hepatocytes, platelets, and leukocytes), and thus redox stress, hepatocyte death, and hepatic inflammation, together with Its administration for four weeks reduces elastin content and aortic stiffness in 27-month-old mice, but has no effect on young mice or age-related collagen synthesis and deposition, and increases proinflammatory cytokine formation.

3.1.4.25. Ageing and Altered Proteostasis

Ageing and age-related diseases are associated with an imbalance in protein production, folding, and degradation, as well as the accumulation of misfolded proteins and proteic aggregates. In CMCs, altered proteostasis can contribute to the development of cardiac hypertrophy, cardiomyopathies, and heart failure.

Hydrotropes are small molecules, usually amphiphilic agents, which dissolve hydrophobic molecules in aqueous solutions. Adenosine triphosphate (ATP), the canonical energy carrier and autacoid, is an energy source for chemical reactions at micromolar concentrations, including muscular contraction, and has the properties of a hydrotrope at physiological millimolar concentrations (5–10 mmol/L) by maintaining protein solubility and preventing molecular aggregation. At relatively high concentrations, ATP increases the solubility of solutes such as nonpolar lipophilic proteins (unlike polar hydrophilic proteins) and organic substances that are nearly insoluble in standard aqueous solutions. Amphiphilic hydrotrope molecules have shorter hydrophobic regions, so they do not self-aggregate in the aqueous phase. ATP prevents the formation of protein aggregates, including prion and amyloid fibers from amyloid-β4 protein. It also helps dissolve previously formed agglutinated masses by dissolving liquid-liquid phase-separated droplets. This keeps the RNA-binding protein fused in sarcoma (FUS) water-soluble and prevents accumulation into separate liquid drops.

The Michaelis-Menten constant of cardiac actin-based nanomotor myosin evolves in the micromolar range (β-myosin encoded by the MYH7 gene: 40 ± 6 µmol/L), while the nucleotide ATP is typically present in millimolar concentrations in the cytoplasm of CMCs. As a result, the discrepancy between the ATP concentration required by ATP-consuming enzymes and its intracellular level can be explained, at least partially, by its hydrotrope activity.

Ageing causes a decrease in intracellular ATP and impaired mitochondrial oxidative phosphorylation. Variant proteins with glutamine repeat expansions (polyQ repeats), or increased polyglutamine motif length, encoded by the DNA nucleotide sequence CAG, can misfold and aggregate, sequestering proteins. Huntington's disease is caused by the expansion of polyQ domains in huntingtin and the deubiquitinase ataxin-3, which results in the loss of striatal neurons and thus changes in mood and personality, defective motor coordination, involuntary movements, and type-3 spinocerebellar ataxia (SCA3), a form of neurodegeneration in the striatum and cerebellum, respectively. PolyQ expansions, as well as the soluble N-terminal huntingtin fragment that includes exon 1, are toxic. Autophagy, which is designed to reduce protein toxicity, removes polyQ-expanded proteins like abnormal huntingtin and ataxin-3.

On the other hand, some polyQ-containing proteins control the degradation of misfolded proteins and autophagy. Ataxin-3 deubiquitinates beclin-1, which then escapes proteosomal degradation and initiates starvation-induced autophagy. Ataxin-3 and beclin-1 can interact thanks to their short polyQ domains. On the other hand, a mutated huntingtin with an expanded polyQ region competes with ataxin-3 for beclin-1 binding, increasing beclin-1 degradation, and disrupting autophagy. Huntingtin also participates in stress-induced autophagy by competing for binding to another autophagic regulator.

The hereditary neurodegenerative disease SCA1 is caused by the expansion of the polyglutamine stretch in ataxin-1 (Atxn1), which is also known as SCA1. The ATXN family consists of proteins with an AXH domain that is involved in protein-protein interactions [25].

Table 3.7. *Ataxins**

Type	Function
Atxn1 (SCA1)	Chromatin-binding factor repressing notch signaling (CBF1 corepressor).
Atxn1L (boat)	Also named chromatin-binding repressor of notch cooperating with Atxn1.
Atxn2 (SCA2)	Inhibition of EGFR internalization.
Atxn2L	Regulation of stress granule and P-body formation.
Atxn3 (SCA3)	Deubiquitinase of proteostasis maintenance.
(MJD1)	Involved in gene transcription, cytoskeleton regulation, and myogenesis.
Atnx3L (MJD1L)	Deubiquitinase.
Atxn7 (SCA7)	Component of the deubiquitination module of the spt-ada-gcn5 acetyltransferase (SAGA) histone acetyltransferase and deubiquitinase complex.
	Histone remodeling for transcriptional regulation.
Atxn7L1 (Atxn7L4), Atxn7L2: Undetermined Role	
Atxn7L3	Component of the transcriptional regulatory SAGA complex.
Atxn8	ND
(SCA8, P1c2)	–
Atxn10 (SCA10)	Survival of cerebellar neurons.

*Atxns; Source: boat brother of ataxin-1, MJDL Machado-Joseph disease protein-like protein.

The deubiquitinase Atxn3L targets the zinc finger-containing transcription factor KLF5, which promotes cell survival and proliferation as well as tumor growth, in part by upregulating the synthesis of fibroblast growth factor-binding protein FGFBP126 and microsomal prostaglandin-E synthase PtgES1. It belongs to the DUB subset of Machado-Joseph disease (MJD) proteic domain-containing peptidases, along with Atxn3 (a.k.a. MJD1 and SCA3), encoded by the gene mutated in MJD, also known as SCA3, and Josephin domain-containing DUBs JosD1 and JosD2 (Table 3.7) [27].

Expansion of the polyglutamine sequence in ataxins causes SCA. Polyglutamine-expanded ataxin-7 aggregates sequester ubiquitin-specific peptidase USP22, rendering it unable to perform its deubiquitination function in the spt-ada-gcn5 acetyltransferase complex, resulting in cytotoxicity and neurodegeneration.

3.1.4.26. Sleeping Disorders

Sleep disorders and short sleep duration (≤ 5 h/night) disrupt neurohormonal regulation and the circadian rhythm of blood pressure, causing a nocturnal decrease in melatonin secretion and favoring hypertension. Sleep deprivation is linked to hypertension, diabetes, and coronary artery disease.

Sleep anomalies have been linked to cardiovascular and metabolic disease (hypertension, atherosclerosis, heart failure, cardiac arrhythmias, obesity, and metabolic syndrome). Sleep modulates the autonomic nervous system, hemodynamics, endothelial and myocardial function, and blood coagulation.

Central sleep apnea (CSA) is caused by a lack of neural input during breathing. Breathing effort is reduced or absent during airflow cessation, which can last 10–30 seconds and occur intermittently or in cycles.

Chemoreceptors control breathing on both the central and peripheral levels. Medullary neurons respond to CO_2 content through shifts in H+ concentration, while carotid body chemoreceptors respond to arterial blood O_2 and CO_2 content. Elevated chemoresponsiveness, combined with blunted chemosensitivity, can disrupt the breathing pattern. In addition, several other homeostatic feedback mechanisms regulate breathing amplitude and frequency to maintain gas exchange, including afferent input from Golgi tendon organs and muscle spindles from respiratory muscles. Ventilatory response to hypoxia and hypercapnia, as well as respiratory load compensation, are reduced while sleeping, particularly during the rapid eye movement stage.

CSA manifestations include high-altitude-induced periodic breathing, idiopathic CSA, narcotic-induced central apnea, obesity hypoventilation syndrome, and Cheyne-Stokes breathing. Nighttime breathing disturbances raise the risk of poor cardiovascular outcomes.

Obstructive sleep apnea (OSA), which causes breathing pauses 5–30 times per hour during sleep due to upper airway obstruction, is associated with respiratory efforts. It can cause hypertension, arrhythmia, stroke, and heart failure. Obstructive sleep apnea is associated with obesity, and the resulting sleep deprivation can promote obesity, creating a vicious cycle.

3.1.4.27. Vascular Tumors and Malformations

Tumors and malformations (direct connections between arteries and veins) are examples of vascular anomalies, which also include infection, trauma, and adverse remodeling.

Vascular congenital tumors include infantile congenital hemangioma, commonly found in girls, as well as tufted angioma, infantile fibrosarcoma, myofibromatosis, and kaposiform hemangioepithelioma.

Vascular malformations that bypass the capillary bed are typically caused by embryogenic errors. However, the majority of arteriovenous malformations are idiopathic. They develop on their own. They differ from those caused by gene mutations in terms of their location and evolution.

The International Society for the Study of Vascular Anomalies classified benign vascular lesions into two groups based on channel type and flow magnitude: (1) vascular tumours, such as infantile hemangioma, and (2) vascular malformations caused by errors in vasculo- and angiogenesis. Vascular malformations usually develop gradually, but they grow faster than the rest of the body, reaching their peak during puberty.

Birth defects may be caused by environmental factors rather than genetics. For example, maternal fever in the first trimester of pregnancy can cause cardiac and craniofacial birth defects. Neural crest cells are the precursors of cells that form the heart and face tissues. Hyperthermia activates TRPV1 and TRPV4 channels in neural crest cells of chick embryos, resulting in cardiac and craniofacial birth defects.

Vascular tumors include non-involuting (NICH) and rapidly involuting (RICH) congenital and infantile hemangiomas, tufted angiomas, kaposiform, spindle cell, and other rare hemangioendotheliomas, as well as dermatologically acquired vascular tumors (e.g., pyogenic granuloma, targetoid, glomeruloid, and microvenular hemangioma).

Slow-flow vascular malformations include venous (blue rubber bleb nevus syndrome, familial cutaneous and mucosal venous malformation, glomuvenous malformation), capillary (telangiectasia and angiokeratoma), and lymphatic malformations (primary lymphedema, micro- and macrocystic lymphatic malformations, as well as combined vascular malformations).

Telangiectasias are small, permanently dilated blood vessels that cause cutaneous red dots, linear or stellate lesions. They frequently progress to form papules, especially on the face.

Angiokeratomas are a diverse group of red-violaceous to black papules caused by vascular dilation in the papillary dermis, often associated with epidermal hyperplasia and hyperkeratosis.

Angiokeratoma corporis diffusum is a diffuse form of angiokeratoma. They are linked with deficiencies in:

Mutations in the *NAGA* gene, which encodes lysosomal α-nacetylgalactosaminidase (NAGα), lead to aspartylglucosaminuria and type-I (infantile) and -II (adulthood) Schindler disease.

Fabry disease is caused by mutations in the *GLA* gene, which encodes lysosomal α-galactosidase-A.

Mutations in the *FUCA1* gene, known as α-fucosidase (Fucα), can lead to severe infantile type-I and milder type-II fucosidosis.

Mutations in the *CTSA* gene, which encodes lysosomal cathepsin-A, cause early and late infantile and juvenile/adult galactosialidosis. CtsA is a protective protein for β-galactosidase and cooperates with neuraminidase-1 and β-galactosidase.

Mutations in the *MANBA* gene, which encodes lysosomal acid α-mannosidase class 2B member 1, can lead to β-mannosidosis.

Mutations in the *GLB1* gene, which encodes acid galactosidase-β1 (Glβ1), can cause GM1 gangliosidosis. This condition occurs when GM1 ganglioside accumulates to toxic levels and cannot be broken down.

Mutations in the *NEU1* gene cause type-I sialidosis (partial deficiency) and type-II sialidosis (severe reduction or elimination of Neu1 activity), respectively. Verrucous hemangioma is not the same as angiokeratoma.

These generally deep lesions are frequently associated with hyperkeratosis.

Fast-flowing vascular malformations include arterial and arteriovenous malformations, arteriovenous fistulas (AVFs), and combined vascular malformations (AVMLMs and CMAVMs).

3.1.4.28. Ectopic Vascular Calcification

Arteries can experience abnormal caliber changes, such as narrowing (stenosis) or enlargement (aneurysm), as well as ectopic calcifications.

Vascular calcification is regulated by bone morphogenetic proteins, tumor-necrosis factor superfamily member TNFSF11, and receptors TNFRSF11a and TNFRSF11b, as well as inflammatory factors and oxidized lipids.

Lipoprotein-A (LPa) transports oxidized phospholipids (OxPLs) that contain phosphocholine and promote inflammation and calcium. In fact, a variety of lipoproteins contribute to the progression from sclerosis to stenosis, with LPa being the preferred OxPL carrier.

3.1.5. Atherosclerosis

Atherosclerotic cardiovascular disease is characterized by subendothelial retention of modified lipoproteins, immunocyte infiltration, maladaptive chronic inflammation of the arterial wall, and vSMC-mediated fibrous cap formation. Atherosclerosis progression is associated with cell death, fibrous cap thinning, plaque rupture, and thrombosis.

Accumulated intracellular cholesterol can be removed through reverse cholesterol transport, which begins with cholesterol egress from cells and ends with elimination from the body, thereby preventing the development and progression of atherosclerosis.

Atherogenesis occurs when there is an imbalance between cholesterol uptake from oxidized or aggregated LDLs through scavenger receptors and cholesterol efflux to apolipoprotein-A and HDLs via ABC transporters.

LDLs can undergo oxidation, glycation, acetylation, ethylation, and methylation. Atherogenesis begins when oxidized and glycated LDLs accumulate in arterial walls. Modifications target LDL components such as ApoB, a surface protein that mediates LDL binding to its receptor. The early stage of atherogenesis is associated with oxidized LDLs that accumulate in the subendothelial space, activating endotheliocytes, which then produce adhesion molecules and chemokines, recruiting inflammatory cells. Attracted monocytes develop into macrophages, which internalise oxLDLs and produce cytokines and ROS, further oxidizing LDLs and attracting medial smooth myocytes to the intima. These smooth myocytes cause atherogenesis through apoptosis and foam cell formation. Non-enzymatic glycation of ApoB lysine residues reduces LDL affinity for its receptor, increasing plasmatic lifetime and glycated LDL uptake by vascular cells and macrophages. Furthermore, glycation makes LDLs more susceptible to oxidation (gl-oxLDLs). After absorbing modified LDLs via scavenger receptors and pinocytosis, macrophages in the arterial intima differentiate into foam cells.

Mitochondria generate ATP and are involved in ion transfer, ROS production, and apoptotic signaling. The mtDNA contains 37 genes encoding subunits of ETCcomplex-I, -III, and -IV, as well as ATP synthase (ETCcomplex-V), ribosomal and transfer RNAs.

Mitochondrial ROS damage mtDNA, a circular molecule connected to the inner mitochondrial membrane; mitochondrial dysfunction and subsequent mitophagy occur before lesion development. The mtDNA damage lowers mitochondrial oxidative phosphorylation. Reduced mitochondrial oxidative phosphorylation thins the fibrous cap through vascular smooth myocyte dysfunction and apoptosis, while macrophage activation increases necrotic core formation.

The MtDNA replisome, made up of the twinkle helicase, MtDNA polymerase, and mitochondrial single-stranded DNA-binding protein, replicates mtDNA.

Mitophagy in plaque vSMCs is increased by reduced MtDNA number and oxidative phosphorylation. However, overexpression of the mtDNA helicase twinkle reduces MtDNA damage but not copy number. Twinkle protects vascular smooth myocytes and macrophages from oxidative stress-induced apoptosis. Overexpressing twinkle in macrophages increases MtDNA copy number without affecting damage. Twinkle overexpression promotes oxidative phosphorylation in both cell types, possibly through increased ETC subunit synthesis, thickening the fibrous cap through increased vSMC proliferation and reduced apoptosis, and inhibiting necrotic core formation through macrophage inactivation.

Atherosclerosis is a chronic disease of the arterial wall involving both innate and adaptive immunity, with inflammation present at all stages of the disease. This inflammatory disease is characterized by lipid accumulation in the arterial intima, monocyte infiltration and proliferation, as well as differentiation into macrophages and other leukocytes, medial smooth myocyte recruitment, and extracellular matrix production and degradation. It is distinguished by hardened arterial segments with narrowed or enlarged lumens (stenoses and fusiform aneurysms).

The German-born French pathologist J. G. C. F. M. Lobstein (1777–1835) described arteriosclerosis, which is the hardening (or stiffening) of normally distensible arteries. It includes atherosclerosis, medial thickening, and medial and intimal calcifications (for example, Mönckeberg medial sclerosis, the most common type of medial calcification in the extremity arteries).

In 2013, atherosclerosis, specifically angina pectoris and myocardial and cerebral infarction (stroke), as well as other types of cardiovascular affections (e.g., arrhythmias, heart failure, and cardiac valvulopathies), accounted for 51% and 42% of deaths in women and men, respectively. In many countries, they cause more than twice as many deaths as cancer. Cancer, on the other hand, kills more men than CVD in at least 10 countries (Belgium, Denmark, France, Israel, Luxembourg, Netherlands, Portugal, Slovenia, Spain, and San Marino), and women in one (Denmark).

Coronary atherosclerosis (also known as coronary artery and heart disease, ischemic heart disease, and cerebrovascular disease) are the leading causes of CVD in Europe, accounting for 20 and 12% of all deaths annually, respectively. Inequalities exist between countries. Low- and middle-income countries now account for about 63% of ischemic and 80% of hemorrhagic strokes.

Acute coronary syndrome refers to unstable angina, ST-elevation myocardial infarction, and non-ST-elevation myocardial infarction caused by atherosclerotic plaque erosion, which can lead to rupture. The resulting intraluminal thrombosis causes sustained myocardial ischemia and infarction due to local partial or complete vascular occlusion or, more commonly, embolisation and subsequent obstruction of downstream arterial segments as platelet aggregates are shed.

Ischemia causes massive cell death, releasing alarmins that activate NFκB, resulting in proinflammatory cytokines. Macrophages consume dead cells and trigger inflammation through IRF3 and type-I interferons. IRF3 initiates a gene expression programme that protects against infection and cancer. Excessive IRF3 activation and type I IFN production are harmful. Myocardial infarction activates IRF3 in a distinct subset of interferon-inducible cardiac macrophages. Type-I interferons act on the IfnAR receptor through both autocrine and paracrine mechanisms. In mice, deficiency in the cytosolic DNA sensor cyclic GMP-AMP synthase (cGAS), its adaptor STING, and the cGAS-STING axis activating IRF3 via TBK1, IRF3, type-I Ifns, or IfnAR improves cell survival. In Irf3−/− mice, myocardial infarction-induced type-I Ifn response is almost completely suppressed. As a result, transient inhibition of the interferon-dependent innate immune response during ischemia can reduce inflammation and limit adverse ventricular remodeling.

Limbs exposed to brief periods of ischemia protect multiple organs, particularly the lung, from ischemia-reperfusion injury. Irisin, a myokine derived from the extracellular portion of fibronectin domain-containing protein FnDC5 in skeletal muscle, targets mitochondria and prevents negative effects of redox stress, resulting in limb remote ischemic preconditioning in the blood. The interaction between irisin and the mitochondrial uncoupling protein UCP2 reduces redox stress caused by ischemia-reperfusion events while preserving mitochondrial function.

3.2. Vasculopathies and Cardiovascular Dysfunction

Heart failure, a complication of coronary atherosclerosis, hypertension, cardiomyopathies, myocarditis, heart defects, and valvular heart disease (also known as heart valve disease), is estimated to affect up to 2% of people in North America and Europe. People over the age of 65 account for 80% of new cases and approximately 11% of deaths. Rheumatic heart disease (RHD) is the fifth and sixth leading cause of CVD-related mortality and disability, particularly in low-income countries (Oceania, Central, South, and Southeast Asia, Sub-Saharan Africa, the Caribbean, and Middle East).

Cardiomyopathies are classified into disease spectra based on aetiology and natural history, which impact medical management. They can be caused by left ventricular stiffening, impaired sensitivity to β-agonists and insulin, depressed autonomic function, endothelial dysfunction, abnormal ionic currents, and disturbed flow in the coronary macro- and microcirculation. The most common types are ischemic and dilated cardiomyopathies.

Dilated cardiomyopathy (DCM) is characterized by left ventricular or biventricular dilation and systolic dysfunction (abnormal ejection fraction) without abnormal loading conditions such as hypertension, valvulopathies, or coronary atherosclerosis. It is a collection of time-varying electrochemical and functional anomalies that can be caused by genetic or acquired disorders. Genetic predisposition may be combined with environmental factors.

DCM can be inherited in an autosomal dominant, recessive, X-linked, or matrilinear fashion. DCM genes include BCL2-associated athanogene-3 (BAG3), lamin-A/C (LMNA), cardiac myosin-binding protein-C (MYBPC3), myosin heavy chain (MYH7), myopalladin (MYPN), phospholamban (PLN), RNA-binding motif protein-20 (RBM20), voltage-gated sodium channel α subunit NaV1.5 (SCN5A), troponin-T (TNNT2), and titin (TTN). DCM may also have a genetic basis within the framework of neuromuscular disorders, such as Becker and Duchenne muscular dystrophy and myotonic dystrophy, which may be linked to mitochondrial diseases and tafazzin. In contrast, DCM can be caused by viral, bacterial, fungal, or parasitic infections, as well as systemic diseases (e.g., polymyositis, sarcoidosis, and systemic lupus erythematosus). It can be a complication of acromegaly, diabetes, hyperthyroidism, Addison and Cushing disease, and pheochromocytoma. Dilated cardiomyopathy can be caused by excessive alcohol consumption, chemotherapeutic and psychiatric drugs, electrolyte disturbances (hypocalcemia and hypophosphatemia), iron overload or deficiency (carnitine, copper, selenium, thiamine, and zinc), anti-heart antibodies, and toxics (e.g., arsenic and cobalt). Autoimmunity, foetal microchimerism, viral infection, stress-activated cytokines, and a toxic prolactin cleavage product are all contributing factors to peri- and postpartum cardiomyopathy.

Hypokinetic nondilated cardiomyopathy (HNDC) is characterized by left ventricular or biventricular systolic dysfunction (ejection fraction <45%) and no dilation.

Ischemic cardiomyopathy is caused by stenosis in large epicardial coronary arteries and/or parietal microcirculation, which is linked to chronic inflammation. Rheumatoid arthritis, systemic lupus erythematosus, and systemic sclerosis all pose a significant risk for myocardial ischemia.

Another type is hypertrophic cardiomyopathy (HCM), which is characterized by abnormal and often asymmetric myocardial thickening, preserved left ventricular function, phenotypic heterogeneity, and incomplete penetrance. Mutations in more than 50 genes, primarily encoding sarcomeric constituents, can cause this autosomal dominant inherited disease. The presence of additional risk factors, particularly hypertension, worsens disease penetrance and severity, as the MYL2 E22K mutation does not cause clinical symptoms in most carriers. Diabetic cardiomyopathy is characterized by decreased diastolic function and increased left ventricular size. Its clinical management is based on appropriate glucose and HbA1c monitoring. However, in people of African ancestry, a particular variant that shortens the lifespan of red blood capsules lowers HbA1c levels.

Diabetic cardiomyopathy is linked to a shift to exclusive FAs as an energetic substrate for CMCs, instead of the usual sources (amino acids, carbohydrates, FAs, ketones, and lactate), due to AMPK at an early stage and then NR1c1 (PPARα) [33]. Endotheliocytes preferentially use glucose (~85%) for ATP synthesis, with the faster rate of glycolysis compensating for the greater amounts of ATP per mole of glucose yielded by mitochondrial oxidative phosphoryla. However, diabetic endotheliocytes have abnormal metabolism. The production of GluT1 is insensitive to hyperglycemia, and glucose egress to the CMC is inadequate. Furthermore, high intracellular glucose concentration generates ROS and inhibits glycolysis, causing glycolytic intermediates to accumulate and be processed by the polyol, hexosamine, and methylglyoxal pathways, which produce ROS, RNS, and AGEs, respectively.

Arrhythmogenic cardiomyopathy is primarily caused by mutations in genes that encode desmosomal elements. It is distinguished by progressive fibroadipose replacement of the myocardium, arrhythmias, and sudden death. Cardiac mesenchymal stromal cells express less plakophilin, have more lipid droplets, and differentiate into adipocytes, all of which contribute to arrhythmogenic cardiomyopathy.

Arrhythmogenic atrial fibrosis, characterized by excess extracellular matrix deposition, fibroblast proliferation, and differentiation into collagen-secreting myofibroblasts, promotes atrial fibrillation (AF), the most prevalent persistent arrhythmia. This cardiac rhythm disorder is the sixth and eighth leading cause of CVD-related mortality and disability, respectively, with the highest prevalence found in North America and the lowest in Asia-Pacific. Excess collagen can impair atriomyocyte bundle continuity, reduce intercellular coupling, and cause longitudinal anisotropy. Furthermore, fibroblasts and myofibroblasts are electrochemically connected to CMCs, modulating their electrical activity, and facilitating re-entry. Re-entrant drivers (or rotors) associated with extensive atrial remodeling contribute to persistent AF by slowing action potential propagation, reducing cell excitability, and causing unidirectional block. These rotors are confined to high-fibrosis-density regions.

1. **Cardiac Wall Remodeling:** Cardiac walls remodel in response to pressure and volume overload or myocardial injury. This can lead to heart failure.

   Heart failure is linked to impaired signaling and pathological cardiac (or ventricular) wall remodeling. Maladaptive cardiac remodeling is defined by structural changes in dimensions, mass, and shape, as well as metabolic remodeling with functional alterations caused by molecular, cellular, and interstitial changes in response to abnormal hemodynamic load and/or damage associated with neurohormonal activation.

   Atrial and ventricular wall enlargement, as well as decreased cardiac contractility and adrenergic responsiveness, are all signs of congestive heart failure. The sympathetic nervous system and the renin-angiotensin-aldosterone axis are activated to compensate for decreased cardiac output, but this promotes heart failure progression through maladaptive wall remodeling.

   Cardiac modifications include cell death, redox stress, inflammation, hypertrophy and/or atrophy, fibrosis, and the development of arrhythmias. Specifically, cardiac fibrosis causes electrical and mechanical dysfunction.

   Heart failure is linked to ion carriers (channels, pumps, and transporters) such as plasmalemmal (sarcolemmal) NaV1.5 and CaV1.2 channels, Na^+–Ca^{2+} and Na^+–H^+ exchangers, KATP channel, sarco(endo)plasmic reticulum ryanodine-sensitive Ca^{2+} channel, and SERCA pump, as well as their regulators (kinases and phosphatases). Heart failure disrupts intracellular sodium regulation, K^+ channel activity, and Ca^{2+} cycling.

2. **Cardiac Wall Hypertrophy:** Sustained hypertension causes adverse left ventricular and arterial wall hypertrophy, as well as associated stiffness. However, hypertension-induced arterial wall hypertrophy in large and medium-sized arteries is not always associated with decreased arterial distensibility. Ageing, on the other hand, has an independent effect on distensibility and blood pressure levels.

   Na^+–K^+ ATPase, also known as the Na^+ pump, is a plasmalemmal αβ dimer. The catalytic ouabain-resistant α1 isoform is expressed in all cell types, with most cells producing a second α isoform (ouabain-sensitive α2-α3, α4 detected in sperm). The catalytic α subunit has Na^+, K^+, ATP, and cardiotonic steroid binding sites. Sodium ATPase β subunit has three isoforms (β1–β3) that support the catalytic activity of the chaperoned α subunit. In cardiac and vSMCs, the β1 subunit is the most important isoform, forming both α1β1 and α2β1 protomers [34]. Arterial smooth myocytes also produce the α2 isoform, which localises to endoplasmic reticulum-plasma membrane contact sites, known as plasmerosomes and controls myogenic tone. However, the α1 subunit has a more uniform distribution.

Sodium pumps are controlled by a variety of factors, including hormones (such as aldosterone, insulin, and catecholamines) and protein phosphorylation. Cardiotonic steroids such as ouabain, digoxin, and bufalin inhibit cation transport via the Na^+ pump mechanism.

The transmembrane regulator phospholemman (Plm), encoded by the FXYD1 gene (FXYD domain-containing ion transport regulator-1), modulates both Na^+ and K^+ affinities. Plm also regulates the activity of the Na^+–Ca^{2+} exchanger NCX1. Unphosphorylated Plm binds to the α2β dimer, decreasing the α2 subunit's affinity for intracellular Na^+ and extracellular K^+ ions. PKA or PKC phosphorylation of cardiac and arterial Plm reduces Na^+ ATPase inhibition and improves Na^+ affinity.

Thus, in arterial smooth myocytes, the Na^+ pump α2 subunit is structurally and functionally linked to NCX1. Other adjacent channels, pumps, and transporters, including TRPC6 and serca2, may influence this crosstalk.

Activation of the renin-angiotensin-aldosterone axis leads to increased ROS generation, glutathionation of the β1 subunit, and inhibition of the sodium pump. Plm promotes Na^+ pump deglutathionation and prevents oxidation in arteries and the heart.

Reduced expression of smooth muscle-specific Na^+ pump α2-subunit increases blood pressure and sensitivity to angiotensin-2 and dietary salt, while overexpression reduces basal BP, Agt2, and NaCl sensitivity. Chronic salt retention increases EOLC, a steroid produced by the adrenal cortex and inhibiting the Na^+ pump. This leads to salt-dependent hypertension mediated by the Na^+–Ca^{2+} exchanger.

Ouabain activates signaling via various effectors, including ERK1, ERK2, PI3Kc1α, PKB, and Src, in addition to NFκB.

Another cardiotonic steroid, marinobufagenin, can be found in human plasma and urine. Prolonged exposure to ouabain or marinobufagenin causes hypertension in normal rats (but not digoxin or digitoxin).

Retention of sodium ions and water leads to increased blood volume and plasmatic EOLC concentration, inhibiting the Na^+ pump. Elevated cytosolic Na^+ concentration increases cytosolic Ca^{2+} concentration through NCX, leading to increased myogenic tone and peripheral vascular resistance to blood flow.

Transaortic constriction-induced hypertrophy in mice is inhibited by immunoneutralizing endogenous ouabain. Endogenous ouabain and its receptor, Na^+ pump α2-subunit, contribute to hypertension-induced cardiac hypertrophy.

In hypertension, circumventricular organs like the subfornical organ activate the brain's RAAA, leading to an increase in sympathetic nerve activity and α-adrenoceptor-mediated arterial constriction. The hypothalamic neurohumoral pathway includes aldosterone production, mineralocorticoid receptor, ENaCs, ouabain release, and Na^+ pump.

Sirtuin-2, a cardioprotective

deacetylase, works through STK11 (LKb1) and AMPK to prevent aging-related and angiotensin-2-induced adverse cardiac hypertrophy. Sirtuin-2 deacetylates STK11 (Lys48), causing STK11 phosphorylation and initiating the STK11-AMPK axis. Cardiac hypertrophy and fibrosis are exacerbated in Sirt2-/- mice (aged 24 months) and Agt2-treated mice. Conversely, cardiac-specific SIRT2 overexpression protects against Agt2-induced cardiac hypertrophy and fibrosis while also restoring cardiac function.

3. **Cardiac Wall Fibrosis:** Fibrosis is a complication of chronic inflammatory conditions. Fibrogenesis begins with the activation of monocytes and their differentiation into profibrotic macrophages. TGFβ promotes the proliferation of myofibroblasts.

   Fibrosis is assessed by its regulators and markers, MMP1-MMP3, MMP7-MMP28, and TIMP1-TIMP4. TIMP1 specifically inhibits MMP9. TIMP1 has been shown to be a strong predictor of CVD death in some populations, including Iceland.

   Fibroblasts differentiate into activated myofibroblasts, producing α-smooth muscle actin and secreting matrix components like type-I α1-procollagen (encoded by the COL1A1 gene). Persistent myofibroblast activation distinguishes pathological fibrosis from wound healing. Myofibroblasts form a feedback loop that maintains fibrosis and extracellular matrix stiffness. Fibroblast-to-myofibroblast differentiation induced by matrix stiffness causes mitochondrial priming in activated myofibroblasts (but not in quiescent fibroblasts). Proapoptotic proteins such as BCL2L11 are activated in myofibroblasts, making them more susceptible to apoptosis; these agents can reverse fibrosis. Myofibroblasts, on the other hand, are dependent on antiapoptotic proteins like BCL2L1 to survive.

   Cardiac fibrosis is defined by the uncontrolled accumulation of extracellular matrix by cardiofibroblasts in the interstitial and perivascular spaces.

   The transcription of typical fibrosis genes, such as Comp and NOX4, which encode cartilage oligomeric matrix protein and the NADPH oxidase subtype NOx4, respectively, is increased.

   Hepatic fibrosis is characterized by the accumulation of matrix proteins, particularly fibrillar collagen-1, which provides mechanical stability. Cartilage oligomeric matrix protein (COMP), also known as thrombospondin-5, activates the ScaRb3 and MAP2K1/2-ERK1/2 pathways, leading to collagen-1 formation and deposition. COMP also supports matrix metallopeptidases MMP2, MMP9, and MMP13, but it does not prevent MMP1 from cleaving collagen 1.

   Cartilage oligomeric matrix protein binds strongly to collagen-1 and collagen-12 on the surface of collagen-1 fibrils. In fact, it binds to the fibril-forming collagens Col1 and Col2, the nonfibrillar fibril-associated collagens with interrupted triple helices (FACIT) collagens (Col9, Col12, and Col14), as well as other matrix proteins like fibronectin and matrilins, and proteoglycans. It also promotes collagen secretion. As a result, in the extracellular matrix, COMP aids in the formation of a collagen fibril meshwork that produces organ rheology, whereas within the cell, COMP facilitates the efficient secretion of collagens into the extracellular space.

This fibrillar collagen assembly regulator is involved in fibrosis in several organs and can thus be used as a fibrosis marker. Cartilage oligomeric matrix protein is synthesized in fibrotic regions and colocalizes with vimentin around SMAD3+ cells. TGFβ1 stimulates fibroblasts, leading to increased COMP production.

NADPH oxidases produce ROS, which regulate cell differentiation. The NOx4 isozyme has been linked to cardiac and pulmonary myofibroblast differentiation. In idiopathic pulmonary fibrosis, fibrogenic lung fibroblasts with high concentrations of the hyaluronan receptor epican variant containing exon 6 (CD44v6) increase NOx4 expression, promoting TGFβ1-induced fibroblast differentiation into myofibroblasts. The synthesis of hyaluronan and epican is increased in many fibrotic organs. The TGFβ1-CD44v6 pathway promotes collagen-1 and Actα synthesis in pulmonary myofibroblasts. It promotes the formation of the early growth response (EGR1). TGFβ1 activates EGR1 and AP1 to produce CD44v6. The ERK-EGR1 axis facilitates CD44v6 splicing. Conversely, CD44v6 maintains ERK signaling, which promotes AP1 activity in pulmonary fibroblasts. The hyaluronan synthase HAS2 is necessary for the colocalization of CD44v6 and Tβ R1. This leads to TGFβ1-CD44v6-ERK1-EGR1 signaling, forming a positive feedback loop that connects TGFβ1 to the myofibroblast phenotype.

TGFβ1, a major profibrotic factor, promotes IL11 synthesis, which acts as a profibrotic effector. Activated fibroblasts produce interleukin-11, which causes cardiac fibrosis. Fibroblasts show the highest expression of the receptor IL11Rα. In these cells, the IL11-IL11Rα couple initiates alternative ERK-dependent autocrine signaling for fibrogenic protein synthesis. Fibroblasts from patients with idiopathic pulmonary fibrosis also produce IL11 at a 100-fold higher level.

Following an acute myocardial injury, cardiofibroblasts release proinflammatory cytokines, causing them to proliferate (feedforward loop) and differentiate into myofibroblasts, which secrete a large amount of proinflammatory and fibrotic agents, as well as matrix components. Adaptive collagen-based fibrotic scarring preserves myocardial structure, but prolonged cardiofibroblast activation results in fibrosis.

Fibroblasts extend their filopodia into the T-tubular lumen. Collagen-6, also known as Col6α1-Col6α2-Col6α3, tetramerizes and forms microfibrils after secretion. Collagen colocalizes with the dystrophin complex in T-tubules, which connects the extracellular matrix to the cytoskeleton's actin microfilaments and microtubules, transmitting stress and strain between the two. Dystrophin localises to the T-tubule periphery and acts as a mechanosensor at the Z disc. Fibrillar Col1 and Col3 deposition stiffens T-tubule membranes, whereas nonfibrillar Col4 and Col6 may anchor fibrillar collagens to the CMC basement membrane.

The endothelium-controlled paracrine couple composed of neuregulin-1 and the receptor protein Tyr kinase human epidermal growth factor receptor (HER) influences cardiac function and adaptation. Neuregulin-1 targets cardiofibroblasts and has an antifibrotic effect in the left ventricle. It reduces myocardial hypertrophy and fibrosis in a mouse model of angiotensin-2-induced myocardial remodeling, as well as pulmonary fibrosis. Furthermore, the Nrg1-HER axis regulates macrophage function. Neuregulin-1 at least partially inhibits macrophages, reduces myocardial macrophage infiltration and cytokine expression, and improves ventricular stiffness. In contrast, mice with myeloid cell-specific deletion of the Her4 gene develop increased myocardial fibrosis in response to Agt2. Neuregulin-1 activates HER4 on macrophages and inhibits the PI3K-PKB pathway as well as STAT3, reducing inflammatory cytokine release.

Myofibroblasts, which are formed by the differentiation of fibroblasts, fibrocytes, and epitheliocytes, are the primary cause of fibrosis. TGFβ1 promotes a hyaluronan-rich pericellular matrix, known as the hyaluronan coat, which is necessary for myofibroblast formation and maintenance [147].

The heparan sulfate proteoglycan epican (CD44) functions as a receptor for hyaluronan, an extracellular matrix constituent that mediates cell-cell and cell-matrix interactions. It is encoded by the Cd44 gene, which has 19 exons. Other ligands include collagens, osteopontin (also known as secreted phosphoprotein SPP1), the soluble galactoside-binding lectin LGalS9, and matrix metallopeptidases. Hyaluronan has several isoforms due to a variable pattern of N- and O-linked glycosylation and the presence of multiple splice variants. All alternatively spliced Cd44 mRNA species contain exons 1–5, 15–17, and 19, which encode the extracellular N-terminus, transmembrane domain, and cytoplasmic region, respectively. The presence of exons 6–14 varies by isoform. Exon 18 is removed before translation in most isoforms due to an early stop codon. Exons v4 to v6 in splice variants (CD44v4, CD44v5, and CD44v6) in mice promote the migration of Langerhans cells (dendrocytes of the skin and mucosa) to lymph nodes. Exons v3 and v6 in rats play a role in FGF-mediated mesenchymal cell proliferation during limb bud development. The standard epican isoform promotes myofibroblast differentiation, which favors fibrosis. However, its alternatively spliced isoform, which contains variant exons v7–v8, CD44v7v8, inhibits myofibroblast differentiation.

Hyaluronan is degraded by hyaluronoglucosaminidases or hyaluronidases, which are encoded by the HYAL1–HYAL4 genes, with Hyal1 and Hyal2 being the most abundant species. Hyaluronidase-2 promotes CD44v7/8 production. Hyaluronidase-2 accumulates in lysosomes, where the acidic environment promotes Hyal activity. However, Hyal2 is a plasma membrane-anchored protein with low enzymatic activity. Hyaluronidase-2 may be enzymatically inactive. It has a non-enzymatic function in regulating epican splicing, which promotes CD44v7v8 production.

When pulmonary fibroblasts are stimulated by BMP7, which prevents or reverses differentiation of cells into myofibroblasts, Hyal2 translocates to the nucleus, where it displaces components of the splicing machinery from the spliceosome, enabling Hyal2, the spliceosomal components U1 and U2 small nuclear ribonucleoproteins, and Cd44 pre-mRNA to complex, whereas arginine- and serine-rich (RS) proteins, which mediate exon exclusion, promote profibrotic st Cd44 pre-mRNA splicing in fibrosis is regulated by SRSF2 and SRSF5, as well as splicing regulators, argonaute-mediated histone modifications, KHDRBS1, and RS-rich splicing factor SFRS10. Hyal2 aids in the inclusion of Cd44 exons 11 and 12, which promote the expression of the antifibrotic CD44v7v8 isoform on the cell surface.

3.2.1. Cardiomyocyte Remodeling

Markers of cardiac remodeling have either an increased expression, such as α-myosin heavy chain isoform (MyH6), GluT1, α-actin (ActC1), natriuretic peptide, galectin, caveolin, nitric oxide synthase (NOS1), angiotensin convertase or decreased production, such as β-MHC (MyH7), GluT4, and serca2a.

3.2.1.1. Energy Metabolism

Cardiac energetics are impaired due to mitochondrial dysfunction and calcium handling, which disrupts myocardial contractility.

Because of contraction-relaxation cycles, the heart produces and turnovers ATP at a rapid pace. Under normoxia, more than 95% of ATP generated in the heart is created by oxidative phosphorylation in mitochondria and the remaining mainly from glycolysis and, to a lesser extent, from the tricarboxylic acid cycle (TCAC; also named citric acid and Krebs cycle). Fatty acid oxidation produces approximately 70–90% of cardiac ATP, with the remainder coming from glucose and lactate oxidation, as well as small amounts from ketone bodies and certain types of amino acids. Sarcomeres use roughly two-thirds of the ATP generated, while ion pumps like endoplasmic reticulum Ca^{2+} ATPase (SERCA) regulate lusitropy.

Substrates are transported from the plasma membrane to the cytosol, where they are metabolized. In oxidative pathways, specific carriers transport metabolic intermediates like pyruvate or acylCoA from glycolysis and β-oxidation across the inner mitochondrial membrane. Anaplerosis occurs within the mitochondrial matrix, where substrates are oxidized or carboxylated and enter the TCAC. This produces reducing equivalents like FADH2 and NADH, which the ETC uses to create a proton gradient for ATP production. The generated energy is either used immediately or stored as phosphocreatine.

Metabolic intermediates act as messengers and regulate multiple pathways beyond ATP production (*see* Table 3.8).

Table 3.8. *Regulators of Metabolic Intermediates**

Metabolic Regulators	Effects
Acylcarnitines	Activate Ca^{2+} channels.
–	Induces insulin resistance.
Acetyl-CoA	Primes cell growth and proliferation, as it promotes histone acetylation.
AMP	Influences metabolism via AMPK.
Ceramides	Activate PP2, PKCζ (insulin inhibition).
–	Trigger mitochondrial and ER stress and apoptosis.
Fatty acids	Activate NR1cs (PPARs).
–	Modulate ion channel activity via palmitoylation.

Hexosamine	Operates via O-GlcNAcylation of regulators.
$NAD(P)^+/NAD(P)H$	Modulate activity of metabolic enzymes.
–	Regulate redox state and sirtuin action.
Pyruvate	Stimulates mitochondrial genesis.
–	Regulates PGC1α expression.
ROS	Determine redox state and enzyme activity.
–	At high levels, induce apoptosis and inflammation.
BCAA	Stimulates protein synthesis.
–	Activates TOR.
–	Inhibits autophagy.

*Source: AMPK, BCAA, CoA, ER, PGC, PKC, PP, ROS, and TOR.

O-GlcNAcylation refers to the O-linked attachment of the monosaccharide βNacetylglucosamine (OGlcNAc).

The myocardial energy pool contains ATP and phosphocreatine (PCr), which functions as an ATP transporter and buffer. Creatine kinase in the mitochondria can transfer the high-energy phosphate bond in ATP to creatine, forming PCr, which can easily diffuse through the mitochondrial membrane into the cytosol, where it can generate ATP from ADP using cytosolic creatine kinase.

Glucose metabolism includes glycolysis and accessory pathways such as glycogen synthesis, pentose phosphate (PPP), and the hexosamine synthetic pathway (HSP). The PPP, which is dependent on glucose 6-phosphate dehydrogenase (G6PDH), is a NADPH source used in lipid synthesis and anaplerosis (i.e., replenishment of the TCAC intermediate pool through pathways other than acetylCoA, as these intermediates are constantly removed from the TCAC for amino and nucleic acid synthesis and must be replaced), as well as redox stress. The hexosamine synthetic pathway (HSP) requires glucose, acetylCoA, and glutamine to produce UDPNacetylglucosamine (GlcNAc), a monosaccharide for protein O-GlcNAcylation. These additional pathways have the potential to play a larger role in the development of CVD.

Fatty acid oxidation is impaired in cardiac hypertrophy and failure, resulting in reduced ATP production. Glucose oxidation can remain constant in compensated hypertrophy while decreasing in heart failure. Non-ATP-producing glucose metabolism pathways (HSP, PPP, and anaplerosis) are stimulated. Metabolic remodeling in HF is characterized by decreased energy production, which is linked to progressive impairment of substrate use, mitochondrial genesis, and function.

3.2.1.2. Ion Carriers

Cardiomyocytic T tubules help to regulate ion fluxes. Bridging integrator BIn1 (also known as amphiphysin Amph2) is a T-tubule protein found in the inner membrane folds that regulates calcium motion. The cardiac-specific splice variant BIn1v13v17 (which contains exons 3 and 17) promotes actin polymerization. It then generates and stabilizes dense T-tubule membrane folds, forming a diffusion barrier for extracellular ions. Its expression is downregulated in heart failure. Cardiofibroblasts affect myocardial function through chemical, electrical, and mechanical interactions with CMCs. Several ion channels (e.g., CaV1, CaV3, BK, SOCE, TRPA1, TRPC1, TRPC6,

TRPM7, NaV1.5, KV4.3, KIR2.1, and volume-sensitive and Ca^{2+}-gated Cl^- channel) influence their fate and activity. They help myofibroblasts differentiate.

Defective ion handling by Ca^{2+}, K^+, and Na^+ channels, pumps, and transporters, along with connexins and nonselective channels, leads to cardiac arrhythmias.

3.2.1.3. Defective Calcium Handling

The endoplasmic reticulum's membrane contains a ryanodine-sensitive Ca^{2+} channel and SERCA pump, which allow for Ca^{2+} release and reuptake. Ca^{2+} binds to troponin-C, allowing for actin-myosin interaction.

The homotetrameric ryanodine receptor at endoplasmic reticulum-transverse tubule junctions plays a crucial role in excitation-contraction coupling via Ca^{2+}-induced Ca^{2+} release (CICR). It is regulated by FKBP1b, a member of the immunophilin family of cis-trans peptidyl-prolyl isomerases, cAMP-dependent protein kinase PKA and its anchoring protein, AKAP6, and protein phosphatases PP1 and PP2. Muscle-selective AKAP6 coordinates a cAMP-sensitive negative feedback loop that includes PKA and the cAMP-selective phosphodiesterase (PDE4D3), with PKA phosphorylating PDE4D3 and increasing its affinity for AKAP6, resulting in increased recruitment of PDE4D3 and faster signal termination.

At the end of systole, RyRs are inactivated and Ca^{2+} is pumped back into the ER by serca2a, regulated by phospholamban, and out of the cell by sarcolemmal NCX, which regulates lusitropy.

Stimulation of β-adrenoceptors increases inotropy. PKA and CamK2 phosphorylate (activate) calcium flux regulators, both of which target CaV1.2 and RyR, as well as phospholamban, which facilitates the process. Failing ventriculomyocytes have reduced contractility. Ca^{2+} transient amplitude reduces, excitation-contraction coupling decreases, and diastolic Ca^{2+} transient decay slows. SR Ca^{2+} levels decrease, serca2a activity decreases, and NCX increases, leading to Ca^{2+} extrusion. Neurohormonal stimulation causes RyR hyperphosphorylation by PKA, and RyR dephosphorylation decays due to defective PP1 and PP2 association and the presence of PDE4d3 in the RyR complex. Increased RyR2 phosphorylation (Ser2808) causes it to dissociate from its regulator FKBP1b, leading to increased Ca^{2+} sensitivity and reduced RyR closing, resulting in diastolic ER Ca^{2+} leak.

Serca2a is inhibited when phospholamban is dephosphorylated by PP1; this inhibition is relieved when PKA (Ser16) and CamK2 (Thr17) phosphorylate it. Heart failure alters the expression of both serca2a and Pln. Furthermore, Pln phosphorylation is reduced, inhibiting serca2a activity.

3.2.1.4. Altered Sodium Control

Heart failure causes increased intracellular Na^+ concentration due to late Na^+ influx and inactivation of some NaV1.5 channels.

Cardiac sodium-hydrogen exchanger SLC9a1 (NHE1) regulates intracellular H+ and Na^+ concentrations by exchanging intracellular H+ for extracellular Na^+. The Na^+–K^+ ATPase's inward gradient drives SLC9a1-mediated H+ extrusion and Na^+ influx. Its activity rises with exposure to ROS, intracellular acidosis, angiotensin-2, endothelin, and α1-adrenoceptor. Increased SLC9a1 activity causes Ca^{2+} overload via the Na^+–Ca^{2+} exchanger.

The Na^+–K^+ ATPase39 transports Na^+ out and K^+ in the CMC. Phospholemman regulates this enzyme's activity. The receptor for cardiac glycosides, such as digoxin and ouabain, has a positive inotropic effect by inhibiting pump activity. This reduces the driving force for Na^+–

Ca^{2+} exchange and increases cellular content and Ca^{2+} release during depolarization.

3.2.1.5. Impaired Potassium Control

Early repolarization relies on the transient outward current (i K, to) through KV4.2 and KV4.3 channels. It decays in heart failure, extending the duration of the action potential.

The mitochondrial KATP channel (KIR6.2) acts as a metabolic sensor, adjusting membrane excitability to meet cellular energy demands. It opens in response to ischemia, physical activity, and stress hormone exposure, reducing the action potential. It can protect the heart from hypertension.

3.2.1.6. Transverse Tubules

In heart failure, abnormal reorganisation of transverse tubules (T-tubules), such as dilation of the lumen and the formation of sheet-like structures, can disrupt Ca^{2+} signaling. Ventriculomyocytes use deep plasma membrane invaginations at Z-line levels to synchronise Ca^{2+} release from the endoplasmic reticulum, leading to contraction. Disrupted Ca^{2+} release reduces contractility in heart failure. Enlarging the T-tubular lumen increases the diffusion space of extracellular ions, specifically Ca^{2+} and K^{+}, which promotes arrhythmia. In addition, losing the T-tubular anchor junctophilin-2 reduces T-tubule density. Furthermore, several collagen isoforms (Col1, Col3-Col4, and Col6) play a role in T-tubule expansion, despite the fact that small amounts of collagen are normally found within T-tubules.

3.2.1.7. Mitochondrion

FunDC1, a FUN14 domain-containing protein found in the outer mitochondrial membrane, induces mitophagy in response to hypoxia. It interacts with the kinesin light chain KLC1 (but not with the motor subunit of kinesin-1 KIF5b or kinesin-2 KIF3a). FunDC1 binds to IP3R2 and localises to mitochondrion-associated endoplasmic reticulum membranes. This promotes communication between mitochondria and the endoplasmic reticulum, modulates Ca^{2+} release, and maintains mitochondrial morphology and function. Overexpression of FunDC1 boosts mitochondrial IP3R2 and Ca^{2+} concentrations. Ablation of the FUNDC1 gene reduces intracellular Ca^{2+} concentration and suppresses the formation of mitochondrial fission protein Fis1. This inhibits CREB binding to the Fis1 promoter, resulting in mitochondrial fission. The FunDC1-CREB-Fis1 axis is inhibited in heart failure patients.

3.2.2. Altered Signaling

Under normal conditions, CMCs and endotheliocytes interact and regulate each other's metabolism. The proper functioning of the cardiovascular system is dependent, at least in part, on interactions between CMCs and endotheliocytes of the cardiac capillaries and endocardium, with dysregulated communication between these two cell types implicated in the development of cardiac structural and functional anomalies, as well as disrupted endothelium-related signaling based on NO and neuregulin in heart failure.

Factor	Signaling	Effect
Apelin	AplnR	Positive inotropy.
–	–	Antihypertrophic.
CTGF	Integrin	Prohypertrophic.
Dkk3	Wnt axis	Antihypertrophic and -fibrotic.
ET1	$ET_{A(B)}$	Positive inotropy and lusitropy.
–	–	Prohypertrophic and -fibrotic.
Fst, FstL	TGFβ axis	Antiapoptotic (FstL1).
–	–	Antihypertrophic (FstL1/3).

MiR146a	Prolactin axis	Induces peripartum cardiomyopathy.
NO	sGC–cGMP	Dose-dependent inotropic effect.
–	–	Positive lusitropy.
–	–	Attenuates cardiac remodeling.
Nrg1	HER4	Reduces contractility.
–	–	Attenuates heart failure progression.
Periostin	Integrin	Profibrotic.
PGi_2	PtgIR	Positive or negative inotropy.
–	–	Antihypertrophic.
Tsp1/2/4	Adhesion molecule	Stretch-mediated contractility (Tsp4).
–	–	Antihypertrophic and -fibrotic.

Endothelial cardioactive factors include angiopoietins, angiotensin-2, apelin, dickkopf-3, endothelin-1, follistatin, neuregulin-1, NO, periostin, prostaglandins like prostacyclin and thrombospondin-1, connective tissue, fibroblast, vascular endothelial growth factor, and endothelial microRNAs (Table 3.9). They can act quickly or over time, and they can work together.

NO and natriuretic peptides initiate the synthesis of cyclic guanosine monophosphate via different effectors, sGC and particulate guanylate cyclase (pGC), and spatially distinct pools, sGC and pGC, which reside in the cytosol and cortex, resulting in different responses. Among the phosphodiesterases that hydrolyze cGMP, PDE2 limits the subsarcolemmal cGMP pool and PDE5 the cytosolic cGMP pool. CGMP produced by pGC and sGC has a positive lusitropic effect, while cGMP produced by sGC blunts the myocardial response to β-adrenoceptor.

At low NO concentrations, the NO-sGC-cGMP axis activates PKG and PKA, increasing Ca^{2+} concentration. Increased NO levels cause a negative inotropic effect by blocking sarcolemmal Ca^{2+} channels and reducing troponin-C sensitivity to Ca^{2+} ions. Additionally, NO has a positive lusitropic effect. Phosphorylation of troponin-I reduces sarcomeric Ca^{2+} sensitivity and promotes cross-bridge detachment. The phosphorylation of titin by PKA and/or PKG improves lusitropy. Furthermore, NO causes vasodilation, thereby reducing afterload.

NO's chronotropic effect is site-dependent, with a positive effect upon cGMP stimulation of a hyperpolarization-activated pacemaker current and a negative effect at the postsynaptic level.

Table 3.9. *Features of Nitric Oxide Synthase (NOS) Isozymes*

Isozyme	NOS1	NOS2	NOS3
Typical site synthesis	Neuron	Macrophage	Endotheliocyte
Other major sites of production	Smooth muscle	Smooth muscle	Smooth muscle
–	Skeletal muscle	Liver	Cardiomyocyte
–	Cardiomyocyte	–	Platelet
NO production magnitude	Moderate	High	Low
–	(n–μ mol/L)	(μ mol/L)	(p–nmol/L)
Function	Neurotransmission	Immunity	Vasodilation
–	Inotropy –	–	Vascular homeostasis
–	Lusitropy +	–	Cardioprotection

NO is produced by NOSs, with NOS1 and NOS3 binding cofactors (FAD, FMN, and BH4), dimerizing, and being stimulated by Ca^{2+}-calmodulin (Table 3.10). NOS3 must also be properly localized to caveolae via HSP90 and caveolin, as well as phosphorylated. In addition to constitutive NOS1 and NOS3, and inducible NOS2, constitutively active MtNOS localises to the inner mitochondrial membrane and modulates the transmembrane potential.

NO mediates parasympathetic endothelial-dependent vasodilation in the vasculature, as well as parasympathetic control of cardiac function, with guanylate cyclase supporting muscarinic agonists on cardiac frequency, atrioventricular conduction, and myocardial contractility.

Endotheliocytes secrete NO, which relaxes vascular smooth myocytes and prevents platelet aggregation, leukocyte-endotheliocyte adhesion, and vascular smooth myocyte proliferation. It also influences CMC contractility via β-adrenergic and muscarinic acetylcholine receptors and controls cardiac substrate utilization. Endotheliocytes have higher NOS3 concentrations than CMCs (40).

Isolated cardiac tissue preparations from Nos3-/- mice show preserved chronotropic and inotropic responses to β-adrenergic and muscarinic agonists, as well as β-adrenergic stimulation and muscarinic inhibition of CaV1.2a current. However, NO produced in CMCs reduces the inotropic and lusitropic responses to stimulation, in addition to basal conditions. NOS3 binds to caveolin-3 at the plasma membrane and interacts with CaV1.2a and β AR, reducing the inotropic response to isoproterenol stimulation. In contrast, NO produced by NOS1 at the CMC endoplasmic reticulum nitrosylates (activates) the ryanodine receptor. Furthermore, NOS1 and NOS1-activating protein (NOS1AP) work together to regulate cardiac frequency.

Young Nos3-/- and Nos3+/+ mice have identical cardiac contractibility. Older Nos3-/- mice have a lower inotropic response to isoproterenol than Nos3+/+ mice of the same age. In contrast, Nos1-/- mice's CMCs contract more and relax slower. Constitutive NOS3 in murine ventriculomyocytes does not significantly affect muscarinic-mediated inhibition of β-adrenergic signaling, nor does it control basal or β-adrenoceptor-stimulated CMC contraction. The myocardial constitutive NOS1 isozyme regulates myocardial inotropy and lusitropy via NO-mediated autocrine regulation.

In addition, NO helps to regulate the metabolism. It inhibits ETC complexes I, II, and IV of the mitochondrial electron transport chain. Acute inhibition of NOS has a reversible effect on cardiac substrate utilization. Cardiac lactate and glucose uptake increases, while free fatty acid uptake decreases, due to a shift to carbohydrate oxidation, with acute NO donor administration cancelling cardiac metabolic changes. As a result, NO inhibits glucose uptake and promotes free fatty acid consumption.

Neuregulin-1, an EGF superfamily member, regulates cardiac adaptation to stress during foetal and postnatal development (41). Endocardial and microvascular endothelial cells release Nrg1. It binds to the receptor protein Tyr kinases HER3 and HER4 receptors, which are found in ventriculomyocytes, with HER4 being the most important in the heart. Nrg1 activates ERK1 and ERK2 (sarcomeric organisation and protein synthesis), the Src-FAK couple (focal adhesion formation), NOS (cardiac function), and the PI3K-PKB axis (CMC survival), which reduces adrenergic stimulation and thus its positive inotropic effect while increasing lusitropy. The Nrg1-HER couple also has an effect on myocardial metabolism, stimulating glucose uptake via PI3K by CMCs and causing Nrg resistance through excess saturated fatty acid exposure.

Hyperglycemia activates notch activation, causing ECs to secrete both inactive latent and lysosomal-stored active forms of heparanase using ATP. These forms liberate VEGFa and VEGFb bound to heparan sulfate proteoglycans (HSPG) of the CMC surface, which serve as a quick auxiliary reservoir for fatty acid transfer by FABP442 and FATPs43. On the other hand, the hexosamine synthesis pathway inhibits angiogenesis. Heparanase also interacts with LPL (lipase-D).

CMCs produce the majority of LPL, which matures with the lipase maturation factor LMF1 and is then secreted by AMPK and P38MAPK, which phosphorylates HSP25. LPL attaches to syndecan-1 at the CMC surface before being detached by heparinase and transported to the luminal endothelial surface. There, it tethers to HSPGs and GPIHBP1, and metabolises the triglyceride core of lipoproteins to FAs, which are then transferred to CMCs.

FoxO activity increases as insulinemia decreases. Increased cardiomyocytic FoxO1 activity increases plasmalemmal ScaRb3 concentration by rearranging the actin cytoskeleton. Endothelial FoxO1 also limits vascular expansion.

Chronic heart failure leads to altered β-adrenoceptor signaling and reduced cAMP formation. Long-term sympathetic stimulation decreases β-adrenoceptor sensitivity, decreases β1AR expression, and increases inhibitory G-protein-coupled receptor kinase (GRK) activity. End-stage heart failure (ESHF) leads to a 30% increase in Gi subunit expression, which inhibits adenylate cyclase via β2AR rather than stimulating it with Gs.

Reduced ventriculomyocytic cAMP concentration and PKA activity, combined with increased phosphatase activity, reduce phosphorylation of key cardiac Ca^{2+}-handling proteins, resulting in decreased Ca^{2+} transient amplitude and CMC contraction efficiency (negative inotropic effect).

Among GRKs, GRK5 is abundant in the myocardium, and its synthesis increases in heart failure. This regulator of cardiac GPCRs exhibits alternative activity in the nucleus following stress, particularly during adverse hypertrophy. IGF1, a regulator of adaptive cardiac hypertrophy, does not cause GRK5 nuclear translocation in CMCs.

Nucleoside diphosphate kinases (NDPKs) are found at the plasma membrane of CMCs in ESHF patients. Group-I NDPKs (NDPKa-NDPKd) contain enzymes. NDPKb, but not NDPKa, interacts with the Gβγ dimer and activates cardiac G proteins independently of

GPCRs. NDPKc can form heterohexamers with NDPKa and NDPKb. Among isozymes, synthesis of NDPKc, which allows for the formation of the NDPKb-NDPKc complex and interaction between NDPK isozymes and G proteins, is upregulated in ESHF patients and rats following long-term stimulation with isoprenaline, which causes NDPKc to translocate to the plasma membrane. Overexpression of NDPKc in CMCs increases cAMP concentration and makes them more sensitive to isoprenaline, which improves contractility. In mice lacking NDPKB, NDPKc production is normal, but prolonged isoprenaline exposure leads to contractile dysfunction and negative cardiac remodeling. In ESHF patients, the amount of the NDPKb-NDPKc complex increases while the NDPKc-Gs interaction decreases, shifting G-protein activation from Gs to Gi2 and contributing to a decrease in cAMP levels. Moderate changes in the Gs/Gi ratio can help identify the G-protein subunit subtypes that bind to NDPKc.

Injuries and stressors can reactivate foetal signaling pathways, including the Wnt-β Ctnn signaling cascade, leading to transcription of genes linked to cardiac fibrosis, a major cause of heart failure.

Connexin-43 location and function are controlled by the plasmalemmal receptor CDO, which is primarily found in intercalated discs (45–46). CDO inhibits Wnt signaling by interacting with the LRP6 coreceptor, preventing abnormal myocardial structure and action potential propagation. Abnormal Wnt signaling is linked to increased Cx43 expression and mislocalization to the CMC's lateral sides.

3.2.3. Interrelationship Between the Heart and Kidney

The cardiovascular system and kidney are inextricably linked in both normal and pathological conditions. The interactions between blood circulation and the kidney are essential for maintaining vasomotor tone and blood volume.

Chronic kidney disease (CKD) frequently accelerates the progression of CVD, whereas cardiac dysfunction causes renal dysfunction, a common complication of CVD.

Renal dysfunction is an independent, significant cardiovascular risk factor. CVD is twice as common in the elderly (age≥66 yr) with CKD (~70%) as in non-CKD patients (~35%), and is linked to a low survival rate.

Acute or chronic dysfunction is bidirectional in nature, with each dysfunctional organ (heart and kidney) causing disease in the other organ. This interaction causes cardiorenal syndrome (CRS), characterized by endothelial and vSMC dysfunction, as well as resistance to natriuretic peptides and diuretics.

Defective renal perfusion and exacerbated vasoconstriction are linked to persistent neurohormonal activation caused by overactivity of arterial baroreceptors and intrarenal sensors, and thus of the sympathetic nervous system, sympathoadrenal and renin-angiotensin-aldosterone axes, adenosine, and vasopressin, dysregulated hydroelectrolytic and calcium-phosphate balance, anemia, inflammation, and redox stress.

Protein-bound uremic toxins (PBUTs), such as indoxyl (IS) and p-cresyl sulfate (pCS), derived from dietary amino acid metabolites by colonic microorganisms, accumulate when renal excretion declines, form large complexes with albumin, and cause renal and cardiovascular damage. These toxins inhibit the proliferation, migration, and senescence of vSMCs and ECs while also causing inflammation, calcification, and oxidative stress.

Calcific uremic arteriolopathy (CUA), also known as calcific obliterative arteriolopathy and calciphylaxis, is typically observed in CKD patients, especially women of Caucasian ethnicity and individuals at end-stage renal disease. Risk factors include malnutrition, insulin resistance, obesity, diabetes mellitus, alcoholic steatohepatitis, secondary hyperparathyroidism (elevated parathyroid hormone concentration), protein-C and/or -S deficiency, and elevated activity.

The uremic environment can lead to metabolic toxicity, redox stress from high ROS levels, inflammation from NFκB and the TNFSF11-TNFRSF11a axis activation, and vasoconstriction from increased endothelin-1 activity.

Arteriolopathy is characterized by endothelial dysfunction, a prothrombotic state, intimal hyperplasia, fibrosis, and vascular smooth myocyte apoptosis and differentiation into osteoblast-like cells, which cause medial calcification.

3.2.4. Ectopic Calcification

Soft-tissue calcification is caused by a combination of tissue injury, exposure to sensitising factors like parathyroid hormone and vitamin D, and a calcium and phosphorus-rich diet. The condition occurs when hypercalcemia, hyperphosphatemia, and hyperparathyroidism are present, while calcification inhibitors like MGP and fetuin-A lose their effectiveness. Hyperglycemia, hyperhomocysteinemia, hyperbeta2microglobulinemia, elevated levels of oxidized low-density lipoprotein cholesterol (LDLCS), and low levels of high-density lipoprotein cholesterol (HDLCS) can increase ROS formation and contribute to vascular calcification.

Calcific aortic valve disease (CAVD) is the leading cause of surgical or transcutaneous valve therapy worldwide. It ranges from mild focal valve thickening without blood flow obstruction (aortic sclerosis), thickening of the valve leaflets, and formation of calcium nodules to end-stage calcification with impaired leaflet motion (aortic stenosis).

Mutations in the genes that encode notch, LDLR, and LPA, an OxPL carrier, have been linked to an increased risk of calcification.

Oxidised phospholipids contribute to the progression of CAVD. ApoB100OxPL and apolipoproteinA (also known as lipoprotein-A) transport these proteins. An increased LPa concentration increases the risk of CoAD. The LPA gene-linked 6q26-27 locus has two heritable variants (rs10455872 and rs3798220) that are strongly linked to higher Lpa concentration. ApoB100OxPL and ApoOxPLA are both associated with CAVD risk.

3.3. Autoimmune Disorders

Giant cell arteritis (GCA), also known as granulomatous arteritis, is a type of autoimmune vasculitis that primarily affects the temporal arteries. GCA can be caused by altered genes, including those encoding classes-I and -II human leukocyte antigens on chromosome 6, as well as PTPN22, NLRP1, IL17A, IL33, and LRRC32. Familial GCA cases are also present.

In GCA, CD4+ effector helper T cells (TH1 and TH17) invade large arterial walls. Adventitial microvascular endotheliocytes regulate the entry of inflammatory leukocytes into the media and intima. In GCA patients, CD4+ T cells activate through the notch-TORC1 pathway and differentiate into vasculitogenic TH1 and TH17 cells.

Because of increased circulating VEGF levels, expression of the notch ligand jagged-1 is upregulated in GCA patients' endotheliocytes. T lymphocytes expressing notch-1 receive abnormal activating signals from jagged-1+ adventitial endotheliocytes.

Vessel walls are involved in inflammatory (autoimmune) disorders like systemic rheumatoid arthritis, disseminated lupus erythematosus, and scleroderma.

Systemic rheumatoid vasculitis causes autoimmune inflammation of small and medium-sized vessels, leading to joint inflammation.

Systemic lupus erythematosus is a connective tissue autoimmune disease that affects the skin, joints, brain, kidney, and lung, with vasculopathy being a common feature.

Scleroderma, also known as systemic sclerosis, is a connective tissue autoimmune disease that causes fibrosis and vasculopathy across multiple organs. Many clinical complications result from dysfunctional microvascular beds, which cause tissue ischemia, as well as medium-sized vessels that can cause endothelial dysfunction and pulmonary arterial hypertension, among other symptoms. Raynaud's syndrome is a type of limited systemic sclerosis.

Raynaud's syndrome is defined as a transient cessation of blood flow in the fingers and toes caused by a vasospasm of the digital arteries in the hands and feet. It can be activated by either cold or emotion. This vasculopathy is associated with myofibroblast proliferation and matrix deposition in the subendothelial layer, which results in obliterative thickening of the vessel walls as well as mononuclear infiltrates. It is characterized by cyanosis and pain caused by sensory nerve ischemia, and it is more common in women. Abnormal vascular reactivity is caused by the hyperactive adrenergic nervous system, α2-adrenoceptors, central stress response, serotonin, endothelin, depressed vasodilatory response to NO, prostaglandin-G/H synthase (cyclooxygenase), the cGMP-PKG signaling cascade, and redox stress.

3.4. Congenital Vascular Malformations

Vascular malformations are localized defects in vascular development that typically affect a small number of vessels in a specific area of the body. The majority of malformations, which appear at birth and grow proportionately with age throughout childhood, are caused by gene mutations. Inherited new lesions can appear, but they are usually small. They are either sporadic with a single lesion or have multifocality in familial forms. Familial vascular malformations have a paradominant inheritance. Somatic mutations in the same genes result in sporadic forms. Table 3.10 lists the major mediators responsible for blood and lymph vessel anomalies and their pathways.

Table 3.10. *Chromosomal Loci and Genes Involved in Vascular Malformations**

Malformation	Locus	Locus Name	Mutated Gene (Protein)
ACDMPV	16q24.1	–	FOXF1 (FoxF1)
AT	11q23	AT1	ATM (ATMK)
BRBNS	–	–	TEK (Tie2)
CCM1	7q21.2	CCM1	KR1T1 (Kr1T1)
CCM2	7p13	CCM2	CCM2 (malcavernin)
CCM3	3q26.1	CCM3	PDCD10 (PdCD10)
CCM4	3q26.3–27.2	CCM4	
CMAVM	5q13.22	CMC1	RASA1
CMVM	9p21	VMCM1	TEK (Tie2)
GVM	1p21.22	VMGLOM	GLMN (glomulin)

*Part 1; Sources: ACDMPV alveolar capillary dysplasia with misalignment of pulmonary veins, AT ataxia–telangiectasia [Louis–Bar syndrome], BRBNS blue rubber bleb nevus syndrome, CCM cerebral cavernous (or capillary) malformation, CMAVM capillary malformation–arteriovenous malformation, CMVM cutaneomucosal venous malformation, GVM glomuvenous malformation, ATMK ataxia telangiectasia mutated kinase, FoxF1 [or ACDMPV] forkhead box-containing transcription factor-F1, KrIT1 ankyrin repeat-containing Krev [Kirsten sarcoma virus Ras-revertant] interaction trapped protein-1 [angiogenesis inhibitor that binds Rap1 (or Krev1)], PdCD10 programmed cell death protein-10 [CCM3 protein], RasA1 [or CMAVM] Ras GTPase-activating protein [RasGAP], TIE protein Tyr kinase with Ig and EGF homology domains [angiopoietin receptor].

Table 3.11. *Chromosomal Loci and Genes Involved in Vascular Malformations**

Malformation	Locus	Locus Name	Mutated Gene (Protein)
HCD	–	–	Idh1/2 (IDH1/2)
HHT1	9q33.34	HHT1	ENG (endoglin)
HHT2	12q11.14	HHT2	Alk1 (ALK1)
HHT3	5q31	HHT3	
HHT4	7p14	HHT4	
JHHT	18q21.1	JPHT	Smad4 (SMAD4)
HLTS	20q13.33	HLT	SOX18 (Sox18)
KTWS	3q26.32	–	PIK3CA ($PI3K_{c1\alpha}$)
LCS	15q	LCSI	
LDS	16q24.3	LD	FOXC2 (FoxC2)
OLEDAID	Xq28	IP2	IKBKG (Iκ BKγ)
PCL	5q35.3	PCLI	FLT4 (VEGFR3)
PHTS	10q23	PHTS	PTEN (PTen)
PPCM	Xp11.3–Xq12		

*Part 2; Sources: [HCD hemangiomatosis chondrodystrophica, HHT hereditary hemorrhagic telangiectasia, HLTS hypotrichosis–lymphedema–telangiectasia syndrome, JHHT juvenile polyposis–HHT syndrome, KTWS Klippel–Trenaunay–Weber syndrome, LCS lymphedema–cholestasis syndrome [Aagenaes syndrome], LDS lymphedema–distichiasis syndrome, OLEDAID osteoporosis, lymphedema, and anhydrotic ectodermal dysplasia with immunodeficiency, PCL primary congenital lymphedema [Milroy disease], PHTS PTEN hamartoma tumor syndrome, PPCM progressive patchy capillary malformation [angioma serpiginosum], ALK1 activin-A type-I receptor-like kinase-1 [AcvRL1], IDH1 soluble cytosolic $NADP^+$-dependent isocitrate dehydrogenase-1, IDH2 mitochondrial $NADP^+$-dependent isocitrate dehydrogenase-2, Iκ BKγ [IKKγ] inhibitor of NFκB kinase subunit-γ, PI3K phosphatidylinositol 3-kinase, PTen phosphatase and tensin homolog deleted on chromosome 10 [phosphatidylinositol 3-phosphatase], SMAD son of mothers against decapentaplegia homolog, Sox sex-determining region Y [SRY]-related high mobility group [HMG] homeobox-derived [DNA-binding domain]-containing transcription factor.

Table 3.12. *Examples of Mediators and Pathways Involved in Congenital Vascular Anomalies*

Cell Type	Pathway (Effect)
BEC	AngPt1/2–TIE2–PI3K–PKB (cell survival)
–	BMP9–ALK1/BMPR2/AcvR2–SMAD–ID1/ID3–EFNB2–EfnB2
–	BMP9–ALK1/BMPR2/AcvR2–HRT1–Vegfr2–VEGFR2
LEC	FoxC2⊖→PDGFb
–	VEGFc–VEGFR3–Sox18–vcam1
vSMC	HGFR–glomulin⊖→FKBP1⊖→Tβ R
–	PDGFb–PDGFRβ (migration)
–	TGFβ–Tβ R–SMADs

Source: BEC blood endotheliocyte, LEC lymph endotheliocyte, vSMC vascular smooth myocyte.

3.4.1. Classification of Congenital Vascular Malformations

Mulliken classifies congenital vascular malformations (CVMs) as high- or low-flow lesions. The Hamburg classification categorises vascular malformations based on their predominant histological components (lymphatic, arterial, and/or venous). Arterial and venous CVMs consist entirely of arteries and veins, respectively. Arterial defect is defined as the absence of an arterial segment, which results in the irrigated organ being perfused by a collateral artery that does not wither. Venous defects produce thin-walled venous lakes or grape-like clusters of lakes.

Arteriovenous shunts can also cause congenital vascular malformations. AVFs refer to a single pair of vessels, while AVMs are a cluster of vessels. Truncular lesions are caused by disruptions in late embryonic angiogenesis from the normal vasculature, while extratruncular lesions occur during early development without a direct connection to the normal vasculature.

Cerebral (CeAVMs) and peripheral arteriovenous malformations (PAVMs) are congenital, localised defects caused by abnormal embryonic angiogenesis that can affect the arterial, venous, and lymphatic circuits. The majority of AVMs are localised. Multiple AVMs are extremely rare lesions that can result in numerous hemorrhagic episodes. Autosomal dominant disorders, such as hereditary hemorrhagic telangiectasia and capillary malformation-arteriovenous malformation syndrome (CMAVM), can cause multifocal AVMs. CMAVM is characterized by small round spots of enlarged capillaries in the dermis, which are most commonly found on the face, arms, and legs.

Capillary malformations may be associated with arteriovenous malformations and fistulas. Type-I CMAVM is caused by mutations in the RASA1 gene, which encodes the RasGAP RasA1. Mutations in the EPHB4 gene, which encodes the receptor protein Tyr kinase ephrin type-B receptor EPHb4, cause Type-II multifocal CMAVM. This receptor is involved in contact-dependent bidirectional signaling between apposed cells. It plays a role in cardiac and angiogenesis, as well as postnatal angiogenesis and vascular remodelling. As a result, AVMs rely heavily on the EPHb4-Ras-ERK pathway.

Ephrin binds to the erythropoietin-producing hepatocyte (EPH) receptors on the adjacent cell's surface, causing EPH aggregation and EPH transphosphorylation (transactivation). Polymerization of the receptor begins with the assembly of monomers into active oligomers (activation phase), which then condensate into large clusters (hundreds of monomers), dampening signaling (inactivation phase), resulting in a fast and transient response. According to the polymerization-condensation model, oligomer coalescence into large aggregates reduces free monomer recruitment by accelerating the formation of large-scale, slowly diffusing clusters, which in turn primes receptor endocytosis and signaling termination.

Arteriovenous malformations are distinguished by lower flow resistance. These shunts connect the high- and low-pressure vascular compartments, bypassing the capillary bed. The resulting arterial steal and venous hypertension are determined by the lesion type and architecture.

Cirsoid AVM, the most common type (>/ 1 cm), has multiple dilated feeding arteries and draining veins with a tortuous shape, resulting in multiple arteriovenous connections. It is next to the collecting circuit.

Angiomatous AVM (size < 1 cm) consists of a single artery feeding multiple distal branches and draining veins.

Aneurysmal AVM has a single feeding artery and draining vein with dilation (diameter > 1 cm), similar to an acquired fistula.

Yakes' AVM classification describes:

- Type I anomalies connect a single artery and vein without a vascular nidus.
- Type II lesions connect arteries to veins directly or indirectly through arterioles and venules, creating a simple network.
- Type III malformations connect multiple arteries to a dilated segment, resulting in one or more veins.
- Type IV anomalies connect arteries and veins through a complex arteriolovenular network.

Coronary arteries can connect to the cardiac chambers (coronary-cameral fistulas) or veins (coronary arteriovenous malformations).

An arteriovenous fistula is an abnormal single direct passage from the artery to a vein. In addition to congenital fistulas, those developed after birth can be caused by infections, degeneration, trauma, or iatrogenic interventions (for example, during angiography, biopsy, bypass grafting, and pacemaker implantation). Secondary hypertension is rarely caused by congenital arteriovenous malformations or acquired AVFs.

3.4.2. Venous Malformations (VMs)

VMs are sporadic, cutaneomucosal (or mucocutaneous), and glomuvenous (GVM). Multiple inherited venous lesions have been identified in venous, glomuvenous, and cerebral cavernous malformations.

Sporadic venous malformations can be bluish or violaceous, solitary or multiple, localised or diffuse, superficial or deep, and typically appear on the head and neck. Venous malformations develop slowly and gradually in the absence of bleeding. Thrombi and calcifications (phleboliths) can form in tortuous veins. Venous nevus, also known as nevus venosus, is a type of venous malformation that occurs sporadically.

Blue rubber bleb nevus (BRBNS), also known as Bean syndrome, is a sporadic syndrome with cutaneous and gastrointestinal VMs of varying sizes and locations. Mutations in the TEK (Tie2) gene can contribute to this condition. Nevi in the intestine can spontaneously bleed, resulting in anemia. Families have autosomal dominant inheritance but also have multifocal venous malformations.

Hemangiomatosis chondrodystrophica, also known as dyschondrodysplasia with hemangiomas, enchondromatosis with multiple cavernous hemangiomas, and Maffucci syndrome, primarily affects bones and skin. It is distinguished by numerous enchondromas (cartilage enlargements), bone deformities, and hemangiomas (tangles of abnormal blood vessels). IDH is caused by mutations in the *IDH1* and *IDH2* genes, which encode NADP+-dependent IDH1 and IDH2, respectively.

Klippel-Trenaunay-Weber syndrome is part of the PIK3CA gene-related overgrowth spectrum (PROS), which also includes megalencephaly, capillary malformation, and polymicrogyria syndrome (MCAP), congenital lipomatous overgrowth, vascular malformations, epidermal nevi, and skeletal/spinal abnormalities (CLOVES) syndrome, hemimegalencephaly, fibroadipose hyperplasia, and epidermal nevus. It affects blood vessel development, resulting in varicose veins and deep vein malformations in the limbs, as well as soft tissue and bone overgrowth. Mutations in the PIK3CA gene, which code for PI3Kc1α, cause this condition.

3.4.2.1. Cutaneomucosal Venous Malformations

Cutaneomucosal venous malformations (in the skin and mucosae) frequently infiltrate the underlying muscles and joints. CMVMs are mostly sporadic (~98% cases), with autosomal dominant inheritance.

Mutations in the TEK gene, which encodes the endothelial-specific receptor protein Tyr kinase TIE2, on chromosomal locus 9p21.22 (e.g., single-nucleotide polymorphisms R849W and Y897S), are to blame. These gain-of-function (GOF) mutations (for example, C2545T in exon 15, A2690G, G2744A, C2752T, G2755T, and G2773T in exon 17, and G3300C in exon 22) increase ligand-independent autophosphorylation of TIE2 without causing endotheliocyte proliferation. TIE2 ligands include angiopoietins AngPt1, AngPt2, and AngPt4 (the latter of which corresponds to mouse AngPt3). AngPt1 exerts a stronger effect than competitive AngPt2, which is thought to be an AngPt1 inhibitor. Once liganded, TIE2 dimerizes and cross-phosphorylates, primarily activating the MAPK module and PI3K pathway, which activates PKB and inhibits apoptosis.

3.4.2.2. Glomuvenous Malformations

Glomuvenous malformations are nodular multifocal lesions on the extremities that involve the skin, subcutis, and, in some cases, the mucosa. They are distinguished by abnormally differentiated vSMCs (glomus cells) in the walls of enlarged veins.

These autosomal dominant disorders are caused by loss-of-function (LOF) mutations in the GLMN gene on chromosomal locus 1p21-22. Glomulin is an essential protein for vasculature development. Glomulin is a ligand for the immunophilins FKBP1a and FKBP4, hence the name FKBP-associated protein. Glomulin synthesis is restricted to vSMCs and plays a role in their differentiation.

TGFβ, which competes with glomulin to bind Tβ R1, is necessary for vSMC differentiation. Glomulin inhibits TGFβ signaling. In contrast, low glomulin levels lead to increased TGFβ activity.

Glomulin also interacts with HGFR; when HGF binds, glomulin is phosphorylated and released, causing S6K phosphorylation and thus influencing protein synthesis.

Glomulin, which interacts with Cul7, can control protein degradation through ubiquitination by the CRL7 complex.

3.4.3. Capillary Malformations

Capillary malformations are cutaneous lesions that most commonly appear in the head and neck. These slow-flowing vascular malformations may include arterioles and postcapillary venules. Except for birthmarks, capillary malformations are gender-neutral. They are usually sporadic, but familial cases can occur.

Megalencephaly capillary malformation syndrome, also known as macrocephaly (megalocephaly) cutis marmorata telangiectatica congenita, is a rare, sporadic congenital capillary malformation characterized by organ overgrowth and cutaneous capillary malformations. These malformations are most commonly unilateral in the lower limbs. Enlarged capillaries increase blood flow near the skin's surface. They can fade away on their own after a few months or years, but they can also last a lifetime. Mutations in the PIK3CA gene, located on chromosome 3q26, cause this disorder.

PTEN hamartoma tumour syndrome (PHTS) is a group of disorders characterized by intramuscular, multifocal hamartomas with ectopic lipid depots. This spectrum includes mutations in the PTEN, SDHB, SDHD, and KLLN genes, which encode PTen, succinate dehydrogenase subunits B and D, and killin, respectively; (2) Bannanyan-Riley-Ruvalcaba syndrome, characterized by macrocephaly and hamartomatous intestinal polyps resulting from mutations in the PTEN gene or partial or complete deletion of this gene; and (3) Proteus and Proteus-like syndrome.

Mutations in the GNAQ gene, which encodes the G protein subunit Gαq, lead to familial multiple nevi flammei. Nevi flammei (nevus flammeus neonatorum) refers to birthmarks. These non-elevated, sharply defined patches fade gradually.

Common birthmarks include salmon patches on the forehead, eyelids, and neck, as well as angel kisses on the back, legs, and arms. Angel kisses are erythematous macules that typically affect the glabella, but can also affect the eyelids, nose, upper lip, and sacral region. Stork bites are erythematous macules that appear on the back of the neck. A port wine stain (nevus flammeus) is a cutaneous firemark caused by an abnormal aggregation of capillaries, resulting in pink to purple macules that resemble port wine. It is most commonly found on the face.

Nevus comedonicus is a rare epidermal nevus that primarily affects the face and neck. It is caused by mutations in the NEK9 gene56 on chromosome 14q24.

Nevus anemicus is a nonhereditary congenital disorder characterized by irregular hypopigmented macules that coalesce to form plaques. It is typically present at birth or develops during the first postpartum days. They concentrate primarily on the chest. This disorder is caused by sustained vasoconstriction caused by vascular hypersensitivity to catecholamines, rather than partial aplasia of dermal blood vessels.

Nevus roseus, also known as "rosé wine stain," has a pale red or pink colour that persists throughout life.

Phacomatosis pigmentovascularis is characterized by both a vascular and extensive pigmentary nevus. The pigmentary anomaly is classified into five types: type I (nevus flammeus and pigmented linear epidermal nevi), type II (nevus flammeus, Mongolian spots, and/or nevus anemicus), type III (nevus flammeus and spilus and/or anemicus), type IV (nevus flammeus, Mongolian spots, and nevus spilus and/or anemicus), and type V (cutis marmorata telangiec). The classification was simplified to include phacomatosis cesioflammea (nevus cesius and flammeus) and spilorosea (nevus spilus and roseus). CMAVM is caused by mutations in the RASA1 gene, which encodes

RasA1, a Ras GTPase-activating protein (RasGAP). AS is a benign cutaneous disease that causes progressive dilation of subepidermal vessels, resulting in clusters of punctate erythematous lesions on the lower limbs. It is both sporadic and autosomal dominant. It can be classified as a capillary nevus. It appears almost exclusively in women. It is caused by mutations at the chromosomal locus Xp11.3-Xq12.

3.4.4. Lymphatic Malformations

There are two types of lymphatic malformations (LMs) that affect the skin: lymphedema and congenital, superficial or deep, solitary or multiple lymphatic malformations. Lymphatic malformations are dilated lymphatic channels or pseudovesicles (lymphangiectasias) that are not part of the lymphatic circuit.

Cystic lesions can be macro- (formerly known as cystic hygromas), microcystic, or mixed. Microcystic lymphatic malformations are also known as lymphangioma, lymphangioma circumscriptum or simplex, verrucous hemangioma, and angiokeratoma circumscriptum. Macrocystic lymphatic malformations typically appear in the neck, axillas, or lateral edges of the trunk. They can be solitary or multiple, as well as interconnected.

Lymphedema, or chronic swelling in the body, usually in the lower extremities, caused by abnormal lymphatic vessels, can be either primary or secondary. Primary lymphedema is classified into several types (Lmph1A-Lmph1D) that are associated with the chromosomal regions 5q35, 6q16.2-q22.1, 1q42, and 4q34.

- Type-IA hereditary lymphedema (Lmph1A), also known as primary congenital lymphedema (PCL) and Milroy disease, typically affects the inferior limbs from the feet to the knees. This autosomal dominant disorder is caused by missense mutations in the *FLT4* gene, which encodes the VEGFR3.
- Type IB hereditary lymphedema (Lmph1B) is caused by anatomical or functional defects in the lymphatic system. It usually appears at birth or in early childhood, but it can happen later.
- Type-IC hereditary lymphedema (Lmph1C) is caused by heterozygous mutations in the GJC2 gene, which encodes gap junction protein-γ2, connexin Cx46.6, or Cx47.
- Type-ID hereditary lymphedema (Lmph1D) is caused by heterozygous mutations in the VEGFC gene, with transmission patterns consistent with autosomal dominant inheritance.
- Type-II late-onset lymphedema (Lmph2), also known as Meige's disease or lymphedema praecox, occurs around puberty. It affects the upper and lower limbs, face, and larynx, and can result in a persistent pleural effusion. It can be caused by truncation or missense mutations in the FOXC2 gene, which is located on chromosome 16q24.3.

Hypotrichosis-lymphedema-telangiectasia syndrome (HLTS) includes lymphedema and cutaneous telangiectasias. Both autosomal dominant and recessive inheritance patterns can be observed. Mutations in the SOX18 gene, which encodes the transcription factor Sox18, an early marker of lymphatic differentiation, cause both dominant and recessive forms. Sox18 interacts with MEF2c and regulates the synthesis of vcam1.

Mutations (e.g., X420W) in the IKBKG gene, which encodes Iκ BKγ, cause osteoporosis, lymphedema, anhydrotic ectodermal dysplasia, and immunodeficiency syndrome (OLEDAID). This reduces NFκB activation [57].

Lymphedema-cholestasis syndrome (LCS),

also known as Aagenaes syndrome, is typically an autosomal recessive disorder, though an autosomal dominant mutation may be present.

3.4.5. Endothelial Signaling in Vasculo- and Angiogenesis

Vasculo- (i.e., de novo blood vessel formation involving differentiation and migration of endothelial precursors), angio- (i.e., development of new blood vessels by capillary sprouting from preexisting vessels), and lymphangiogenesis construct (1) the vascular closed circuit, which is formed from arteries downstream from the heart, capillaries perfusing the body's tissues, and veins upstream from the heart, and (2) vascular walls, which are composed of vECs and mural cells. Blood and lymph vessels are made up of a single layer of endotheliocytes surrounded by pericytes or a variable number of layers of vascular smooth myocytes separated by elastic laminae in the microvasculature (capillaries and upstream lymphatics) and macrovasculature, respectively. The proper organisation of the vascular circuit necessitates the controlled activity of multiple types of messengers that regulate vessel formation, vascular branching, elongation and pruning, capillary fusion, vascular stability and anastomosis, and arterial and venous differentiation of endotheliocytes, which separates arteries and veins.

A transcriptional programme in endotheliocytes regulates vascular development and maintenance by integrating both extracellular and intracellular signals.

Aside from hemodynamic stress, a variety of signaling cascades control vascular and angiogenesis. The initiation and formation of new blood vessels, known as sprouting angiogenesis, is primarily controlled by the messengers VEGFa and Notch.

Angiogenesis is controlled by endothelial tip cells, which form the vascular front and are followed by proliferating stalk cells. Tip cells detect several extracellular pro- and antiangiogenic signals and migrate to the hypoxic region.

In mice and cardiac organ culture, coronary vessels develop from angiogenic sprouts of the sinus venosus, which is the vein that returns blood to the embryonic heart. As they migrate over and into the myocardium, sprouting venous endotheliocytes dedifferentiate. Intramyocardial ECs redifferentiate into arterial and capillary cells, while epicardial ECs differentiate into venous cells.

Endotheliocyte differentiation into arterial and venous cells is genetically determined in both vessel types. It precedes the start of blood circulation. Arterial and venous angioblasts separate at the start of vasculogenesis. A group of messengers (such as notch, SHh, and VEGF) regulate arterial identity acquisition. The acquisition of the venous phenotype is dependent on the nuclear receptor NR2f2, which inhibits notch signaling. Ephrins and their receptors (such as the transmembrane ligand ephrin-B2 and its cognate receptor EPHb4) also play a role in determining arterial and venous identity.

The susceptibility to certain vasculopathies varies between arteries and veins. The intracellular receptor NR2f2 regulates pathophysiological processes in adult blood vessels. It acts as an antiatherogenic and anti-osteogenic agent, inhibiting the formation of inflammatory factors while increasing the formation of antithrombotic agents and suppressing the osteogenic transcriptional programme and endothelial-to-mesenchymal transition. It regulates the TGFβ pathway by controlling the production of TGFβ2 and BMP4, which help endotheliocytes convert into mesenchymal stem cell-like cells and undergo osteogenic differentiation.

3.4.5.1. Notch, FoxC, SoxF, and NR2F2

The notch receptor (notch-1-notch-4) binds to one of two ligands: jagged proteins (Jag1-Jag2) and delta-like ligands (DLL1-DLL3). Jag1, Jag2, and DLL4 are only expressed in arterial endotheliocytes in the early embryo of mice.

Notch cleavage allows the notch intracellular domain (notchICD) to enter the cytosol. NotchICD interacts with RBPJκ, a transcriptional repressor in the absence of notch signaling, and Mastermind (Mam), a transcriptional coactivator. NotchICD moves to the nucleus and activates RBPJκ, leading to the synthesis of bHLH transcription factors HESs59 and HRTs60. In zebrafish, notch signaling is downstream of the SHh and VEGF pathways in arterial specification.

Notch-1 and notch-4 are required to maintain vessel identity. Notch signaling overcomes ALK1 loss by restoring EfnB2 expression in endotheliocytes. Notch signaling is also involved in tip-to-stalk cell conversion.

SOXF61 proteins work together with RBPJκ in endotheliocytes in mouse and zebrafish embryos. They are activated prior to notch signaling. Sox17 activates notch signaling by binding to the promoters of multiple genes involved in the notch pathway.

Three SOXF genes, SOX7, SOX17, and SOX18, encode transcription factors of the SOXF group that are expressed in vascular endotheliocytes during blood circulation development, with only Sox18 being involved in lymphangiogenesis. Sox7 and Sox18 work together to specify arterial and venous identities.

Single-nucleotide polymorphisms at the SOX17 chromosomal locus can cause intracranial aneurysms.

High VEGF concentrations cause tip cells to produce the delta-like ligand DLL4, which activates the notch on adjacent endotheliocytes, conferring stalk cell identity. In adult venous endotheliocytes, VEGFa inhibits EPHb4, a venous marker, while stimulating DLL4, an arterial marker.

DLL4 is responsible for initiating the arterial programme, whereas DLL1 is required for arterial identity maintenance. DLL1 formation in mouse embryos is limited to arterial endotheliocytes after embryonic day 13. DLL1 activates notch signaling, which regulates neuropilin-1 (Nrp1) synthesis, and VEGF controls it.

Among the forkhead box transcription factors implicated in cardiovascular system development, FoxC1 and FoxC2, which are expressed in both arteries and veins of the mouse embryo, play an overlapping role. They help to regulate the formation of arterial-specific genes (such as Dll4 and Hrt2) and the remodelling of primitive blood vessels. They use a FoxC-binding element (FBE) located upstream of notch signaling to directly activate Dll4 gene transcription.

In mice lacking FOXC1 and FOXC2, AVMs form, endotheliocytes do not express DLL4, and other arterial markers (notch-1, notch-4, Jag1, HRT2, and EfnB2) are reduced in expression. Although FoxC1 and FoxC2 are required for DLL4 synthesis, deletion of the forkhead-binding element on the Dll4 promoter does not attenuate Dll4 gene transcription by the FoxC factors, notch1ICD and notch4ICD, using the RBPJ-binding site. FoxC2 and notchICD synergistically act on the Hrt2 gene promoter, suggesting they may also collaborate on the Dll4 gene promoter.

In endotheliocytes, FoxC1 and FoxC2 regulate HRT2 expression via the Hrt2 promoter, which contains two FBEs. Furthermore, Foxc2 binds to the RBPJ (or Csl) gene promoter while FoxC1 does not. Foxc2 interacts with CSL and NotchICD to initiate HRT2 synthesis. In endotheliocytes, VEGF stimulates FoxC production of DLL4 and HRT2.

NR2f2, a genetic determinant of venous specification, is expressed specifically in venous endotheliocytes and acts upstream from EPHb4 in mice, inhibiting Nrp1 and notch formation. However, it works in conjunction with other factors to determine the fate of venous cells. Furthermore, it works with Prox1 to activate lymphatic gene expression.

Notch regulates endothelial cell responsiveness to BMP2 and BMP6 via the inhibitory SMAD6, which is involved in neovessel branching formation.

The notch- and ALK1-mediated signaling cascades interact and can partially compensate for one another. Sequestration of BMP9 and BMP10, followed by ALK1 inhibition and notch blockage, results in a hyperfused and hypersprouting vascular plexus in a neonatal mouse retina model. Many notch-targeted genes have SMAD1/5/8 binding sites in their regulatory regions (for example, HES1 and HRT1-HRT2).

3.4.5.2. Wnt and Sox

Wnt signaling controls many biological processes, including angiogenesis, inflammation, and tumorigenesis. Wnt morphogens are secreted by cysteine-rich palmitoylated glycoproteins that are critical for cell fate determination, tissue homeostasis, and embryo and foetus development.

Canonical Wnt signaling promotes vascular invasion of the central nervous system. Wnt and Norrin messengers target Frizzled receptor, LRP5 and LRP6 coreceptors, tetraspanin-12 and GPR124 coactivators, and β-catenin effectors. In the absence of any of these Wnt signaling mediators, vascular cerebral network formation fails, despite the hypoxic organ's high VEGF concentration.

Norrin (or Norrie disease protein) is an atypical Wnt ligand that secretes a cysteine-rich, cystine knot-like growth factor from a precursor encoded by the NDP gene. It activates the canonical Wnt signaling pathway through Fzd4 and LRP5, which work together with TSpan12 to activate Fzd4, independent of Wnt. Norrin, like Wnt, can tether and activate frizzled by assembling a molecular platform that includes Fzd4, its LRP5-LRP6 coreceptor complex, auxiliary TSpan12, and an associated HSPG. It then initiates the Ctnnβ1—LEF/TCF axis. Norrin keeps the blood-retina and blood-brain barriers intact while also controlling angiogenesis in the eye, ear (cochlea), brain, and female reproductive organs (uterus). Norrin also connects to secreted frizzled-related proteins (sFRPs).

The production of Sox17 in retinal arterioles, capillaries, and veins is dependent on frizzled-4 and norrin. Members of the SOXF group help to regulate the development of the blood and lymph vasculature, as well as arterial and venous identity (i.e., vascular differentiation), remodelling, and maintenance in a functionally redundant manner (strong but partial redundancy), compensating for any SOXF factor's defective activity. Each SOXF factor has a distinct pattern of production among the various types of retinal blood vessels. Sox7 and Sox18 show similar temporal expression patterns. They are primarily produced in endothelia during the early stages of endothelial differentiation, but their synthesis is differentially regulated. They also localise to specific vessels in zebrafish.

Both Sox7 and Sox18 are unnecessary for the initial specification and positioning of the major trunk vessels. On the other hand, Sox17 is primarily formed during gastrulation. Vascular endotheliocytes express all three SOXF group members simultaneously. SOXF members are regulated in a reciprocal manner in the developing blood vasculature. In mice, Sox17 and Sox18 play redundant roles in postnatal angiogenesis, whereas Sox7 and Sox18 have overlapping expression profiles. Sox7, Sox17, and Sox18 are functionally redundant in mouse retinal vasculature development (cell differentiation and vessel growth), as well as mature vasculature maintenance. Sox7 and Sox17 have overlapping functions and gene expression is regulated reciprocally, therefore, deleting a single SOXF member gene has little or no effect on vascular architecture or differentiation. At the start of retinal angiogenesis, combined deletion of Sox7, Sox17, and Sox18 results in a dense capillary plexus with nearly complete loss of radial arteries and veins, whereas the presence of a single Sox17 allele restores arterial identity with vSMC coverage. Indeed, Sox17 is critical for vSMC coverage of the radial retinal arteries. In the developing retina, all three SOXF genes are downregulated in the absence of canonical Wnt signaling mediated by norrin and frizzled-4, but are unaffected by reduced VEGF signaling after the NRP1 gene is deleted. In adulthood, Sox7, Sox17, and Sox18 perform redundant functions in blood vessel maintenance. Despite nearly normal vascular architecture, adult-onset vascular endothelial-specific deletion of all three SOXF genes causes massive edoema.

Endotheliocytes upregulate the production of GPR124, also known as tumour endothelial marker TEM5,63 during both physiological and tumour angiogenesis. Rac induces its synthesis during the formation of capillary networks, and it inhibits endotheliocyte proliferation.

3.4.5.3. Hedgehog

Sonic hedgehog signals are secreted and transmitted to recipient cells via the transmembrane receptors patched (Ptc) and smoothened (Smo). It can cause arterial cell fate in zebrafish angioblasts. Zebrafish embryos lacking SHh lose arterial expression of ephrin-B2, which causes the formation of VEGF, which activates notch.

In mice, defective Shh signaling does not result in severe vascular defects, but vascularization in the developing lung is reduced, and the formation of the dorsal aorta and remodelling of the yolk sac vasculature are altered. Murine SHh signaling may be sufficient for arterial and venous specification.

3.4.5.4. Vascular Endothelial Growth Factor

In angiogenesis, VEGF is responsible for the specification of tip and stalk cells. High VEGF concentrations induce DLL4 synthesis in tip cells, which activates notch signaling on adjacent endotheliocytes, conferring stalk cell identity.

In mice, arterial development in the retina requires lower-molecular-weight isoforms, diffusible VEGFa120 and intermediate VEGFa164 rather than VEGFa188.

Neuropilin-1, a VEGFa164 coreceptor, works alongside VEGFR2 to initiate signaling. In mice, impaired Nrp1 activity impairs arterial differentiation.

Vascular endothelial growth factor activates the PI3K pathway and induces the synthesis of notch-1 and DLL4, resulting in the VEGF-DLL4-notch-HRT2 cascade, which promotes arterial cell determination. It regulates FoxC activity based on the balance of PI3K and ERK activity. High VEGF concentrations (~50 ng/mL) activate arterial marker genes, while low VEGF concentrations (≤10 ng/mL) increase expression of the venous marker NR2f2. Depending on the level, VEGF signaling may preferentially activate the PI3K or ERK pathway.

The protein Tyr phosphatase receptor, or PTPRJ, is involved in arterial specification. It interferes with VEGFR2-primed signaling in endotheliocytes.

CalRLR is a G-protein-coupled receptor for adrenomedullin that coordinates with the VEGF and notch pathways during arterial differentiation in mouse embryos. CalRLR is expressed in the somite and arterial progenitors of zebrafish after VEGF exposure, with VEGF activity regulated by SHh. CalRLR promotes arterial gene expression, including ephrin-B2 and notch-5.

Neuropilin-2 is found in both venous and lymphatic endotheliocytes. VEGFR3, which is first detected in early embryonic blood vessels, is eventually restricted to venous and then lymphatic endotheliocytes.

VEGFc, a VEGFR3 ligand, is predominantly expressed in mesenchymal cells surrounding embryonic veins. Prox1+ VEFR3+ lymphatic endothelial progenitors then bud and migrate from veins via paracrine VEGFc-VEGFR3 signaling, thereby initiating developmental lymphangiogenesis.

As a result, a subset of venous endotheliocytes gradually synthesize the transcription factors Sox18 and Prox1 and develop a lymphatic endothelial phenotype. Sox18 is first detected in a subpopulation of the cardinal vein, before Prox1 synthesis begins. Sox18 activates Prox1 expression via two Sox18-binding sites on the Prox1 promoter. Sox18 is required for lymphatic differentiation but not for maintaining the lymphatic phenotype. Prox1 is a master regulator of lymphatic endothelial identity, inducing the expression of lymphatic markers such as VEGFR3 and LyVE1. Prox1 works with NR2f2 to promote the synthesis of FGFR3, VEGFR3, and integrin-α9, which regulates lymphatic endotheliocyte migration triggered by VEGFc.

FoxC1 and FoxC2 may help regulate lymphatic vessel development, pericyte recruitment to lymphatic vessels, and lymphatic valve formation in a paracrine fashion.

3.4.5.5. Ephrin-B2 and the EPHb4 Receptor

Venous and arterial endotheliocytes express the Tyr kinase receptor EPHb4 and its ligand ephrin-B2 (EfnB2), respectively (Table 3.13). They support but are not required for arterial and venous specification.

Table 3.13. *Regulators of Arterial, Venous, and Lymphatic Specification*

Factor	Effects
Arterial Identity	
CalCRL	Synthesized under control of the SHh–VEGF axis.
EfnB2	Segregates arteries from veins.
FoxC1/2	Regulate DLL4 and HRT2 expression.
Notch (notch-4)	SHh and VEGF effector.
	DLL1 maintains arterial identity.
	DLL4 elicits arterial specification.
Nrp1	Involved in a positive feedback loop of VEGF signaling.
PTPRJ	Acts upstream from PI3K in arterial specification.
SHh	VEGF affector.
Sox7/17/18	Control arterial and venous identity.
VEGF	SHh effector.

–	Activates notch via the PLCγ–ERK pathway.
Venous Identity	
EPHb4	Segregates arteries from veins.

Source: CalCRL calcitonin receptor-like receptor, Efn ephrin [EPH receptor interactor], EPH erythropoietin-producing hepatocyte receptor kinase, Fox forkhead box-containing transcription factor, NR nuclear receptor [transcription factor], Nrp neuropilin [VEGFR coreceptor], Prox Prospero homeodomain-containing transcription factor, PTPRJ protein Tyr phosphatase receptor type J, SHh sonic hedgehog, Sox sex determining region-Y box (SOX) homeodomain-containing transcription factor, VEGF vascular endothelial growth factor.

EfnB2 and EPHb4 expression is clearly visible in the primary vascular plexus before circulation begins in the developing embryo. Arterial-venous identity is genetically predetermined, but it is influenced by hemodynamic forces that allow for remodelling and EC phenotype change.

Bidirectional signals mediated by both proteins are critical in vascular development. EfnB2 and EPHb4 are differentially expressed in arterial and venous endotheliocytes of the mouse embryo, and are thus thought to be markers of arterial and venous identity during development. EfnB2 forward signaling via EPHb4 (EfnB2-EPHb4 axis) inhibits cell adhesion and migration while suppressing cell proliferation, whereas EPHb4 reverse signaling via EfnB2 (EPHB4-EfnB2 axis) promotes cell attachment and migration.

EfnB2-EPHb4 plays a role in embryonic vascular circuit development, vascular remodelling, as well as neovascularization, arteriovenous differentiation, and tumoral angiogenesis in adults. Veins and arteries in hemorrhagic (hCeAVMs) and nonhemorrhagic cerebral arteriovenous malformations (nhCeAVMs) are coated by EPHb4+ and EfnB2+ endotheliocytes, respectively. EPHb4 and EfnB2 content are higher in hCeAVMs than in nhCeAVMs, whereas endotheliocytes in the normal superficial temporal artery express neither EPHb4 nor EfnB2.

Arterial specification is dependent on VEGF, which promotes the expression of notch and DLL4, as well as the transcription factors FoxC1 and FoxC2, which regulate DLL4 synthesis. Notch stimulates HRT1 and HRT2, which promotes arterial differentiation.

On the other hand, the nuclear receptor NR2f2 is a determinant of venous specification because it inhibits the expression of arterial specification genes such as Nrp1 and notch.

A subset of venous endotheliocytes gradually expresses the transcription factors Sox18 and Prox1, gaining lymphatic fate and differentiating into lymphatic endotheliocytes.

A functional vasculature is formed when the developing arteries and veins coordinate their sizes. In mouse embryos, the developing dorsal aorta and cardinal vein are proportionately balanced. Gain-of-function notch mutations result in enlarged aortas and small cardinal veins, whereas loss-of-function mutations produce small aortas and large cardinal veins.

The dorsal aorta emerges before the cardinal vein when endotheliocytes form the dorsal aorta primordium, a transient capillary plexus. The dorsal aorta is formed through the remodelling of this primitive structure. The cardinal vein appears slightly later, at a point when transient capillaries form between the dorsal aorta and cardinal vein. Ephrin-B2 is expressed specifically in arterial endotheliocytes prior to the onset of blood circulation, but it does not determine endothelial arterial specification. Notch regulates the proportion of endotheliocytes in the dorsal aorta and cardinal vein by promoting arterial specification and controlling both artery and vein size. The interdependence of arterial and venous size is based on a balanced allocation of endotheliocytes between these vessel types. Notch regulates endotheliocyte allocation by determining arterial specification and thus the ratio of arterial to venous endotheliocytes.

Loss of EfnB2 or EPHb4 causes enlarged aortas and small cardinal veins. However, endotheliocytes with venous identities mislocalize in the aorta. EfnB2-EPHb4 signaling may function independently from notch, sorting arterial and venous endotheliocytes into their respective vessels.

EPHb4+ endotheliocytes cover arterioles and venules. EPHb4+ capillaries in sprouts contain significantly more EphB4 than capillaries connecting arterioles and venules. As a result, EPHb4 is not an arterial or venous-specific marker in adult rat microvasculature, but rather an indicator of capillary sprouting.

3.4.5.6. Transforming Growth Factor (β Group)

The transforming growth factor-β superfamily, including bone morphogenetic proteins, is crucial for embryo and foetal development and organ function. TGFβ and BMP group members alter signaling in endotheliocytes, leading to diffuse malformations. Deregulated TGFβ/BMP signaling can lead to aortic aneurysms.

The TGFβ signaling cascade includes:

Several messengers, including three TGFβ subtypes (TGFβ1-TGFβ3), BMPs, growth differentiation factors (GDFs), activins, nodal, and inhibins.

There are seven type-I receptors (ALK1-ALK7), with ALK5 corresponding to Tβ R1, ALK3 and ALK6 to BMPR1a and BMPR1b, and ALK2, ALK4, ALK7, and ALK164 to AcvR1a, AcvR1c, and AcvRL1, respectively.

There are five type II receptors: Tβ R2, BMPR2, AcvR2a-AcvR2b, and AMHR2.

Endoglin, a coreceptor found on endotheliocytes, cryptic, and β-glycan (Tβ R3) modulate the activity of types-I and -II receptors.

Various ligand-receptor combinations result in distinct TGFβ/BMP signaling. For example, ALK2, which primarily transmits the BMP6 signal, can also act as a BMP9 receptor. In the endothelium, heterotetrameric receptors composed of types-I and -II receptors stimulate specific SMAD signaling cascades. ALK1 signals through SMAD1, SMAD5, and SMAD8, while ALK5 signals through SMAD2 and SMAD3.

BMP9 (GDF2), BMP10, and TGFβ1 all weakly activate ALK1, a transmembrane receptor. The ALK1-Eng-Tβ R2 complex phosphorylates cytosolic SMAD1, SMAD5, and SMAD8 after binding to ALK1.

ALK1 signaling within cells has been linked to various diseases. Endothelium-specific ALK1 stimulates arterial endothelial maturation and quiescence. In mice, the deletion of genes encoding ALK1, endoglin, and MAP3K7 results in embryonic lethality and altered vascular circuit morphogenesis due to impaired arterial endothelial differentiation.

Phosphorylated SMADs form complexes with common SMAD4 and move to the nucleus, where they activate or suppress transcription of specific target genes. Smad6 and Smad7 are inhibitory SMADs that interact with ALK1 and ALK5, respectively (self-regulatory loop). They compete for binding type-I receptors and recruiting specific ubiquitin ligases and phosphatases for receptor degradation or dephosphorylation. Proangiogenic BMP2 and BMP6 are dominant in the early stages of blood vessel formation, signaling through ALK2 or ALK3. Antiangiogenic BMP9 and BMP10, two major ALK1 ligands, primarily signal through ALK1 during vascular remodelling and maturation. Both BMP9 and BMP10 reduce EC proliferation and migration. Endoglin and ALK1 are involved in vasculo- and angiogenesis during embryogenesis. ALK1 synthesis decreases during mouse postnatal development, except in the lung endothelium, but remains high enough to keep the adult vasculature quiet via BMP9-ALK1 signaling. ALK1 production, which is associated with angiogenesis, increases during wound healing and tumourigenesis.

On the one hand, the BMP9-ALK1 couple stimulates the formation of notch-related mediators such as HES1 (bHLHb39), HRT1 (bHLHb31), HRT2 (bHLHb32), and Jag1, as well as endoglin, ephrin-B2, transmembrane protein TMem100, and endothelin-1. On the other hand, it inhibits the expression of E-selectin, CXCR4, and apelin.

TMem100 is an embryonic endothelium-enriched intracellular transmembrane protein that is primarily found in the endoplasmic reticulum (but not in the plasma membrane). BMP9 and BMP10 activate its synthesis via the ALK1 receptor. TMem100 may aid in post-translational protein modification and intracellular sorting.

In neurons, TMem100 regulates the interaction of ankyrin-like and vanilloid TRP channels TRPA1 and TRPV1, disconnecting them and increasing Ca^{2+} influx. Both TRPA1 and TRPV1 are found on endotheliocytes; TRPV1 helps to regulate vasomotor tone, whereas TRPV4 promotes arteriogenesis.

Calcium signaling upstream from NFATc1 is impaired in TMEM100-/- embryos. Bmp10-/- mice exhibit impaired cardiac growth without angiogenesis defects. Among ALK1 targets, TMEM100 ablation produces a phenotype similar to Alk1 mutants (though not identical). Both Alk1-/- and TMEM100-/- mice exhibit heart defects, failed vascular remodelling, abnormal dorsal aortic dilation and narrowing, and detachment of endo- and mesodermal layers in the yolk sac. Ablation of TMEM100 postnatally causes AVMs in the lung and intestine, but not injury-induced cutaneous AVMs, as seen in Alk1-/- mice.

In utero, TMEM100-/- and ECTMEM100-/- mice die due to impaired signaling from ALK1, notch, and PKB, resulting in abnormal arterial endothelial differentiation and vascular morphogenesis.

Calcium forms the notch heterodimer, and the transplasmalemmal gradient in Ca^{2+} concentration plays a role in activating the notch in endotheliocytes. When extracellular calcium levels are low, notch subunits dissociate, promoting cleavage.

Notch and its ligands are abundant in the arterial (but not venous) endothelium of mouse embryos. Notch-1, notch-4, DLL4, CSL65 (or RBPJκ), HRT1, and HRT2 all affect arterial cell fate. ALK1, notch, and TMem100 signaling changes influence vascular smooth myocyte recruitment or differentiation during arterial maturation. PKB and presenilin-1, which interact with the notch pathway, are repressed in TMEM100-/- and Alk1-/- mouse embryos. The PKB kinase promotes PS1-mediated notch cleavage. PS1 peptidase activates PKB in the opposite direction. PKB activity is impaired by altered presenilin-1, resulting in apoptosis.

ALK1 synthesis is dependent on blood flow, which promotes endoglin-ALK1 association, making endotheliocytes sensitive to low BMP9 concentrations. In ALK1-deficient mice, arteriovenous malformation, enlarged veins, and hyperbranching of the capillary plexus in the retina are seen. Retinal arteriovenous malformations are more common in areas of high blood flow. Endotheliocytes also migrate. Although pericyte coverage is normal at the retina's migration front, the central region of the capillary plexus has less pericyte coverage in its capillaries. Endotheliocytes from AVMs express the venous marker EPHb4, but lack the arterial marker Jag1.

Endoglin-deficient endotheliocytes are incapable of sensing and adapting to applied wall shear stress. This vascular endothelial glycoprotein has a strong affinity for TGFβ1. It aids in the regulation of angiogenesis, which includes tip cell selection, endotheliocyte proliferation and migration, mural cell recruitment, lumen formation, anastomosis, neovessel expansion, and pruning.

Endoglin is linked to Tβ R3, encoded by the TGFBR3 gene, which retains TGFβ for presentation to signalling receptors. It functions as a TGFβ coreceptor, contributing to BMP9 signaling in endotheliocytes.

Endoglin is involved in the regulation of VEGFR2 signaling. Endoglin and VEGFR2 colocalize in intracellular vesicles. Endoglin influences VEGFR2 transfer and recycling, and thus the balance of endotheliocyte proliferation and migration following VEGFa stimulation, favouring PKB activation. Furthermore, PKB phosphorylation favours venous differentiation at the expense of arteriogenesis.

Hereditary hemorrhagic telangiectasia (HHT), also known as Osler-Weber-Rendu syndrome, and cerebral cavernous malformation (CCM) are caused by decreased and increased signaling from TGFβ/BMP receptor complexes, respectively.

Endoglin works with CCM pathway components KRIT166 (or CCM1) and ALK1 (or HHT2) to inhibit angiogenesis. The CCM complex consists of CCM1 (KRIT1), CCM2 (OSM67 and malcavernin), and CCM3 (PdCD10) [68].

Loss-of-function mutations in the ENG and ACVRL1 genes result in abnormal regulation of angiogenesis processes. Although LOF ENG mutations result in a mild hyperbranching phenotype, LOF ACVRL1 mutations promote tip cell potential and branching. Cells with LOF ENG mutations do not respond adequately to migratory signals provided by the direction of blood flow.

3.4.6. Hereditary Hemorrhagic Telangiectasia

Hereditary hemorrhagic telangiectasia is an autosomal dominant disorder that affects less than 2 out of 10,000 people. It is characterized by AVMs, capillary overgrowth, and fragile vessels.

AVMs bypass capillaries; blood flows directly from some arteries to veins, which then experience increased stress and strain, causing them to enlarge (enlarged shunts).

Telangiectasias, or focal dilations of postcapillary venules with excess vSMCs, occur near the skin. Cutaneomucosal telangiectasias produce bleeding (epistaxis). AVMs develop in the lungs, liver, and brain.

Several types of HHT are distinguished primarily by their genetic cause rather than by symptoms. Type-I (HHT1) patients experience symptoms earlier than type-II (HHT2) and are more likely to exhibit vascular malformations in the brain and lung. The incidence of pulmonary AVMs is higher in HHT1 than in HHT2.

Mutations in the Smad4 gene cause juvenile polyposis combined with HHT, a syndrome characterized by AVMs that grow and regress throughout life as well as polyps in the gastrointestinal tract. Two additional chromosomal loci, 5q31 and 7p14, are associated with other types, HHT3 and HHT4. Heterozygous LOF autosomal dominant mutations in the ENG69 and Alk1 genes, which encode TGFβ receptors primarily found on endotheliocytes, result in HHT1 and HHT2, respectively. Arteriovenous malformations can occur in the brain, spinal cord, lung, gastrointestinal tract, and liver.

In endotheliocytes, LOF mutations in the ENG gene, which encodes endoglin, result in type-1 HHT (HHT1) that is favoured by VEGFa, and arteriolar endotheliocytes develop venous characteristics. Endotheliocytes overexpressing endoglin act as tip cells, primarily in the arterial compartment. Deletion of the ENG gene alters VEGFa-VEGFR2 signaling while priming the PI3K-PKB pathway.

HHT2 results from mutations in the ACVRL1 gene, which encodes ALK1. Arterial endotheliocytes produce EfnB2, which is involved in vascular development. Its concentration decreases in ACVRL1−/− mice. The ALK1 ligand BMP9 stimulates EfnB2 production in endotheliocytes via ALK1 and its coreceptors BMPR2 and AcvR2.

BMP9 activates DNA binding inhibitors ID1 and ID3 (bHLHb24-bHLHb25), which are required for EfnB2 formation. ID1 and ID3 inhibit DNA binding by forming heterodimers with other bHLH transcription factors, including E-proteins (TcFE2α, TcF4, and TcF12) and ALK1 and notch signaling effectors (HES1 (bHLHb39) and HRT1 (bHLHb31), which repress cell differentiation but promote cell proliferation (70). In addition, IDs downstream of SMAD1 and SMAD5 promote the stalk cell phenotype during angiogenesis, preventing excessive tip cell formation.

Loss of ALK1 or EfnB2, which target the EPHb4 receptor involved in venous specification, results in arteriovenous anastomosis, whereas loss of ALK1 (but not EfnB2) stimulates VEGFR2 production and capillary sprouting. In contrast, BMP9 inhibits endothelial sprouting via the ALK1-BMPR2-AcvR2 receptor complex, as well as ID1 and ID3. HHT markers include VEGF, TGFβ, soluble endoglin, angiopoietin-2, clotting factor FVIII, and von Willebrand factor, as well as microRNAs like miR27a, which promotes angiogenesis, miR205, which inhibits SMAD1 and SMAD4, and miR210.

The BMP9-ALK1 pathway targets the GJA5 gene, which encodes the gap junction protein connexin-40 in human aortic endotheliocytes, which may explain the heterogeneity and severity of HHT2. GJA5 haploinsufficiency in ACVRL1+/− mice results in arterial vasodilation and capillary bed rarefaction, similar to AVMs in HHT2 patients. Reduced Cx40 concentration also causes ROS production, resulting in vessel remodelling. Capillaries form transient arteriovenous shunts, which can develop into large malformations when exposed to stressors.

Although some idiopathic AVMs have been linked to increased notch signaling (notch-1 and notch-4, as well as Jag1 and DLL4), notch activity in HHT decreases. Both GOF and LOF notch signaling cause abnormal arterial and venous specification, resulting in artery-vein fusion. In adult mice, constitutively active notch-4 causes AVMs in the brain, liver, skin, and uterus, which can be reduced by inhibiting notch-4 activity. Endotheliocyte-specific, constitutively active notch-1 also causes AVMs. AVMs grow in HHT patients due to endotheliocyte proliferation, which expands the arteriovenous shunt, whereas idiopathic AVMs are caused by endotheliocyte hypertrophy. Decayed notch signaling promotes endotheliocyte proliferation and may explain at least some of the vascular enlargement seen in HHT-related AVMs.

3.4.7. Cerebral Cavernous Malformations

Cerebral cavernous (or capillary venous) malformations are made up of dilated capillary-like vessels (cavernomas) combined with large saccular vessels with thickened walls in the cerebral parenchyma. Endotheliocytes lack tight junctions and are therefore separated by gaps.

These disorders occur in sporadic and familiar forms, with single and multiple lesions, respectively. Four chromosomal loci are linked to the condition: (1) 7q11.22 with mutations in the KRIT1 gene (Ccm1; ~40% cases), (2) 7p13 with mutations in the Ccm2 gene (encoding malcavernin, a stabiliser of endotheliocyte junctions, also abbreviated CCM2), (3) 3q26.1 with mutations in the PDCD10 gene (Ccm3), and (4) 3q26.3-27.2.

These disorders are classified as pseudodominant diseases. Although patients are heterozygous for Ccm gene mutations, biallelic mutations have been observed locally in lesions. Biallelic Ccm mutation is also found in lesions of patients with sporadic CCM.

Mutations in the KRIT1 gene, which produces KrIT1 in neurons, astrocytes, epitheliocytes, and endotheliocytes, can cause hyperkeratotic cutaneous capillary venous malformations, as well as CCMs. KrIT1 connects to microtubules and interacts with Itgβ1BP1, which regulates cell adhesion and migration, ultimately controlling EC fate. Itgβ1BP1 can trap KrIT1 in the nucleus. Malcavernin can sequester KrIT1 in the cytoplasm. PdCD10 may be involved in the same pathway.

Gain-of-function mutations in CCM genes can lead to increased TGFβ/BMP signaling, endothelial-to-mesenchymal transition, and cerebral cavernomas. TGFβ and KLF4-induced BMP2 and BMP6 formation disrupts cellular junctions, increases vascular permeability, and leads to hyperproliferation and mesenchymal marker acquisition, resulting in AVMs and multilumen cavernomas. The transcription factor KLF4 facilitates the endothelial-to-mesenchymal transition. Early after Ccm gene ablation, both KLF2 and KLF4 are overexpressed. BMPs stimulate KLF4 synthesis in cultured human umbilical vein ECs. However, the MAP3K3-MAP2K5-ERK5 pathway can also activate KLF4, which stimulates the transcription factors MEF2a and MEF2c and thus increases KLF4 production. In addition, KLF4 can initiate BMP6 formation, resulting in a positive feedback loop.

3.5. Summary

Diseases of the cardiovascular system, encompassing a wide range of conditions affecting the heart and blood vessels, are a leading cause of morbidity and mortality worldwide. This group includes coronary artery disease (CAD), hypertension (high blood pressure), heart failure, arrhythmias, and valvular heart diseases, among others.

Coronary artery disease, the most common type of heart disease, is caused by the buildup of plaque in the heart's arteries, leading to reduced blood flow to the heart muscle and potentially resulting in a heart attack. Hypertension, another prevalent condition, increases the risk of developing heart disease, stroke, and other complications due to the persistent elevation of blood pressure against artery walls. Heart failure, a condition where the heart cannot pump enough blood to meet the body's needs, can result from untreated coronary artery disease, hypertension, and other cardiac conditions. Arrhythmias refer to irregular heartbeats, which can affect the heart's efficiency in pumping blood throughout the body. Valvular heart diseases involve malfunctions of one or more of the heart valves, affecting the flow of blood within the heart.

Prevention and management of CVDs involve lifestyle modifications such as healthy eating, regular physical activity, avoidance of tobacco use, and managing stress levels. Medications, surgical interventions, and other treatments may also be necessary depending on the specific condition and its severity. Therefore, CVDs are complex conditions with varied etiologies, manifestations, and treatment approaches. Advances in medical research continue to provide insights into their pathophysiology, enabling the development of more effective prevention, diagnostic, and treatment strategies. The focus on early detection and management, along with public health efforts to address risk factors, is crucial in reducing the impact of these diseases on individuals and healthcare systems globally.

A Closer Look

Lymphatic Malformations

Lymphatic malformations (LMs) are rare, congenital anomalies in the lymphatic system, characterized by benign cyst-like structures filled with lymphatic fluid. These malformations arise from the improper development of lymphatic vessels, forming localized masses that can vary in size and affect various body parts, most commonly the head, neck, and extremities. Although benign, LMs can cause significant functional and aesthetic issues, particularly when they compress nearby organs or disrupt normal physiological processes.

LMs are classified based on their size and structure into macrocystic, microcystic, or combined types. Symptoms depend on the size and location of the malformation, ranging from visible swelling to complications such as respiratory distress, infection, and pain. Some cases may remain asymptomatic until a secondary infection or trauma occurs, causing the lesion to enlarge and become symptomatic.

Diagnosis of lymphatic malformations is primarily achieved through imaging techniques like ultrasound, MRI, and CT scans. These methods help define the size, extent, and relationship of the malformation to surrounding structures, guiding the treatment approach. Histopathological examination may further confirm the diagnosis.

Treatment options vary depending on the size, location, and symptoms. Surgical resection is a common treatment, although complete removal may be challenging in complex cases due to the risk of damaging nearby structures. Sclerotherapy, where a sclerosant is injected to shrink the malformation, is another effective option, particularly for macrocystic lesions. More recently, targeted therapies involving drugs like sirolimus have shown promise, offering a non-invasive alternative with fewer side effects for managing extensive or recurrent LMs.

Given the impact of LMs on quality of life, research into innovative and less invasive treatments is ongoing. Supportive care and multidisciplinary management remain essential to improving the quality of life for affected individuals, particularly children, who may experience developmental challenges due to LMs.

References

1. Banerjee, I., Fuseler, J. W., Price, R. L., Borg, T. K., et al., (2007). Determination of cell types and numbers during cardiac development in the neonatal and adult rat and mouse. *Am. J. Physiol. Heart Circ. Physiol. 293,* H1883–H1891.
2. Bang, C., Batkai, S., Dangwal, S., Gupta, S. K., et al., (2014). Cardiac fibroblast-derived microRNA passenger strand-enriched exosomes mediate cardiomyocyte hypertrophy. *J. Clin. Investig. 124,* 2136–2146.
3. Bansal, S., Sharma, M., Ranjithkumar, R., & Mohanakumar, T., (2018). The role of exosomes in allograft immunity. *Cell Immunol. 331,* 85–92.
4. Bennett, V., & Baines, A. J., (2001). Spectrin and ankyrin-based pathways: Metazoan inventions for integrating cells into tissues. *Physiol. Rev. 81,* 1353–1392.
5. Benz, P. M., Merkel, C. J., Offner, K., Abesser, M., et al., (2013). Mena/VASP and alphaII-Spectrin complexes regulate cytoplasmic actin networks in cardiomyocytes and protect from conduction abnormalities and dilated cardiomyopathy. *Cell Commun. Signal. 11,* 56.
6. Borosch, S., Dahmen, E., Beckers, C., Stoppe, C., et al., (2017). Characterization of extracellular vesicles derived from cardiac cells in an in vitro model of preconditioning. *J. Extracell Vesicles 6,* 1390391.
7. Broughton, K. M., Wang, B. J., Firouzi, F., Khalafalla, F., et al., (2018). Mechanisms of Cardiac Repair and Regeneration. *Circ. Res. 122,* 1151–1163.
8. Cosme, J., Guo, H., Hadipour-Lakmehsari, S., Emili, A., et al., (2017). Hypoxia-Induced Changes in the Fibroblast Secretome, Exosome, and Whole-Cell Proteome Using Cultured, Cardiac-Derived Cells Isolated from Neonatal Mice. *J. Proteome Res. 16,* 2836–2847.
9. Davis, J., & Molkentin, J. D., (2014). Myofibroblasts: Trust your heart and let fate decide. *J. Mol. Cell Cardiol. 70,* 9–18.
10. Emanueli, C., Shearn, A. I., Angelini, G. D., & Sahoo, S., (2015). Exosomes and exosomal miRNAs in cardiovascular protection and repair. *Vasc. Pharmacol. 71,* 24–30.
11. Feng, G., Bajpai, G., Ma, P., Koenig, A., et al., (2022). CCL17 Aggravates Myocardial Injury by Suppressing Recruitment of Regulatory T Cells. *Circulation 145,* 765–782.
12. Frangogiannis, N. G., (2019). Cardiac fibrosis: Cell biological mechanisms, molecular pathways and therapeutic opportunities. *Mol. Aspects Med. 65,* 70–99.
13. Fu, X., Khalil, H., Kanisicak, O., Boyer, J. G., et al., (2018). Specialized fibroblast differentiated states underlie scar formation in the infarcted mouse heart. *J. Clin. Investig. 128,* 2127–2143.
14. Gourdie, R. G., Dimmeler, S., & Kohl, P., (2016). Novel therapeutic strategies targeting fibroblasts and fibrosis in heart disease. *Nat. Rev. Drug Discov. 15,* 620–638.
15. Gundelfinger, E. D., Kessels, M. M., & Qualmann, B., (2003). Temporal and spatial coordination of exocytosis and endocytosis. *Nat. Rev. Mol. Cell Biol. 4*, 127–139.
16. Habibie, H., Adhyatmika, A., Schaafsma, D., & Melgert, B. N., (2021). The role of osteoprotegerin (OPG) in fibrosis: Its potential as a biomarker and/or biological target for the treatment of fibrotic diseases. *Pharmacol. Ther. 228,* 107941.
17. Hohn, J., Tan, W., Carver, A., Barrett, H., et al., (2021). Roles of Exosomes in Cardiac Fibroblast Activation and Fibrosis. *Cells 10,* 2933.

18. Huang, Z., Chen, X. J., Qian, C., Dong, Q., et al., (2016). Signal transducer and activator of transcription 3/microRNA-21 feedback loop contributes to atrial fibrillation by promoting atrial fibrosis in a rat sterile pericarditis model. Circ. *Arrhythm Electrophysiol. 9,* e003396.

19. Humeres, C., & Frangogiannis, N. G., (2019). Fibroblasts in the Infarcted, Remodeling, and Failing Heart. *JACC Basic Transl. Sci. 4,* 449–467.

20. Hund, T. J., Snyder, J. S., Wu, X., Glynn, P., et al., (2014). betaIV-Spectrin regulates TREK-1 membrane targeting in the heart. *Cardiovasc. Res. 102,* 166–175.

21. Ibrahim, A. G., Cheng, K., & Marban, E., (2014). Exosomes as critical agents of cardiac regeneration triggered by cell therapy. *Stem Cell Reports. 2,* 606–619.

22. Kanisicak, O., Khalil, H., Ivey, M. J., Karch, J., et al., (2016). Genetic lineage tracing defines myofibroblast origin and function in the injured heart. *Nat. Commun. 7,* 12260.

23. LaFramboise, W. A., Scalise, D., Stoodley, P., Graner, S. R., et al., (2007). Cardiac fibroblasts influence cardiomyocyte phenotype in vitro. *Am. J. Physiol. Cell Physiol. 292,* C1799–C1808.

24. Lindner, D., Zietsch, C., Becher, P. M., Schulze, K., et al., (2012). Differential expression of matrix metalloproteases in human fibroblasts with different origins. *Biochem. Res. Int. 2012,* 875742.

25. Liu, N., Xie, L., Xiao, P., Chen, X., et al., (2022). Cardiac fibroblasts secrete exosome microRNA to suppress cardiomyocyte pyroptosis in myocardial ischemia/reperfusion injury. *Mol. Cell Biochem. 477,* 1249–1260.

26. Lyu, L., Wang, H., Li, B., Qin, Q., et al., (2015). A critical role of cardiac fibroblast-derived exosomes in activating renin angiotensin system in cardiomyocytes. *J. Mol. Cell Cardiol. 89,* 268–279.

27. Machnicka, B., Grochowalska, R., Boguslawska, D. M., Sikorski, A. F., et al., (2012). Spectrin-based skeleton as an actor in cell signaling. *Cell Mol. Life Sci. 69,* 191–201.

28. Martin, T. P., Lawan, A., Robinson, E., Grieve, D. J., et al., (2014). Adult cardiac fibroblast proliferation is modulated by calcium/calmodulin-dependent protein kinase II in normal and hypertrophied hearts. *Pflugers Arch. 466,* 319–330.

29. Nagaraju, C. K., Dries, E., Popovic, N., Singh, A. A., et al., (2017). Global fibroblast activation throughout the left ventricle but localized fibrosis after myocardial infarction. *Sci. Rep. 7,* 10801.

30. Nassal, D. M., Patel, N. J., Unudurthi, S. D., Shaheen, R., et al., (2021). Ca2+/calmodulin kinase II-dependent regulation of betaIV-spectrin modulates cardiac fibroblast gene expression, proliferation, and contractility. *J. Biol. Chem. 297,* 100893.

31. Parkinson, N. J., Olsson, C. L., Hallows, J. L., McKee-Johnson, J., et al., (2001). Mutant beta-spectrin 4 causes auditory and motor neuropathies in quivering mice. *Nat. Genet. 29,* 61–65.

32. Patel, N. J., Nassal, D. M., Greer-Short, A. D., Unudurthi, S. D., et al., (2019). betaIV-Spectrin/STAT3 complex regulates fibroblast phenotype, fibrosis, and cardiac function. *JCI Insight 4,* e131046.

33. Piriya Ananda Babu, L., Wang, H. Y., Eguchi, K., Guillaud, L., et al., (2020). Microtubule and actin differentially regulate synaptic vesicle cycling to maintain high-frequency neurotransmission. *J. Neurosci. 40,* 131–142.

34. Shah, H., Hacker, A., Langburt, D., Dewar, M., et al., (2021). Myocardial Infarction Induces Cardiac Fibroblast Transformation within Injured and Noninjured Regions of the Mouse Heart. *J. Proteome Res. 20,* 2867–2881.

35. Sorkin, R., Huisjes, R., Boskovic, F., Vorselen, D., et al., (2018). Nanomechanics of Extracellular Vesicles Reveals Vesiculation Pathways. *Small 14,* e1801650.

36. Tallquist, M. D., & Molkentin, J. D., (2017). Redefining the identity of cardiac fibroblasts. *Nat. Rev. Cardiol. 14,* 484–491.

37. Taylor, J., Patio, K., De Rubis, G., Morris, M. B., et al., (2021). Membrane to cytosol redistribution of alphaII-spectrin drives extracellular vesicle biogenesis in malignant breast cells. *Proteomics 21,* e2000091.

38. Travers, J. G., Kamal, F. A., Robbins, J., Yutzey, K. E., et al., (2016). Cardiac fibrosis: The fibroblast awakens. *Circ Res. 118,* 1021–1040.

39. Trifaro, J., Rose, S. D., Lejen, T., & Elzagallaai, A., (2000). Two pathways control chromaffin cell cortical F-actin dynamics during exocytosis. *Biochimie 82,* 339–352.

40. Unsain, N., Stefani, F. D., & Caceres, A., (2018). The actin/spectrin membrane-associated periodic skeleton in neurons. *Front. Synaptic Neurosci. 10,* 10.

41. Unudurthi, S. D., Greer-Short, A., Patel, N., Nassal, D., et al., (2018). Spectrin-based pathways underlying electrical and mechanical dysfunction in cardiac disease. Exper*t Rev. Cardiovasc. Ther. 16,* 59–65.

42. Unudurthi, S. D., Nassal, D., Greer-Short, A., Patel, N., et al., (2018). betaIV-Spectrin regulates STAT3 targeting to tune cardiac response to pressure overload. *J. Clin. Investig. 128,* 5561–5572.

43. Weisheit, C. K., Kleiner, J. L., Rodrigo, M. B., Niepmann, S. T., et al., (2021). CX3CR1 is a prerequisite for the development of cardiac hypertrophy and left ventricular dysfunction in mice upon transverse aortic constriction. *PLoS ONE 16,* e0243788.

44. Wu, L. G., & Chan, C. Y., (2022). Multiple Roles of Actin in Exo- and Endocytosis. Front. *Synaptic Neurosci. 14,* 841704.

45. Yang, L., Dun, A. R., Martin, K. J., Qiu, Z., et al., (2012). Secretory vesicles are preferentially targeted to areas of low molecular SNARE density. *PLoS ONE. 7,* e49514.

Chapter

CHRONIC KIDNEY DISEASES

4

Contents

Introduction

Chronic kidney disease (CKD), which is considered to be a "silent epidemic" disease, is considered to be one of the major causes of mortality. This is in addition to the fact that its primary complication, cardiovascular disease (CVD), is a factor that contributes to the poor prognosis of these patients. It has been established that inflammation is an essential component of CKD, and it is closely associated with cardiovascular complications. It is possible that the early detection of renal diseases could be improved through the identification of novel biomarkers through the use of omics technologies, which are continuously advancing. In addition to identifying accurate inflammatory biomarker panels, which play an important part in disease monitoring and follow-up, omics approaches, which include proteomics, have the potential to offer novel insights into the mechanisms underlying disease. Recent research has shed light on the hypothesis that the microbiota in the gut are a significant contributor to inflammation in kidney diseases. In CKD, there is a growing body of evidence that demonstrates the interaction between the microbiota and the host. Furthermore, gut dysbiosis may be an underappreciated cause of inflammation, which could ultimately result in malnutrition, accelerated CVD, and the progression of CKD. This chapter discusses the connection between inflammation and CKD, as well as the novel approaches that have been proposed regarding the involvement of microbiota in the pathology of CKD, and as well as the potential of these approaches to facilitate improvements in quality of life.

Orientation and Directional Terms

Term	Definition	Illustration
Kidney	Bean-shaped organs that filter waste from the blood, balance bodily fluids, and regulate various physiological functions.	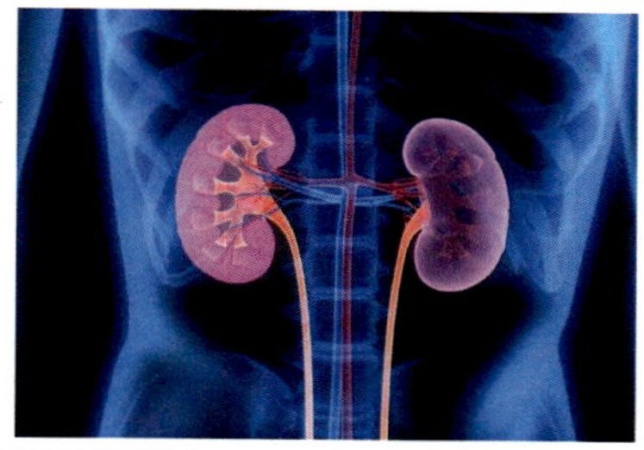
Inflammation	The body's immune response to injury or infection, characterized by redness, swelling, pain, and heat, which can be acute or chronic.	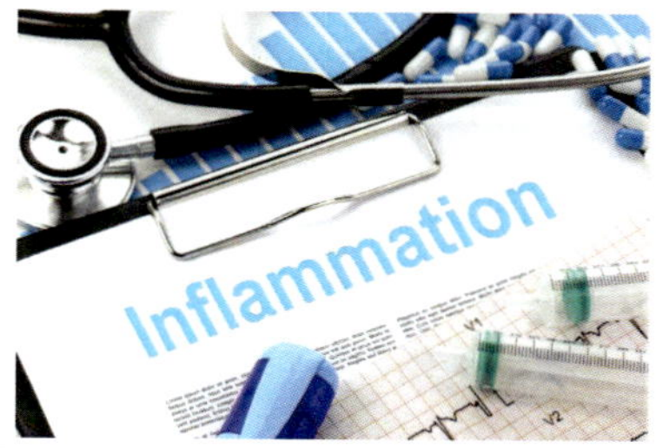
Omics Technologies	Advanced scientific methods used to study the various 'omics' layers (genomics, proteomics, metabolomics) to understand complex biological processes, especially in disease research.	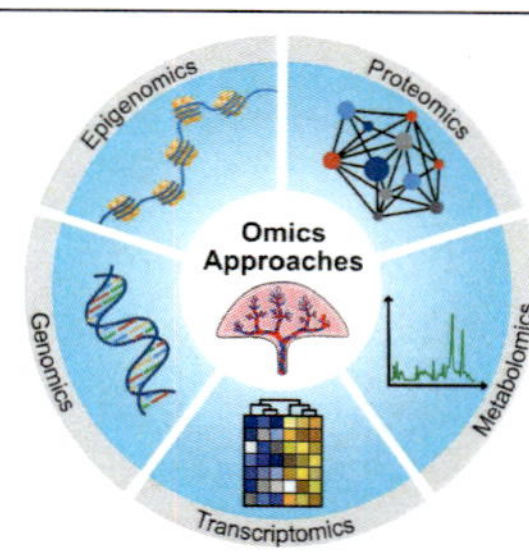
Renal Diseases	Disorders affecting the kidneys, including acute and chronic kidney disease, which impair the kidneys' ability to filter blood and maintain bodily homeostasis.	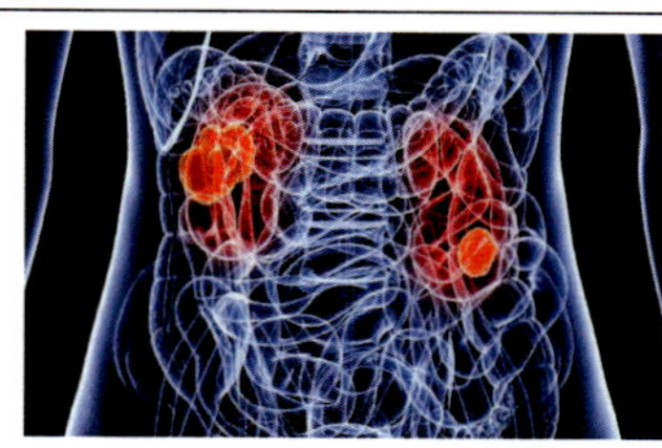
Gut Microbiota	The community of microorganisms living in the digestive tract, which plays a vital role in digestion, immunity, and overall health.	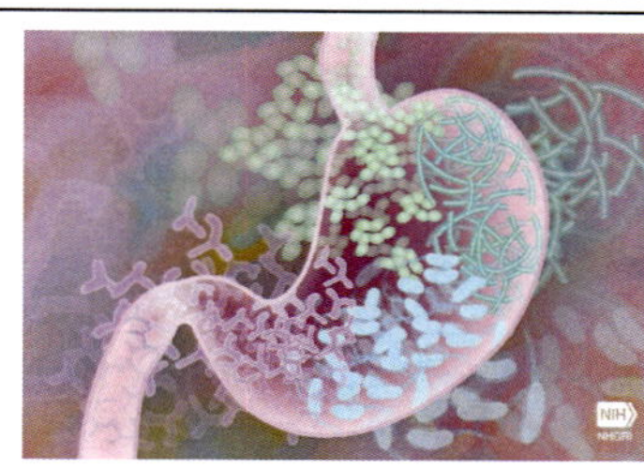

4.1. Chronic Kidney Disease: An Overview

Chronic kidney disease (CKD) is defined, according to KDIGO 2017 Clinical Practice Guideline Update for the Diagnosis, Evaluation, Prevention, and Treatment of Chronic Kidney Disease–Mineral and Bone Disorder (CKD-MBD), as "abnormalities of kidney structure or function, present for more than 3 months, with implications for health." CKD is classified based on pathological cause, glomerular filtration rate category (from G1, normal, to G5, kidney failure), and albuminuria category (from A1, <30 mg/g, to A3 > 300 mg/g). If it is not managed in such a way that addresses treatment of the underlying condition, diagnosis and treatment of the pathologic manifestations, and timely planning for long-term renal replacement therapy, it will inexorably lead to end-stage renal disease. The majority of cases of CKD are in stage 3, according to a recent systematic review and meta-analysis of observational studies. The prevalence of CKD is estimated to be between 11 and 13% worldwide. There are a multitude of risk factors that contribute to the complexity of CKD pathogenesis. These risk factors include genetic and epigenetic age, low birth weight, socioeconomic status, obesity, smoking and/or hypoxia, and vascular factors, which are induced by atherosclerosis, hypertension, and diabetes atherosclerosis. Furthermore, the complications of this disease have an impact that extends beyond the kidneys, with cardiovascular burden (including coronary artery disease, congestive heart failure, arrhythmias, and sudden cardiac death) being a significant mark. In addition, CKD is linked to an increased formation of atherosclerotic plaques. Other complications include endocrine dysfunctions, which involve hormones that control the balance of calcium and phosphate, as well as the metabolism of vitamin D, and consequently, bone mineralization defects. Patients undergoing hemodialysis are at an increased risk for cardiovascular complications. These complications include vascular overload, which can result in arterial stiffness, and ischemia, which can be induced by repeated episodes of hypovolemic hypoperfusion that occur during hemodialysis in a seemingly paradoxical manner (Figure 4.1).

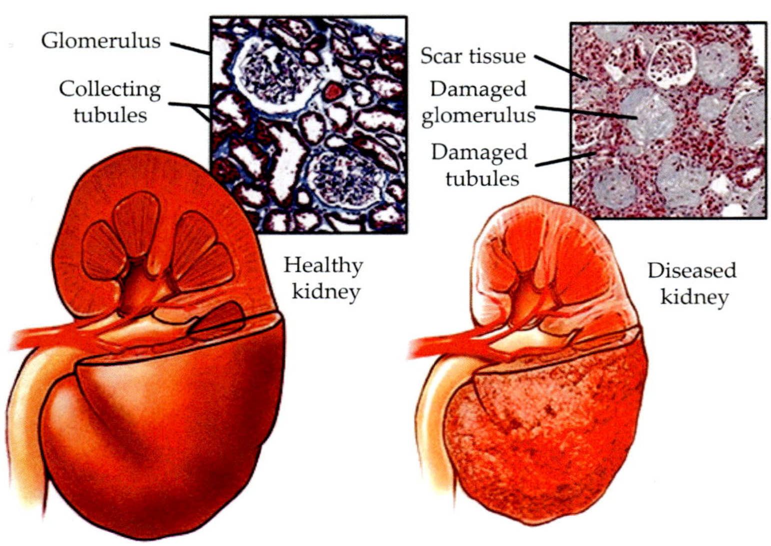

Figure 4.1. *Illustration of kidney disease.*

Source: mayoclinic.org/-/media/kcms/gbs/patient-consumer/images/2016/06/08/06/mcdc7_diseased_kidney-8col.jpg.

As inflammation has been recognized as an essential component of CKD since the late 1990s, it is now considered to be a well-established risk factor for this pathology, in addition to other renal pathologies. As a matter of fact, inflammation is now recognized as a significant factor in a variety of major pathologies, including neurodegeneration, CVD, and the progression and survival of cancer. Chronic systemic inflammation, which is also known as low-grade chronic inflammation, is characterized by a two- to threefold increase in the levels of circulating inflammatory mediators (including interleukins-1, 6 tumor necrosis factor, and their soluble receptors), a slow development, a persistent nature, and the presence of multiple factors of origin, and it can be difficult to identify at times. According to recent research, chronic systemic inflammation is linked to changes in the microbiota of the gut, which is constantly communicating with the immune system. This cross talk is necessary for the maintenance of a tolerant immune response toward commensal flora as well as the elimination of pathogens. A number of factors, including the production of toxic metabolites, excessive consumption of energy, and molecular mimicry of host proteins, contribute to the negative effects of intestinal dysbiosis on health. These factors extend beyond the environment of the intestinal tract. The purpose of this chapter is to present the most recent findings concerning chronic systemic inflammation and CKD, with a particular focus on the involvement of gut dysbiosis and the question of whether or not intervention on gut microbiota could be discovered to be beneficial for the outcome of this fatal disease.

4.2. An Update on Inflammation and Its Influence on the Progression of Chronic Kidney Disease

Inflammation that is persistent and of low grade is considered to be an essential component of CKD, as it plays a significant role in the development of mortality from all causes that is associated with renal disease. There has been a growing interest in the role that inflammation plays in CKD and end-stage renal disease (ESRD), which has resulted in a shift in the perception of inflammation as a risk factor for CKD morbidity and mortality that is no longer considered to be novel. A challenging theory regarding the direct effect of inflammation on the progression of CKD and CVD was developed with the assumption of association between markers of inflammation, changes in glomerular filtration rate (GFR), and nutrition habits in elderly individuals. It was discovered that an increase in the number of markers of inflammation and thrombosis was associated with a decline in renal function, which was characterized by changes in glomerular filtration rate (GFR), urea amount, and creatinine levels. CKD is a condition that accelerates premature aging through a variety of mechanisms in the internal milieu. These mechanisms include DNA damage, inflammation, low Klotho expression, redox perturbations, toxicity, and local signaling of growth factors. This speeding up of the aging process is independent of the genetic background of the individual. When the conditions are normal, it is common knowledge that the intrarenal vasculature is distributed in a heterogeneous manner, and that the medulla is the only part of the kidney that is affected by hypoxia. An onslaught of mediators, including hormones, autocoids, and vasoactive substances, such as medullipin, prostaglandins, endothelins, nitric oxide, angiotensin II, kinins, and adenosine, are involved in the complex processes that are involved in the bypassing of energy deprivation in the parts of the kidneys that have a deficiency in pO2 production (Figure 4.2).

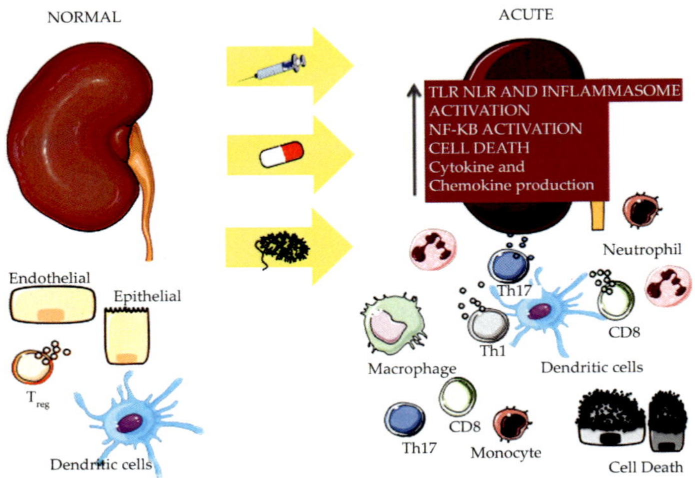

Figure 4.2. *Inflammation in renal diseases: New and old players.*

Source: https://www.frontiersin.org/files/Articles/452338/fphar-10-01192-HTML-r1/image_m/fphar-10-01192-g001.jpg.

A state of persistent inflammation has the potential to alter the microvascular feedback to its regulators. It also has the potential to activate the reaction of a variety of tubular toxins, including ROS, which can lead to additional renal failure. The highly reactive ROS have the potential to alter various structures and functional pathways within cells. As a consequence, a vicious circle is created, in which inflammatory cells are stimulated by cell damage caused by ROS, resulting in the emergence of a state of oxidative stress. The common oxidant "imbalance" theory has been remarkably completed with recent advancements regarding the cross talk between oxidants and antioxidants. The rationale behind antioxidant therapies is therefore based on the idea that they are able to repair the imbalances that exist in the redox environment of cells. There is a continuous enrichment of the old theory that proposes oxidative stress as a "unifying concept of CVD in uremia." Additionally, novel molecules that belong to the family of paraoxonases are being proposed as potential biomarkers. It is believed that paraoxonase-1 has a protective effect against lipoprotein oxidation, and the expression of this enzyme, which serves as a marker for antioxidant status, is decreased in patients with CKD. The development of specific redox proteomic techniques will make it easier to implement new preventative and therapeutic strategies in the fight against metabolic diseases such as atherosclerosis and other metabolic conditions.

There is a possibility that proteomic biomarkers could provide an accurate and earlier detection of renal pathology in comparison to the clinical markers that have been established for a long time. In some populations, the circulating creatinine levels fall into normal ranges despite the loss of more than 50% of renal function. As a result, additional biomarkers of renal function are desired. This is despite the fact that the "breaking point" could be different for each individual patient. According to the findings of recent research, CKD is characterized by a cross-talk between inflammation, bone, vasculature, and renal function. It was observed that there was an increase in the expression of a panel of proteomic biomarkers during the early stage 2 of CKD. These biomarkers include IL-6, TNF-α, osteoprotegerin, osteocalcin, osteopontin, and FGF-23. This observation, at first glance, highlights the hope of improving the management of patients with CKD beginning with the early stages. This is an area that will be the focus of research in the near future. Plasma levels of IL-1β, IL-1RA, IL-6, TNF-α, hs-CRP, and fibrinogen were found to be higher among participants with lower levels of estimated glomerular filtration rate (GFR) in another study that evaluated the association between kidney function, albuminuria, and biomarkers of inflammation in a large cohort of CKD patients. An additional finding was that patients with a lower estimated GFR and a higher urine albumin to creatinine ratio (UACR) had a higher inflammation score. According to these findings, biomarkers of inflammation were found to have a negative correlation with measurements of kidney function, while they had a positive correlation with albuminuria testing. Within the population of adolescents, it has been demonstrated that the erythrocyte sedimentation rate, which is a nonspecific measure of inflammation, can accurately predict the presence of end-stage renal disease. The level of the pro-inflammatory cytokine IL-2 was found to be higher in hemodialysis patients who experienced uremic pruritus, which is a common symptom that causes these patients a great deal of discomfort, when compared to hemodialysis patient controls who did not experience irritation. The findings that were obtained from a number of studies indicate that tumor necrosis factor-like weak inducer of apoptosis (TWEAK) plays a significant part in kidney injury that is associated with inflammation and that it promotes both acute and CKD. Several studies are currently being conducted to investigate the potential of various nanoconjugates to prevent TWEAK-induced cell death and inflammatory signaling in a variety of cell types, including renal tubular cells. When comparing patients with a pattern of high T-cell regulatory or anti-inflammatory parameters (IL-2, IL-4, IL-5, IL-12, CH50, and T-cell number) to those with a specific pattern of high pro-inflammatory cytokines (IL-1, IL-6, and TNF-α), the findings of a study that investigated hemodialysis patients revealed that the group of patients with a specific pattern of high pro-inflammatory cytokines had a higher mortality of compared to patients with a pattern of high T-cell regulatory or anti-inflammatory parameters.

With the availability of omics multiplex technology, there was the possibility of shifting the focus from the analysis of a single individual marker to the evaluation of cytokine panels. An inflammatory panel was described, which included pro-inflammatory cytokines such as IL-1, IL-6, and TNF-α, as well as anti-inflammatory cytokines such as IL-2, IL-4, IL-5, IL-12, and CH50. This panel was found to have a significant impact on the survival rate of CKD patients. Recent years have seen a significant increase in the amount of focus placed on the potential role that adipokines, including pro-inflammatory leptin, apelin, omentin, visfatin, resistin, and anti-inflammatory adiponectin, play in CKD. Leptin levels that are higher than normal have been shown to be associated with CKD, according to the findings of the National Health and Nutrition Examination Survey (NHANES). In addition, the expression of adiponectin was found to be significantly higher in patients with ESRD when compared to healthy individuals.

As a result of the fact that atherosclerosis is now considered to be a chronic inflammatory disease, CVD is a significant complication of CKD. Because of this, inflammation and CKD create a vicious cycle. Complex mechanisms that involve a cross talk between lymphocyte T helper type 1 and subendothelial macrophages as antigen presenting cells are responsible for the acceleration of atherosclerosis found in CKD. Alterations in lipid metabolism and the accumulation of plasma lipoproteins in the subendothelial space are the factors that set off this reactive cellular response. An inflammatory response is produced when lymphocytes that have been recruited locally react to autoantigens that are derived from the apolipoprotein B100 protein of LDL. The prevalence of inflammation is growing among patients with CKD who are undergoing pre-dialysis, and it is an important indicator of both the patient's current health and their potential future outcomes. The process of hemodialysis itself may be a contributor to the pro-inflammatory state that is associated with ESRD, and the various types of dialysis membranes may be responsible for determining an inflammatory response.

On the other hand, hemodialysis is not the only cause of inflammation on account of the fact that patients with CKD who are not undergoing hemodialysis already exhibit a certain inflammatory state. An ongoing inflammatory state in CKD is not only associated with cardiovascular complications, but it is also one of the primary contributors to the development of malnutrition and protein-energy wasting, which ultimately results in the malnutrition-inflammation-cachexia syndrome in patients with CKD and ESRD. It was also described that circulating levels of IL-1 and IL-6 could suppress the secretion of PTH in a group of patients who were undergoing dialysis. This, in turn, may be indicative of the malnutrition-inflammation-cachexia syndrome rather than the low bone turnover disease. Depending on factors such as racial or ethnic background, as well as genetic characteristics, the pathophysiology of inflammation may be completely different. The results of recent studies indicate that dietary habits may contribute a peculiar signature to the composition of the gut microbiota, and intestinal dysbiosis may therefore interfere with the inflammatory mechanisms in the population of people with CKD.

In conclusion, chronic low-grade inflammation has been identified as a significant component of the CKD scenario. It plays a significant role in the pathophysiology of the disease and has a significant impact on the complications that have been associated with it. On the other hand, additional research is required in order to determine the role that inflammation plays in the population of people with CKD, particularly in the early stages.

4.3. The Role That Inflammation Plays in the Progression of Cardiovascular Diseases in Chronic Kidney Disease

As a result of the fact that the early stages of CKD are significantly correlated with an increased risk of subsequent coronary heart disease, CVD is one of the primary factors that contributes to the poor prognosis of CKD. It has been established through a number of clinical studies that approximately 50% of patients who have CKD experience an increase in mortality as a consequence of cardiovascular complications. These complications include advanced calcific arterial and valvular disease. Despite this, the mechanisms that involve the accelerated calcification that occurs in CKD remain uncertain, and as a result, there are no specific therapies that have been developed to target the prevention of the disease.

The current guidelines for CKD recommend screening for vascular calcification (VC). This is due to the fact that VC is a cardiovascular risk factor, and it is associated with an increased risk of morbidity and mortality in the CKD group, culminating in CKD stage 5. It is now generally accepted that vascular calcification is an active process that involves a large number of proteins, which could serve as potential candidate markers. Numerous studies have shed light on a variety of circulating biomarkers that have been identified in individuals with CKD. These biomarkers have the potential to play significant roles in extra-skeletal calcification and mineral metabolism alterations, both of which are considered to be characteristics of CKD-mineral bone disorder (CKD-MBD). As a consequence of these findings, it has been established that CKD with myocardial infarction (CKD-MBD) is characterized by abnormalities in the laboratory and bone, as well as vascular calcification, and it has a negative impact on clinical outcomes. Nevertheless, these processes are interconnected, and it is necessary to investigate them in conjunction with CVDs.

However, cardiovascular calcification is an exceptional marker of chronic inflammatory status in CKD, and it has a strong correlation with morbidity and mortality. Confoundingly, CKD has been shown to hasten the progression of atherosclerosis, and it has also been demonstrated that CKD causes an increase in vascular inflammation and calcification. Recent developments have brought to light the possibility that matrix vesicles, which are secreted by macrophages, play a role as key molecules in alternative processes that are independent of osteogenic differentiation. Through the process of deciphering the association between these mechanisms and signaling pathways, it is possible that novel insights into the mechanistics of calcification will be brought about. Additionally, it is possible that new therapeutic strategies that target CVD in CKD will be developed. Taking into consideration the fact that several loci were linked to coronary arterial calcification, these findings are in agreement with the genetics, and it was demonstrated that 40% to 50% of cases of coronary calcification could be linked to genetic predisposition. The involvement of single polymorphisms located at the 9p21 locus, which is close to the cyclin genes, was proposed as a genetic mechanism of this pathology. The genes that are being discussed could be generally associated with cellular senescence and inflammation, although the precise DNA sequences that are responsible for this pathology are still unknown. Recent evidence suggests that the overlap between CKD and CVD is due, on the one hand, to the dynamic cross talk between these organs, which results in cardio-renal syndrome, which is becoming increasingly recognized. While on the other hand, it could be linked to the common etiologies of these major diseases (hypertension and diabetes mellitus), an increasing number of people are becoming aware of this phenomenon. At the same time, it has been investigated as a potential common disorder of the kidneys and the heart, in which acute or chronic dysfunction in one organ can cause acute or chronic dysfunction in the other organ. Despite this, a comprehensive picture of the mechanisms that are involved in these processes is still lacking. ROS, which stands for highly ROS, have the potential to disrupt a variety of structural and functional pathways within cells. As a result, the inflammatory cells are activated by the cell damage that is produced by ROS; consequently, a vicious circle of chronic disturbance is continuously perpetuated. The oxidant imbalance theory encompasses a number of significant pathways, and the cross-talk between oxidants and antioxidants has also been the subject of investigation in the context of cell metabolism. However, the hypothesis that antioxidant therapies could target and reconstruct the disturbances in the redox environment of cells is necessary for the purpose of understanding the role that oxidative stress plays in the pathogenesis of CKD. For the purpose of reducing oxidative stress in models of CKD and CVD, various therapeutic approaches have been considered. One of these approaches is to propose a low oxidant intake in various dietary approaches. As people get older, they experience an increase in oxidative stress and inflammation, and both of these conditions are linked to kidney failure in its early stages as well. In both the case of normal aging and CKD, there is evidence to suggest that a diet that is supplemented with oxidants may produce increased serum levels of oxidative stress and inflammatory mediators. The reduction of oxidative stress and inflammation in patients with CKD and in the elderly population with decreased kidney function is one of the novel therapeutic strategies that could be offered by dietary intervention, as reported.

As many inflammatory mediators, such as cytokines and immune cells, circulate in the body, it is tempting to hypothesise that the immune system might play important roles in organ interactions and might be responsible for mediating the reciprocal dysfunction that is observed in cardio-renal syndromes.

4.4. The Incorporation of Proteomics into Clinical Settings: The Role of Omics Technologies and the Clinical Significance of Proteomic Biomarkers in Renal Diseases

An increasing progression of omics approaches has occurred over the course of the past decade, accompanied by a remarkable improvement in methodologies and analytical instruments. This progression is based on the idea that a comprehensive characterization of a complex system, which provides novel perceptions into functional pathways and regulatory networks, could be deciphered within the framework of these omics. The access that scientists have to the data that they have experimentally observed regarding the fundamental biochemical and pathological mechanisms has been facilitated as a result of recent advancements in bioinformatics and biostatistics on platforms that are considered to be state-of-the-art. It is possible that proteomic biomarkers in kidney disease, along with traditional markers such as serum creatinine and urinary albumin, could be considered valuable tools in clinical diagnosis due to the fact that they have the potential to facilitate accurate clinical implementation. Furthermore, proteomic biomarkers may also be useful in determining which therapeutic targets are the most appropriate for a particular patient or disease setting.

This significant advancement was made possible by combining liquid chromatography and mass spectrometry, which made it possible to identify proteins without targeting specific proteins. In addition, capillary electrophoresis has also undergone a rapid development in recent years, and it is now capable of rapidly separating analytes in a manner that is highly reproducible. Additionally, the matrix-assisted laser desorption/ionization (MALDI) platform has pushed the boundaries further, allowing for the evaluation of tissue specimens with a high resolution in order to differentiate between individual cells. The use of this method has the potential to detect particular biomarkers and provide detailed information pertaining to CKD. Recent research indicates that MALDI has the potential to produce molecular signatures of both primary and secondary kidney injury. One particular signal, which has been identified as serine/threonine-protein kinase MRCK gamma, is found to be overexpressed in the glomeruli of primary membranous nephropathy. These findings have the potential to serve as future targets for the ongoing process of further stratification of these patients. Other research places an emphasis on the role that omics technologies, such as MALDI, play in the generation of molecular signatures that are able to differentiate between normal kidneys and pathological kidneys. These signatures include specific signals that could be indicators of the development of CKD. The Kidney and Urinary Pathway Knowledge Base is an open-source resource that encourages the exploration of multi-omics data and the generation of new in silico theories through the utilization of a novel approach that is founded on semantic web software. Furthermore, CKDdb is the most comprehensive molecular information resource regarding the characterization of CKD-related experiments and model systems. It has the potential to be useful in the design of disease models, thereby avoiding the challenges associated with the handling and integration of heterogeneous enormous data.

By identifying novel biomarkers that could improve, in real time, the early diagnostics, monitoring, and prognostics, the emerging knowledge that is generated by the application of omics (genomics, proteomics, and metabolomics) in major diseases, such as CKD, could provide new insights into the pathophysiology of the disease. As a result, omics will have a significant impact on the field of personalized medicine.

4.5. Gut Microbiota as a Source of Inflammation in CKD: A Bidirectional Relationship

As evidence has accumulated over the past few years, it has become clear that chronic inflammation is a nontraditional risk factor in the population of people with CKD. Furthermore, it has been discovered that the gastrointestinal tract is a significant contributor to the systemic inflammation that occurs in CKD. It is essential for the regulation of both local and systemic immunity, and the gut microbiota is responsible for maintaining the symbiotic relationship with the host under normal circumstances. However, in recent years, an imbalance in the gut microbiota has been linked to a number of diseases. Alterations in the functions or signaling pathways of the commensal flora have been found to contribute to the pathogenesis of a variety of diseases, including chronic inflammation and renal disorders. Additionally, bacterial DNA fragments from the gut have been found in the blood of patients who are undergoing chronic hemodialysis as well as those who are predialysis for CKD. The decisive role that the biochemical milieu plays in shaping the gut microbiota, in terms of structure, composition, and function, was also described. This milieu has the potential to promote a proinflammatory activity, and it also has the potential to restrict the beneficial effects that are offered by a microbiota that is in balance. These conditions could result in a change in status, which would target inflammation, uremic toxicity, and other complications that are present within patients with CKD. The interactions are bidirectional: on the one hand, uremia negatively interferes with the microbiota, altering the composition and metabolism and, on the other hand, the microbiota dysbiosis releases compounds that are normally excreted by the kidneys but could be considered as potential uremic toxins, both conditions further leading to a toxin avalanche exposure, due to the disruption of the epithelial barrier with an increased intestinal permeability, often referred to as "leaky gut," a condition that has been reported in CKD.

The condition known as uremia appears to compromise the function of the intestinal barrier and to promote inflammation throughout the entire gastrointestinal tract. In a prospective and observational study, the baseline concentration of indoxyl sulfate, a uremic toxin that has the potential to have predictive power in the progression of CKD, was investigated. Other uremic toxins, such as p-cresol sulfate and trimethylamine N-oxide, were evaluated in relation to kidney function (estimated GFR), and the findings led the researchers to the conclusion that elevated expression was associated with an increased risk for mortality from any cause in patients with experimentally induced ESRD. CKD and kidney failure are both conditions that can be accompanied by a condition known as uremia. Toxins that originated in the intestine or were introduced into the body through the intestine, such as glycation metabolites, phenols, and indoles, may all play significant roles in the pathophysiology of CKD. Consequently, because of this, it is biologically plausible, but not widely accepted, that the microbiota in the gut is a significant participant in the toxic scenario of CKD.

Understanding the composition, function, and homeostasis of the gut microbiota within each individual is necessary in order to decipher the role that the gut microbiota plays in the progression of CKD. Both Gram-negative Bacteroidetes and Gram-positive low-GC Firmicutes make up the majority of the gut microbiota, as was to be expected. The composition of the gut microbiota demonstrates significant variations, each of which represents a distinctive signature that is specific to the individual. When CKD is present, there is a correlation between gut dysbiosis and an increase in pathogenic flora in comparison to symbiotic flora. This, in conjunction with increased intestinal permeability, leads to an increase in the absorption of endotoxins, which can have detrimental effects on the organism. Both an increased inflammatory state and oxidative stress, which are constant features of advanced CKD and have a significant impact on its complications, have been correlated with the gut-derived uremic toxins. Additionally, an expanded permeability of the intestinal barrier has also been found to be associated with these toxins. There may be a connection between the dysbiotic intestinal microflora and the edema and ischemia of the intestinal wall, as well as a dysfunctional epithelial barrier in the colon. Several circulating metabolites that are derived from the metabolism of gut microbiota have been suggested to have a possible connection to the systemic immunoinflammatory response as well as kidney damage, according to recent evidence. It has been demonstrated that short-chain fatty acids, also known as SCFAs, are significant players in the modulation of immunity, blood pressure, glucose, and lipid metabolism. SCFAs are metabolites that are essentially derived from the fermentation of dietary fiber in the gut. In addition, short-chain fatty acids (SCFAs) have been shown to "modulate different cell signal transduction processes via G-protein–coupled receptors and act as epigenetic regulators by the inhibition of histone deacetylase and as potential mediators involved in the autophagy pathway." Despite the fact that they are controversial, SCFAs have the potential to be considered as potential therapeutic targets and appear to be the link between kidney damage and the inflammatory response. Inflammation of the gut is common in CKD, and it plays a role in systemic inflammation as a result of disruptions in the epithelial tight junction. This disruption causes endotoxin and bacterial translocation, and it is associated with a dysfunctional Nrf2 pathway. In a study that was carried out on rats, oral administration of Nrf2 activator was found to have reestablished the epithelial tight junction protein expression, thereby alleviating arterial hypertension and rehabilitating the markers of kidney function. This was based on the fact that Nrf2 is a protein that regulates the expression of antioxidant proteins that protect against oxidative damage that is caused by injury and inflammation.

In a nutshell, there is a growing body of evidence that suggests that dietary fiber has the potential to reverse gut dysbiosis and eliminate microinflammation. This finding is in agreement with epidemiological evidence that suggests correlations between higher dietary fiber intake, improved kidney function, and decreased inflammation, at least in the general population.

Numerous researchers are in agreement that enhancing the health of the intestines and reestablishing the integrity of the intestinal wall will be among the most significant objectives in the process of enhancing the quality of life of people who have CKD.

4.6. Restoring Microbiota Balance: The Exploration of Novel Therapeutic Avenues in Renal Diseases

Intestinal inflammation and dysbiosis of the gut microbiota are now recognized as important contributors in chronic inflammation and other complications associated with CKD. This provides an explanation for the novel gut-therapeutic avenues that are taken into consideration when designing interventions for CKD.

There are a variety of metabolites that are derived from microbiota dysbiosis that are engaged in distinct physiology pathways that are linked to renal dysfunction. The microbiota can be considered a recently discovered "organ," as it is involved in many pathological axes and is related to almost every organ, including the kidneys. Many studies have pointed out that there is a two-way connection between the microbiota in the gut and CKD. Additionally, the effect of CKD on the structure of the gut, which can then lead to dysbiosis (Figure 4.3), has also been mentioned. These enterotypes have a significant correlation with long-term diets, particularly the level of proteins and animal fats (Bacteroides) as opposed to carbohydrates (Prevotella). Bacteroides, Prevotella, and Ruminococcus are the bacterial groups that predominate in the abundance of specific bacterial groups in the gut microbiota of normal individuals. However, the gut microbiota of patients with CKD is altered, particularly with a decreased amount of Lactobacillaceae and Prevotellaceae families, as well as with an increased amount (more than 100 times higher) of Enterobacteria and Enterococci, which are species that are typically found in lower concentrations in healthy individuals. The "supplementary organ" has also an important contribution to digestion, using two different catabolic pathways: saccharolytic (fermentation), with a high prevalence of Bifidobacteria and Lactobacilli, having short-chain fatty acids as end products, and the second, proteolytic (putrefaction) pathway, involving some species within Clostridium, Bacteroides, Enterobacterium, Bifidobacterium, and Lactobacillus that leads to short or branched-chain fatty acids and other cometabolites, considered as microbial uremic toxins. Another controversial mechanism that has been linked to microbial dysbiosis in patients with CKD is the elevated secretion of urea from the gastrointestinal tract. This leads to significant amounts of ammonia, which in turn contributes to the disturbance in the commensal bacteria. As a result, targeting the composition of the gut microbiota could be a promising approach in the monitoring and follow-up of CKD. Since it is generally accepted that a microbiota that is in balance is primarily saccharolytic, it follows that diet plays a beneficial role in the process of modulating the composition of the microbiota that is found in the gut.

A special diet, such as the Mediterranean diet (detailed in Table 4.1), that is high in nondigestible carbohydrates and is subject to fermentation by the microbiota in the gut, and that contains low quantities of proteins or fats, is considered to be one of the most important mechanisms for maintaining the balance of the gut microbiota to be preserved. The dietary content and its metabolites, such as advanced glycated end products (AGEs), which are types of uremic toxin that are produced as a result of the glycation process, were also found to have the potential to have a close connection to CKD. Uremic toxin absorbents and inhibitors of AGEs or the receptor for AGEs are examples of promising therapeutic targets that are based on nutrition-based approaches. Additionally, certain types of amino acids, such as d-serine, or fatty acids, such as palmitate, have been discovered to be associated with the progression of CKD. However, these findings are preliminary, and additional research is required to confirm their effectiveness. Dietary interventions have the potential to improve the quality of life of patients with CKD, although the specific effects of these interventions on mortality, cardiovascular events, and ESRD are not yet fully understood. The importance of maintaining a healthy diet was established through the use of large retrospective cohort studies. These studies demonstrated that the mortality rate in patients undergoing penile dialysis who were under the supervision of a dietitian was reduced by 19% when compared to patients who were not receiving any dietary treatment. However, to demonstrate that this hypothesis is correct, randomized clinical trials are required. The conclusion that was reached is that nutritional care in the early stages of CKD could have a better prognosis on survival.

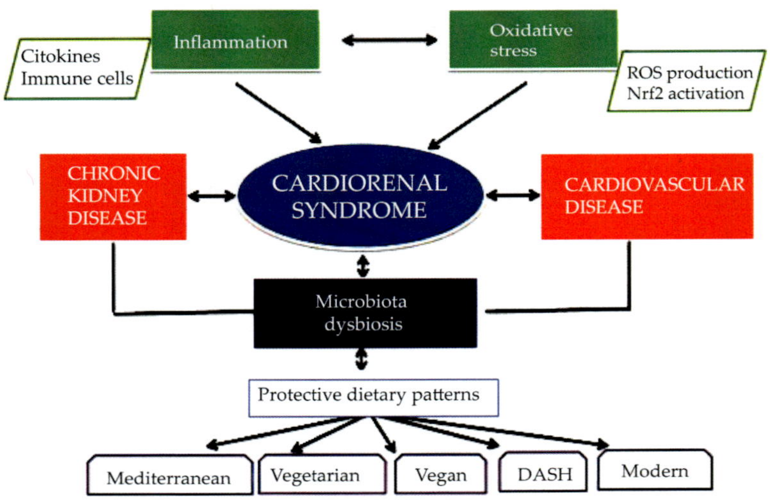

Figure 4.3. *The crosstalk between CKD and inflammation in correlation with microbiota dysbiosis modulation.*

Source: https://www.researchgate.net/figure/The-crosstalk-between-CKD-and-inflammation-in-correlation-with-microbiota-dysbiosis_fig1_323332634.

Table 4.1. *Different Dietary Patterns Assessed in Association with CKD*

Dietary Type	Diet Summary	Effects on CKD
Mediterranean diet	Carbohydrates, basically unrefined grains, fruits and vegetables, nuts, olive oil, fish, and a moderate consumption of red wine, dairy products, and red meats.	Protective: Potentially restoring microbiota balance, ameliorating CKD conditions, slow down disease progression.

Vegetarian diet	Fruits and vegetables, olive oil.	Additional Benefits: Reduce the burden of uremic toxins; attention must be paid to serum potassium levels.
Vegan diet	Fruits and vegetables, olive oil.	Positive: The addition of inulin modulates microbiota metabolism and the high fiber intake of vegan diet may have favorable effects on intestinal microbiota.
DASH diet	Consistent with a dietary approach to hypertension.	Protective: Decreased risk of rapid eGFR decline.
Modern dietary pattern.	High intake of fruit, soy milk, egg, milk, and deep-fried products.	Protective: Inversely associated with CKD.
Western diet	Excessively rich in protein and low in fruit and vegetables, grains, and fibers.	Detrimental: Increased risk of rapid eGFR decline.
Southern diet	Fried foods, organ meats, sweetened beverages Rice, pork, and vegetables, and low intake of wheat.	Detrimental: Independently associated with mortality in persons with CKD.
Modern dietary pattern, with increased cadmium intake.	High intake of fruit, soy milk, egg, milk, and deep-fried products, with cadmium contamination in parts of the food supply.	Detrimental: Directly associated with CKD.
DGA diet	Diet based on Dietary Guidelines for Americans (DGA)	Detrimental: Rapid kidney function decline.
DAL diet	Diet enriched in dietary acid load.	Detrimental: Increased risk of ESRD and mortality.

The administration of prebiotics and probiotics, as well as the combination of the two therapies into "synbiotic" preparations, is another area of potential beneficial therapies that could be utilized in patients with CKD.

"Probiotics" are defined as "live microorganisms that confer a health benefit on the host when administered in adequate amounts when they are administered in adequate amounts." *Bifidobacteria* species, *Lactobacilli*, and *Streptococci* are the two most common types of probiotic bacteria. Probiotics are made up of living bacteria that have the ability to alter the microbiota in the gut, which in turn can have an effect on the inflammatory status. A study conducted on mice revealed that treatment with *Lactobacillus acidophilus* could potentially reduce the development of atherosclerotic lesions in mice by lowering the levels of oxidative stress and the inflammatory response. This was discovered through the researchers' investigation of the mice. On the other hand, the optimal dose of the bacteria that is necessary to achieve an impeccable engraftment and the questions regarding whether or not these bacteria will be resistant in the uremic environment continue to be a matter of debate. The treatment with a proprietary formulation of S for a period of half a year was described in a multinational trial that included patients with CKD stages 3 and 4 of the thermophilus, *L. acidophilus*, as well as B. A significant decrease in the levels of urea nitrogen that are circulating in the blood has been induced by longum over, which has also resulted in an improvement in the quality of life scores of these patients. There is still a lack of clarity regarding whether the interventions that have been described have the potential to alter the integrity of the gut tight junction barrier; consequently, additional research is required to expand the knowledge in this particular field.

Moreover, prebiotics, which are specialized plant fibers that encourage the growth of beneficial bacteria in the digestive tract, play a significant part in preventing the progression of CKD. Candidates for the role of prebiotics include inulin, fructo-oligosaccharides, galacto-oligosaccharides, soya-oligosaccharides, xylo-oligosaccharides, and pyrodextrins. These prebiotics have the potential to stimulate the growth of *Bifidobacteria* and *Lactobacilli* species. Prebiotic oligofructose-enriched inulin, also known as p-inulin, has been shown to improve metabolic function, reduce inflammation, and also facilitate weight loss, according to recent research. Other prebiotic studies have described the role that supplements containing fructo-oligosaccharides and/or inulin play in modulating the microbiota in the gut, as well as the potential role that these supplements play here. There was a correlation between the supplementation of prebiotics with fructo-oligosaccharides and a decrease in proteolytic metabolites. This suggests that potential prebiotics like AXOS could significantly disrupt the ratio of protein to carbohydrates that are fermented, leading to changes in the profile of fermentation metabolites. However, the modifications that are related to the composition of the microbiota are still unknown.

Synbiotics are a dual approach that comprises combining a probiotic with a prebiotic. They have been the subject of a number of studies regarding their effectiveness. Synbiotics Easing Renal Failure by Improving Gut Microbiology Study was a single-center, double-blind, placebo-controlled, randomized cross-over trial that tested the effects of synbiotics in CKD patients who were in moderate to severe stages of the disease. In this study, preliminary findings indicated that the administration of synbiotic therapy did result in a significant reduction in the levels of nephrovascular uremic toxins that were circulating in the bloodstream. This was accompanied by a significant modification of the microbiome of the stool (particularly with an increase in *Bifidobacterium* and a deficiency of *Ruminococcaceae*) in patients with CKD who were not receiving antibiotics. Both indoxyl sulfate and p-cresyl sulfate, which are important uremic nephrovascular toxins, are released as a result of the alteration of the gut microbiota that occurs in CKD. Emerging evidence suggests that the modulation of the gut microbiota through the consumption of pre- and/or probiotics as a dietary supplement may play a significant role in the prevention of the production of key nephrovascular toxins.

In light of the fact that all of these preparations have the potential to alter the expression of uremic toxin and also to delay the progression of CKD, the investigation of these novel therapeutic avenues may provide essential insights into this nutritional therapy that is not offensive.

4.7. Summary

Persistent, low-grade inflammation has recently been accepted as a potential hallmark of CKD. This inflammation plays an essential role in the pathophysiology of CKD and is also involved in the cardiovascular complications and poor prognosis that these patients experience for all causes. The perception of inflammation as a risk factor for CKD morbidity and mortality has shifted as a result of the increasing interest in the role that inflammation plays in CKD and ESRD. This shift has resulted in the perception of inflammation as no longer being a new risk factor.

As a result of the development of proteomics, genomics, and other omics, as well as the advancements in state-of-the-art technologies for the identification of novel biomarkers in renal diseases, the growing body of evidence concerning the close relationship between inflammation and kidney function has become pathophysiologically relevant in patients who have CKD. The complex mechanisms that are involved in the development and progression of CKD would necessitate the evaluation of a panel of biomarkers rather than a single marker to enhance all of the different types of alterations that are characteristic of such a complicated and sneaky disease.

Recently, a number of novel interventions have been proposed with the intention of targeting inflammation in CKD. It appears that in the not too distant future, the conventional biomarkers may be able to be proficiently improved or even replaced with novel ones. However, to confirm their efficacy, sensitivity, and specificity, it will undoubtedly be necessary to conduct clinical trials that are randomized, controlled, and adequately interventional.

There is a growing body of evidence suggesting that the microbiota in the gut can be regarded as a recently discovered "organ," as it is involved in various pathological axes and is related to almost every organ, including the kidneys. A number of recent discoveries suggest that gut dysbiosis is associated with unanticipated health risks. Within the context of renal diseases, the gut-kidney axis has established itself as a novel therapeutic avenue that has a great deal of potential in the near future. There is a growing body of evidence that suggests a possible connection between dysbiosis and a wide variety of diseases. However, the imbalance of the gut microbiota represents the plausible missing link between nutrition and health, with a particular emphasis on CKD. The prognosis of CKD, as well as the high risk of cardiovascular complications, uremic toxicity, and inflammation, have all been linked to changes in the microbiota of the gut and a wide variety of responses from the host. In CKD, there is a vicious circle in which, on the one hand, toxic gut microbiota metabolites are the major circulating uremic toxins, and on the other hand, their aggregation deteriorates gut dysbiosis and promotes the progression of CKD.

This innovative and promising field of research may, in the not-too-distant future, will lead to the development of remarkably personalized nutritional procedures, with the goal of designing the most convenient dietary strategy for each individual.

A Closer Look

Renal Diseases

Renal diseases, encompassing a range of conditions that impair kidney function, are a critical global health concern affecting millions worldwide. Kidneys play a pivotal role in maintaining overall health by filtering waste, balancing electrolytes, and regulating blood pressure through hormonal control. When kidney function is compromised, either acutely or chronically, it can lead to a spectrum of diseases such as acute kidney injury (AKI), chronic kidney disease (CKD), and end-stage renal disease (ESRD).

Chronic Kidney Disease (CKD) is the most prevalent form of kidney dysfunction, characterized by a gradual decline in kidney function over time. Causes of CKD are multifaceted, including diabetes, hypertension, glomerulonephritis, and genetic conditions like polycystic kidney disease. CKD progresses in stages, and without timely intervention, it can advance to ESRD, requiring dialysis or kidney transplantation. Regular monitoring, through serum creatinine levels and glomerular filtration rate (GFR), enables early detection and management. Treatment often involves lifestyle changes, medication to manage blood pressure, and interventions to control diabetes or hyperlipidemia, all aimed at slowing disease progression.

Acute Kidney Injury (AKI), in contrast, is a sudden decline in kidney function often triggered by events like severe infections, drug toxicity, or physical trauma. AKI can frequently be reversible if treated promptly; however, it is also a significant risk factor for CKD if left untreated. Key challenges in AKI management include rapid identification of the underlying cause, prevention of further kidney damage, and ensuring adequate hydration and electrolyte balance.

Innovative Research and Treatment Advances in renal diseases have provided new insights. Recently, regenerative medicine approaches like stem cell therapy and renal tissue engineering have shown promise in promoting kidney regeneration. Furthermore, artificial intelligence in nephrology assists in predicting disease progression, identifying risk factors, and optimizing treatment plans. Additionally, immunotherapy and gene editing for genetic renal diseases are under investigation, holding the potential to transform the renal disease treatment landscape. As renal disease prevalence continues to rise, ongoing research and personalized medicine approaches remain essential in advancing patient outcomes.

References

1. Ainsworth, B. E., Haskell, W., Leon, A., David, D. R., Jacobs, J., Montoye, H., Sallis, J. F., et al., (1993). Compendium of physical activities: classification of energy costs of human physical activities. *Med Sci Sport Exerc. 25,* 71–80.

2. Alberti, K. G. M. M., Eckel, R. H., Grundy, S. M., Zimmet, P. Z., Cleeman, J. I., Donato, K. A., et al., (2009). Harmonizing the metabolic syndrome: A Joint Interim Statement of the International Diabetes Federation Task Force on Epidemiology and Prevention; National Heart, Lung, and Blood Institute; American Heart Association; World Heart Federation; International Atherosclerosis Society; and International Association for the Study of Obesity. *Circulation. 120,* 1640–5.

3. Beltrán-Sánchez, H., Harhay, M. O., Harhay, M. M., & McElligott, S., (2013). Prevalence and trends of metabolic syndrome in the adult US population, 1999–2010. *J Am Coll Cardiol. 62,* 697–703.

4. Brenner, H., Gefeller, O., & Greenland, S., (1993). Risk and rate advancement periods as measures of exposure impact on the occurrence of chronic diseases. *Epidemiology. 4,* 229–236.

5. Bruno, G., Merletti, F., Biggeri, A., Bargero, G., Ferrero, S., Runzo, C., et al., (2004). Metabolic syndrome as a predictor of all-cause and cardiovascular mortality in type 2 diabetes The Casale Monferrato Study. *Diabetes Care. 27,* 2689–94.

6. Discacciati, A., Andrea, B., Nicola, O., & Sander, G., (2016). On the interpretation of risk and rate advancement periods. *Int J Epidemiol. 45,* 278–284.

7. Dun, Y., Thomas, R. J., Smith, J. R., Medina-Inojosa, J. R., Squires, R. W., Bonikowske, A. R., et al., (2019). High-intensity interval training improves metabolic syndrome and body composition in outpatient cardiac rehabilitation patients with myocardial infarction. *Cardiovasc Diabetol. 18,* 104.

8. Elosua, R., Garcia, M., Aguilar, A., Molina, L., Covas, M. I. M., & Marrugat, J., (2000). Validation of the Minnesota leisure time physical activity questionnaire in Spanish women. *Med Sci Sport Exerc. 32,* 1431–7.

9. Elosua, R., Marrugat, J., Molina, L., Pons, S., & Pujol, E., (1994). Validation of the Minnesota leisure time physical activity questionnaire in Spanish men. *Am J Epidemiol. 139,* 1197–209.

10. Estruch, R., Martínez-González, M. A., Corella, D., Salas-Salvadó, J., Ruiz-Gutiérrez, V., Covas, M. I., et al., (2006). Effects of a Mediterranean-style diet on cardiovascular risk factors a randomized trial. *Ann Intern Med. 145,* 1–11.

11. Expert Panel on Detection. (2001). Evaluation and T of HBC in an Executive summary of the third report of the National Cholesterol Education Program (NCEP) expert panel on detection, evaluation, and treatment of high blood cholesterol in adults (adult treatment panel III). *JAMA. 285,* 2486–2497.

12. Ford, E. S., (2005). Risks for all-cause mortality, cardiovascular disease, and diabetes associated with the metabolic syndrome: A summary of the evidence. *Diabetes Care. 28,* 1769–1778.

13. Galassi, A., Reynolds, K., & He, J., (2006). Metabolic syndrome and risk of cardiovascular disease: a meta-analysis. *Am J Med. 119,* 812–819.

14. Gami, A. S., Witt, B. J., Howard, D. E., Erwin, P. J., Gami, L. A., Somers, V. K., et al., (2007). Metabolic syndrome and risk of incident cardiovascular events and death. A systematic review and meta-analysis of longitudinal studies. *J Am Coll Cardiol. 49,* 403–414.

15. Grundy, S. M., Cleeman, J. I., Daniels, S. R., Donato, K. A., Eckel, R. H., Franklin, B. A., et al., (2005). Diagnosis and management of the metabolic syndrome: An American Heart Association/National Heart, Lung, and Blood Institute scientific statement. *Circulation. 112,* 2735–52.

16. Guallar-Castillón, P., Pérez, R. F., López García, E., León-Muñoz, L. M., Aguilera, M. T., Graciani, A., et al., (2014). Magnitude and Management of Metabolic Syndrome in Spain in 2008–2010: The ENRICA Study [magnitud y manejo del síndrome metabólico en España en 2008–2010: Estudio ENRICA]. *Rev Esp Cardiol. 67,* 367–373.

17. Inchiostro, S., Fadini, G. P., de Kreutzenberg, S. V., Citroni, N., & Avogaro, A., (2007). Is the metabolic syndrome a cardiovascular risk factor beyond its specific components? *J Am Coll Cardiol. 49,* 2465.

18. Isomaa, B. O., Almgren, P., Tuomi, T., BjoB, Forsén, B., Lahti, K., et al., (2001). Cardiovascular Morbidity and Mortality Associated With the Metabolic Syndrome. *Diabetes Care. 24,* 683–9.

19. Ju, S. Y., Lee, J. Y., & Kim, D. H., (2017). Association of metabolic syndrome and its components with all-cause and cardiovascular mortality in the elderly. *Medicine (Baltimore). 96,* e8491.

20. Kazlauskiene, L., Butnoriene, J., & Norkus, A., (2015). Metabolic syndrome related to cardiovascular events in a 10-year prospective study. *Diabetol Metab Syndr. 7,*102.

21. Kim, G., Lee S-E, Jun, J. E., Lee Y-B, Ahn, J., Bae, J. C., et al., (2018). Increase in relative skeletal muscle mass over time and its inverse association with metabolic syndrome development: a 7-year retrospective cohort study. *Cardiovasc Diabetol. 17,* 23.

22. Klein, B. E. K., Klein, R., & Lee, K. E., (2002). Components of the metabolic syndrome and risk of cardiovascular disease and diabetes in Beaver Dam. *Diabetes Care. 25,* 1790–4.

23. Kyu, H. H., Abate, D., Abate, K. H., Abay, S. M., Abbafati, C., Abbasi, N., et al., (2018). Global, regional, and national disability-adjusted life-years (DALYs) for 359 diseases and injuries and healthy life expectancy (HALE) for 195 countries and territories, 1990–2017: A systematic analysis for the Global Burden of Disease Study 2017. *Lancet. 392,* 1859–922.

24. Lawlor, D. A., Smith, G. D., & Ebrahim, S., (2006). Does the new International Diabetes Federation definition of the metabolic syndrome predict CHD any more strongly than older definitions? Findings from the British Women's Heart and Health Study. *Diabetologia. 49,* 41–48.

25. Li, G., Esangbedo, I. C., Xu, L., Fu, J., Li, L., Feng, D., et al., (2018). Childhood retinol-binding protein. 4(RBP4) levels predicting the 10-year risk of insulin resistance and metabolic syndrome: the BCAMS study. *Cardiovasc Diabetol. 17,* 69.

26. Liese, A. D., Hense, H.-W., Brenner, H., Löwel, H., & Keil, U., (2000). Assessing the impact of classical risk factors on myocardial infarction by rate advancement periods. *Am J Epidemiol. 152,* 884–888.

27. Lohman, G. T., Roche, A. F., & Martorell, R., (1988).Anthropometric standardization reference manual. Champaign, IL: Human Kinetics Books.

28. Martínez-González, M. A., Gea, A., Ruiz-Canela, M., (2019). The Mediterranean diet and cardiovascular health. *Circ Res. 124,* 779–798.

29. Martínez-Larrad, M. T., Fernández-Pérez, C., Corbatón-Anchuelo, A., Gabriel, R., Lorenzo, C., Serrano-Ríos, M., (2011). Revised waist circumference cut-off points for the criteria of abdominal obesity in the Spanish population: Multicenter nationwide Spanish population based study. *Av en Diabetol. 27,* 168–174.

30. McNeill, A. M., Rosamond, W. D., Girman, C. J., Golden, S. H., Schmidt, M. I., East, H. E., et al., (2005). The metabolic syndrome and 11-year risk of incident cardiovascular disease in the atherosclerosis risk in communities study. *Diabetes Care. 28,* 385–390.

31. Ministry of Health, Social Services and Equality. (2015). Annual Report on the National Health System of Spain. Ministry of Health, Social Services and Equality. https://www.mscbs.gob.es (accessed on 29 May 2020).

32. Moreno-Iribas, C., Sayon-Orea, C., Delfrade, J., Ardanaz, E., Gorricho, J., Burgui, R., et al., (2017). Validity of type 2 diabetes diagnosis in a population-based electronic health record database. *BMC Med Inform Decis Mak. 17,* 34.

33. Mottillo, S., Filion, K. B., Genest, J., Joseph, L., Pilote, L., Poirier, P., et al., (2010). The metabolic syndrome and cardiovascular risk: A systematic review and meta-analysis. *J Am Coll Cardiol. 56,* 1113–32.

34. Mozaffarian, D., Hao, T., Rimm, E. B., Willett, W. C., & Hu, F. B., (2011). Changes in diet and lifestyle and long-term weight gain in women and men. *N Engl J Med. 364,* 2392–404.

35. Nanri, A., Miyaji, N., Kochi, T., Eguchi, M., Kabe, I., & Mizoue, T., (2020). Eating speed and risk of metabolic syndrome among Japanese workers: the Furukawa Nutrition and Health Study. *Nutrition. 78,* 110962.

36. O'Neill, S., O'Driscoll, L., (2015). Metabolic syndrome: a closer look at the growing epidemic and its associated pathologies. *Obes Rev. 16,* 1–12.

37. Richter-Stretton, G. L., Fenning, A. S., & Vella, R. K., (2020). Skeletal muscle—a bystander or influencer of metabolic syndrome? *Diabetes Metab Syndr Clin Res Rev. 14,* 867–875.

38. Roth, G. A., Abate, D., Abate, K. H., Abay, S. M., Abbafati, C., et al., (2018). Global, regional, and national age-sex-specific mortality for 282 causes of death in 195 countries and territories, 1980–2017: a systematic analysis for the Global Burden of Disease Study 2017. *Lancet. 392,* 1736–1788.

39. Royston, P., & Lambert, P. C., (2011). Flexible parametric survival analysis using stata: beyond the cox model. 1st ed. College Station, TX: Stata Press.

40. Sattar, N., McConnachie, A., Shaper, A. G., Blauw, G. J., Buckley, B. M., de Craen, A. J., et al., (2008). Can metabolic syndrome usefully predict cardiovascular disease and diabetes? Outcome data from two prospective studies. *Lancet. 371,* 1927–35.

41. Sayon-Orea, C., Moreno-Iribas, C., Delfrade, J., Sanchez-Echenique, M., Amiano, P., Ardanaz, E., et al., (2020). Inverse-probability weighting and multiple imputation for evaluating selection bias in the estimation of childhood obesity prevalence using data from electronic health records. *BMC Med Inform Decis Mak. 20,* 9.

42. Schröder, H., Fitó, M., Estruch, R., Martínez-González, M. A., Corella, D., Salas-Salvadó, J., et al.,

(2011). A short screener is valid for assessing Mediterranean diet adherence among older spanish men and women. *J Nutr. 141,* 1140–5.

43. Simmons, R. K., Alberti KGMM, Gale, E. A. M., Colagiuri, S., Tuomilehto, J., Qiao, Q., et al., (2010). The metabolic syndrome: Useful concept or clinical tool? Report of a WHO expert consultation. *Diabetologia. 53,* 600–5.
44. Tanaka, M., Okada, H., Hashimoto, Y., Kumagai, M., Nishimura, H., & Fukui, M., (2020). Trunk muscle quality and quantity predict the development of metabolic syndrome and the increase in the number of its components in individuals without metabolic syndrome. *Nutr Metab Cardiovasc Dis. 30,* 1161–8.
45. Tenenbaum, A., & Fisman, E. Z., (2011). "The metabolic syndrome... is dead": These reports are an exaggeration. *Cardiovasc Diabetol. 10,* 11.
46. van Herpt, T. T. W., Dehghan, A., Hoek, M., Ikram, M. A., Hofman, A., Sijbrands, E. J. G. G., et al., (2016). The clinical value of metabolic syndrome and risks of cardiometabolic events and mortality in the elderly: the Rotterdam study. *Cardiovasc Diabetol. 15,* 69.
47. Viñes, J. J., Díez, J., Guembe, M. J., González, P., Amézqueta, C., Barba, J., et al., (2007). Estudio de Riesgo Vascular en Navarra: Objetivos y Diseño. Prevalencia del Síndrome Metabólico y de los Factores Mayores de Riesgo Vascular [Study of Vascular Risk in Navarre: Objectives and Design. Prevalence of Metabolic Syndrome and of Vascular Risk Factors]. *An Sist Sanit Navar. 30,* 113–124.
48. Wilkins, E., Wilson, L., Wickramasinghe, K., Bhatnagar, P., Leal, J., Luengo-Fernandez, R., et al., (2017). European Cardiovascular Disease Statistics 2017. Brussels: European Heart Network, https://researchportal.bath.ac.uk/en/publications/european-cardiovascular-disease-statistics-2017. Accessed 1 March 2020.
49. WONCA International Classification Committee. (1999). ICPC-2. International Classification of Primary Care. Second Edition. Barcelona: Masson.
50. World Health Organization (1999). Definition, Diagnosis and Classification of Diabetes Mellitus and its Complications. Report of a WHO Consultation. Part, 1, Diagnosis and Classification of Diabetes Mellitus. World Health Organization. https://apps.who.int/iris/handle/10665/66040. Accessed 1 May 2020.
51. Younis, A., Younis, A., Tzur, B., Peled, Y., Shlomo, N., Goldenberg, I., et al., (2016). Metabolic syndrome is independently associated with increased 20-year mortality in patients with stable coronary artery disease. *Cardiovasc Diabetol. 15,* 149.

Chapter

DISEASES OF THE GASTROINTESTINAL SYSTEM

5

Contents

Introduction

Gastrointestinal diseases in tropical regions constitute a significant public health challenge, exacerbated by factors such as climate, sanitation, and dietary practices. According to Smith & Johnson (2018), these conditions predominantly affect the digestive tract, including vital organs such as the stomach, intestines, liver, and pancreas, leading to a wide array of symptoms and health complications. Diarrhea, identified by Gupta et al. (2019) as one of the most prevalent symptoms, poses a particularly severe risk of dehydration and nutrient loss, notably in vulnerable populations like young children and the elderly. The etiology of diarrhea encompasses a diverse range of pathogens, including bacteria, viruses, and parasites, thriving in the humid and warm climates characteristic of tropical regions (Brown, 2020).

Abdominal pain, as highlighted by Martinez & Rivera (2021), is another common manifestation of gastrointestinal diseases resulting from infections, inflammations, or obstructions within the digestive system. The impact of abdominal pain ranges from mild discomfort to debilitating cramps, severely affecting individuals' quality of life (Chen & Kumar, 2022). Furthermore, abnormal abdominal weight gain can indicate serious underlying conditions such as liver disease or intestinal blockage, with the potential to lead to ascites, primarily associated with liver cirrhosis or heart failure (Wilson et al., 2018).

Intestinal blockage represents a critical concern within this spectrum of diseases, caused by factors like foreign bodies, tumors, or severe constipation, impeding the normal digestive processes and presenting symptoms like severe abdominal pain and vomiting (Singh & Patel, 2019). Another significant syndrome is gastrointestinal lacrimation, which involves the excessive secretion of fluids by the gastrointestinal tract, leading to potential dehydration and electrolyte imbalance (Diaz & Lopez, 2017). This condition typically responds to gastrointestinal tract irritation or infection, necessitating immediate medical intervention to mitigate serious health implications.

The case of cholera, as discussed by Thompson & Sanders (2020), exemplifies the severe impact of waterborne diseases prevalent in tropical regions. Caused by the bacterium *Vibrio cholerae*, cholera can result in acute diarrhea and dehydration, posing a life-threatening risk without prompt treatment. This underscores the critical need for improved access to clean water and sanitation, alongside effective public health strategies to combat gastrointestinal diseases in these climates.

In conclusion, addressing the challenges posed by gastrointestinal diseases in tropical regions demands an integrated approach. As advocated by experts like Smith & Johnson (2018); Gupta et al. (2019); and Thompson & Sanders (2020), efforts must focus on enhancing sanitation, ensuring access to clean water, educating the public on health practices, and expanding medical care availability to mitigate the widespread impact of these conditions.

Orientation and Directional Terms

Term	Definition	Illustration
Diarrhea	A condition characterized by frequent, loose, or watery stools, often due to infection, food intolerance, or gastrointestinal disorders.	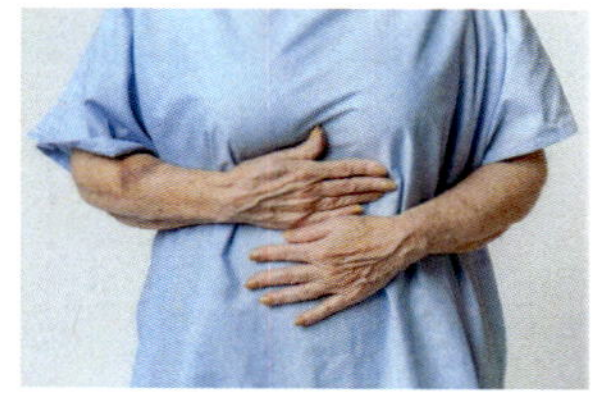
Esophagus	A muscular tube connecting the throat to the stomach, responsible for transporting swallowed food and liquids.	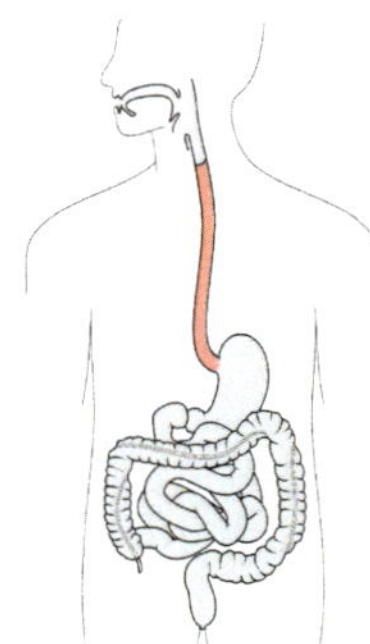
Antibiotics	Medications that kill or inhibit the growth of bacteria, used to treat bacterial infections.	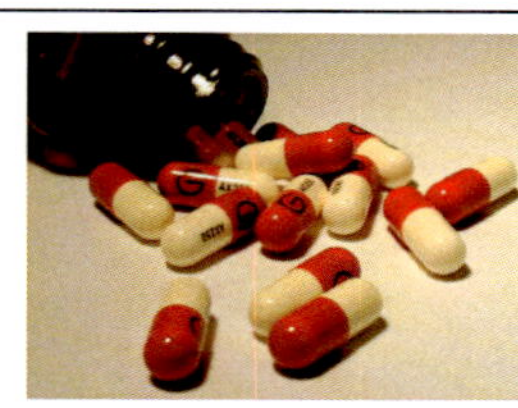
Small Bowel	The part of the gastrointestinal tract between the stomach and the large intestine, responsible for nutrient absorption and digestion.	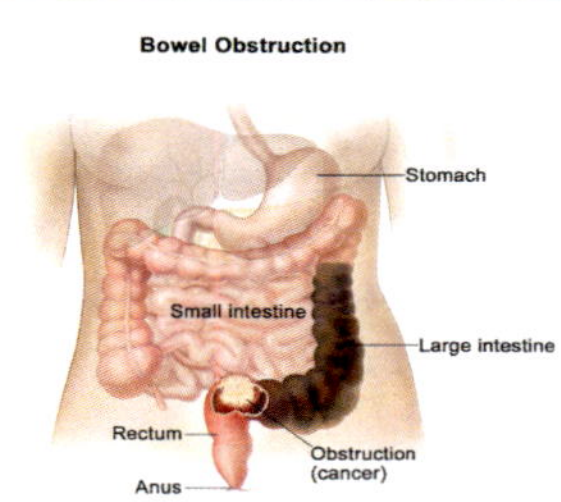
Antimicrobial Agents	Substances that kill or inhibit the growth of microorganisms, including bacteria, fungi, and viruses.	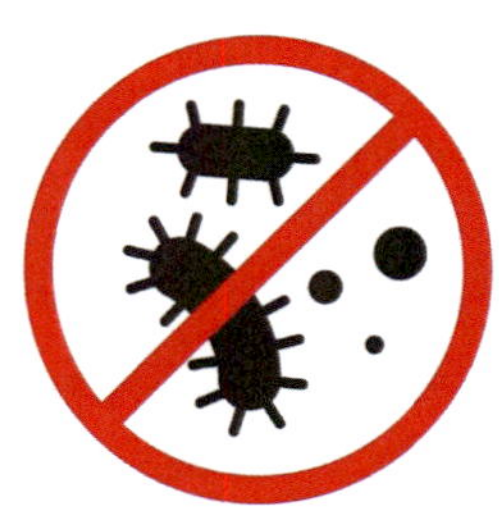

5.1. Diarrhea

Diarrheal diseases are a significant contributor to illness and death in tropical and subtropical regions. Diarrhea primarily affects children, resulting in 1.8 million deaths annually among children under the age of five. Dehydration is the primary factor leading to mortality, while malnutrition is the primary factor contributing to illness.

5.1.1. The Etiology and Distribution

Rotavirus is the predominant etiological agent responsible for the exacerbation of diarrhea in infants and young children on a global scale. Norovirus is identified as the second most prevalent etiological agent of viral gastroenteritis. Enterotoxigenic *Escherichia coli* (ETEC) is the predominant bacterial pathogen that impacts both indigenous inhabitants and tourists in developing nations. *Salmonella* is a prevalent etiological agent of foodborne illnesses in developed nations, with varying occurrences documented in tropical regions. The species *Campylobacter* and *Shigella*. These pathogens exhibit a global distribution and are prevalent etiological agents of infectious diarrheal diseases across various age cohorts. E. The dysenteric illness caused by *E. coli* O157 bears a striking resemblance to shigellosis. Cholera continues to be prevalent in numerous regions across Africa, Asia, as well as Central and South America.

5.1.2. Transmission and Epidemiology

The transmission of infection takes place through the consumption of microorganisms present in food and water that have been contaminated by fecal matter originating from either a human or an animal. The presence of this contamination is linked to insufficient public sanitation and subpar levels of personal hygiene. The occurrence of defecation in close proximity to pools and streams, which serve as water sources for domestic purposes, is a prevalent phenomenon. Additionally, rudimentary sewage disposal systems frequently release fecal matter into the community's domestic water supply. Infection can also be transmitted through person-to-person contact. The transmission of gastroenteritis-causing viruses, *Vibrio cholerae* and *V. parahaemolyticus*, is facilitated by seafood, such as shellfish, mussels, and crabs. Bacteria are transmitted by flies through various routes, including feces, mouthparts, and legs. Inadequate kitchen hygiene standards in both residential and public dining settings also promote the spread of intestinal infections. The prolonged heating of precooked food has the potential to transmit various gut pathogens and contain enterotoxin produced by staphylococci that thrive in warm food. The consumption of poultry and eggs constitutes significant reservoirs of nontyphoidal salmonellae and campylobacter. Bottle-feeding with powdered milk solution instead of breastfeeding is a significant and preventable cause of intestinal infection in infants. The presence of unsterile bottles, nipples, and contaminated water significantly increases the likelihood of acquiring a gut infection.

5.1.3. Pathogenesis

Diarrhea is characterized by an elevation in the moisture content of fecal matter. From a physiological standpoint, the potential causes of this condition can be attributed to several factors. Firstly, the small intestine may secrete a greater amount of fluid than it is able to reabsorb. Secondly, the absorption of solutes in the small intestine may be hindered, resulting in the retention of fluid in the gut lumen due to impaired osmotic load. Thirdly, the volume of fluid entering the colon may surpass its capacity for water absorption. Fourthly, the colon's ability to reabsorb water and electrolytes may be diminished due to enterotoxigenic infections like cholera. Lastly, the water-reabsorbing capacity and motility of the colon may be altered due to localized or generalized inflammation and ulceration. Diarrhea is induced by infectious agents through the induction of one or more of the following effects. Bacteria that produce enterotoxins encompass *V. cholerae* and enterotoxigenic E. Gram-negative bacteria such as *E. coli*, *Staphylococcus aureus*, *Shigella*, and *Salmonella* spp. *Shigella*, *Salmonella*, and *Campylobacter* spp. are examples of enteroinvasive bacteria.

5.2. The Clinical Manifestations

The onset of symptoms can exhibit a range of durations, spanning from a few hours following the consumption of food containing preformed toxins to several days following the ingestion of bacterial pathogens and potentially extending to two or more weeks in cases of parasitic infections. The classification of acute infectious diarrhea encompasses two main types: watery diarrhea and bloody diarrhea, also known as dysentery (Box 5.1).

Noninfectious factors contributing to acute diarrhea are less prevalent in tropical regions. However, it is important to take into account causes such as toxin-induced diarrhea (e.g., organophosphate poisoning), medication-related diarrhea, and ischemic colitis. The primary physical indicators to be obtained pertain to the evaluation of hydration (Box 5.2); it is advisable to measure the patient's weight upon initial presentation, as any changes in weight can serve as a valuable indicator of the efficacy of rehydration (Figure 5.1).

Causes of Acute Infectious Diarrhea

- Intoxication
  - Staphylococcus aureus
  - Clostridium perfringens
  - Bacillus cereus
  - Botulism (uncommon)
- Infection
  - Viruses
  - Rotaviruses
  - Noroviruses
  - Enteric adenoviruses
  - Coronaviruses
- Bacteria
  - Escherichia coli (enterotoxigenic, enteropathogenic, enteroadherent, enterohemorrhagic, enteroinvasive)
  - Campylobacter spp.
  - Salmonella spp.
  - Shigella spp.
  - Vibrio cholerae, V. parahaemolyticus
  - Yersinia enterocolitica, Y. pseudotuberculosis
  - Clostridium difficile
  - Aeromonas spp.
  - Plesiomonas spp.
- Protozoa
  - Cryptosporidium hominis/ parvum
  - Giardia lamblia
  - Entamoeba histolytica
  - Cyclospora cayetanensis

Box 5.1

Nausea, vomiting, and diarrhea that occur quickly after eating are typically caused by consuming a preexisting toxin produced by *Staphylococcus aureus*, *Bacillus cereus*, or *Clostridium perfringens*.

Excessive watery diarrhea suggests a cause in the small intestine, such as *V. cholerae* or enterotoxigenic E. infections caused by coli and rotavirus. The occurrence of secretory diarrhea induced by toxins persists regardless of the consumption of food. Carbohydrate malabsorption in the small intestine results in the fermentation of unabsorbed substances by bacteria in the colon. This can lead to symptoms such as bloating, excessive rectal gas, and frothy stools, which are all typical of giardiasis. Cryptosporidiosis has the potential to affect both the small and large intestines, resulting in transient and self-limiting diarrhea. Nevertheless, individuals with compromised immune systems may experience an extended duration of infection. The pathogen *Cyclospora cayetanensis* has the potential to induce both acute and chronic diarrhea, accompanied by disruptions in intestinal absorption.

Dehydration Assessment

Mild dehydration

- Decreased urine output

Moderate dehydration (25% volume loss)

- Irritability
- Delayed capillary refill time
- Tachycardia
- Orthostatic hypotension
- Deep respirations
- Decreased skin turgor
- Dry mucous membranes
- Sunken eyes
- Sunken fontanelle (infants)

Severe dehydration (≥10% volume loss)

- Decreased consciousness
- Hypotension
- Deep respirations with an increase in respiratory rate
- Cool extremities
- Peripheral cyanosis

Box 5.2

The presence of regular bowel movements characterized by reduced stool volumes and the expulsion of blood and mucus indicates the possibility of a colonic infection. Bloody diarrhea, also known as dysentery, can be attributed to the presence of invasive bacteria, such as *Campylobacter* spp. and enterohemorrhagic *Escherichia coli*, *Salmonella*, *Shigella*, and *Yersinia* spp. are among the bacterial pathogens responsible for the infection. Nonbacterial causes of the disease include *Entamoeba histolytica* (amebic dysentery) and Balantidium coli, which can be transmitted through close proximity to pigs. Colicky abdominal pain is a prevalent symptom observed in numerous gastrointestinal infections, with particular severity observed in cases of campylobacteriosis and yersiniosis, which bear resemblance to acute appendicitis. Infection by invasive organisms is typically accompanied by fever, chills, and generalized myalgia. These patients exhibit symptoms of illness and experience widespread abdominal tenderness.

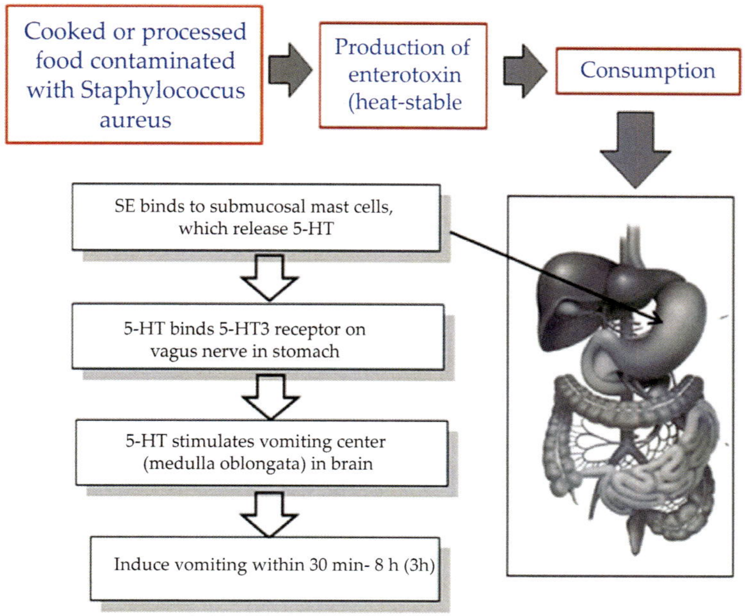

Figure 5.1. *Staphylococcal food poisoning (SFP)–Staphylococcus aureus enterotoxins.*

Source: https://microbenotes.com/wp-content/uploads/2021/07/Symptoms-and-complications-of-Staphylococcal-food-poisoning.jpg.

5.2.1. Colitis Caused by Antibiotics

Antibiotics have the potential to induce diarrhea through various mechanisms, with pseudomembranous colitis resulting from infection with cytotoxigenic *Clostridium difficile* being a prevalent etiological factor. Initially documented in individuals who had undergone clindamycin treatment. The presence of *C. difficile* infection has been observed to pose challenges in the treatment of various antibiotic classes, particularly fluoroquinolones. The prevalence of *C. difficile* infection in North America and Europe has experienced a significant rise following the emergence of a highly virulent strain in 2003. The exact incidence of this infection in other regions of the world remains uncertain, although it seems to be on the rise. Patients experience symptoms such as fever, diarrhea, and significant leukocytosis. The results of sigmoidoscopy indicate the presence of an inflamed mucosa punctured by pseudomembranous plaques. Management involves the cessation of superfluous antibiotics, administration of metronidazole or oral vancomycin, and, in cases where life is at risk, colectomy.

An example of antibiotic-associated colitis is antibiotic-associated hemorrhagic colitis, characterized by the presence of C. Difficulty is not present, is linked to the administration of penicillin, and has been identified as a result of *Klebsiella oxytoca* infection (Figure 5.2).

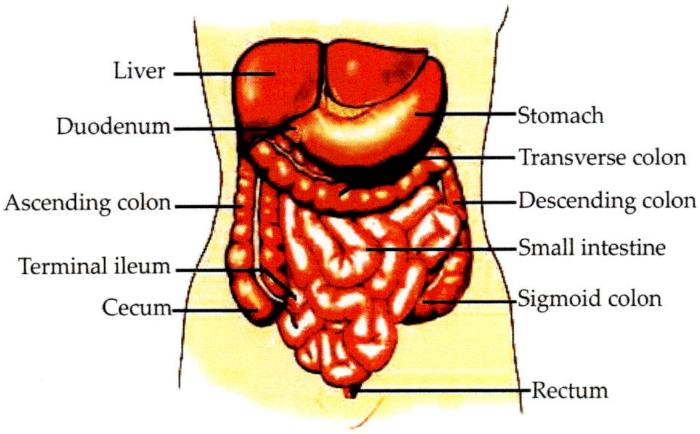

Figure 5.2. *Antibiotic-associated colitis clostridium difficile.*

Source: https://www.healthyatra.com/wp-content/uploads/2018/02/Antibiotic-associated-Colitis-C-difficile.jpg.

5.2.2. Chronic Diarrhea

The resolution or resolution of most acute gut infections typically occurs within a period of two weeks. Repeated infection and persistent infection are the primary etiologies of chronic diarrhea. Parasitic infections, such as those caused by protozoa (*Giardia lamblia*, *Entamoeba histolytica*, *Isospora belli*, *Cyclospora cayetanensis*, *Cryptosporidium hominis/parvum*, microsporidia) and helminths (*Strongyloides stercoralis*, *Capillaria philippinensis*) are frequently responsible for persistent infections (Box 5.3). Malabsorption is characterized by the presence of frequent, pale, and offensive stools in patients. Mucosal malabsorption can be attributed to noninfectious factors such as celiac disease, tropical sprue, Crohn's disease, and small bowel neoplasms. Intraluminal maldigestion, resulting from pancreatic exocrine insufficiency and bacterial overgrowth of the small intestine, can also lead to malabsorption. Additional factors contributing to the development of chronic diarrhea encompass the impact of medication, endocrinopathies such as hyperthyroidism and diabetes mellitus, as well as hormone-producing neoplasms.

Causes of Persistent/Chronic Diarrhea

- Infection
- Parasitic

Giardia lamblia

- Entamoeba histolytica
    - Isospora belli
    - Cyclospora cayetanenis
    - Cryptosporidium hominis/parvum (immunodeficient)
    - Microsporidia
    - Strongyloides stercoralis
    - Capillaria philippinensis
- Mycobacterial

Mycobacterium avium-intracellulare

- Mycobacterium tuberculosis

- Malabsorption
- AIDS enteropathy
- Inflammatory bowel disease

Box 5.3

5.2.3. Complications

Dehydration emerges as the primary cause of mortality among individuals experiencing acute diarrhea, necessitating expeditious replenishment of fluids and electrolytes. The nutritional status of children frequently experiences a decline due to factors such as anorexia, impaired nutrient absorption, and the practice of withholding nourishment from children experiencing diarrhea. Hypolactasia is a consequence of numerous gastrointestinal infections and can lead to chronic diarrhea. Severe local complications, such as hemorrhage, toxic megacolon, and bowel perforation, can be observed in cases of dysentery. Furthermore, the presence of invasive organisms can lead to systemic manifestations such as hemolytic uremic syndrome, which can complicate infections caused by *Shigella dysenteriae* and *Escherichia coli* O157. Additionally, reactive arthritis may occur as a result of shigellosis, salmonellosis, campylobacteriosis, yersiniosis, and *C. difficile* infection. Furthermore, Guillain-Barré syndrome, also known as campylobacteriosis, can also affect the body.

5.2.4. Diagnosis

The diverse array of laboratory tests and specialized knowledge required to establish a precise microbiologic diagnosis in the majority of patients suffering from diarrhea necessitates facilities that are not commonly accessible in tropical regions. Basic tests can be beneficial in the majority of situations. It is crucial to analyze the stool sample for the presence of blood. Direct microscopy should be employed to examine a smear of fluid stools for the presence of trophozoites of *Entamoeba histolytica*, as well as trophozoites and cysts of *Giardia lamblia*. When examining the smear, it is important to observe for any cellular exudate. The presence of polymorphonuclear leukocytes indicates infection with enteroinvasive bacteria, while a predominance of red cells may suggest amebic dysentery. The bacteriologic diagnosis is determined through the culture of stool samples or rectal swabs. In patients with persistent dysentery, it is advisable to perform a proctosigmoidoscopy. This procedure is recommended when there is widespread inflammation, ulceration, and bleeding of the rectal mucosa. In cases where the mucosa is ulcerated or bleeding, it is important to scrape the material and promptly examine it for the presence of amebic trophozoites.

5.2.5. The Management and Prognosis

The implementation of timely interventions to address and sustain adequate hydration is expected to result in a reduction in mortality rates associated with dehydrating diarrheal diseases.

5.2.6. Treatment of Dehydration

Upon evaluating the extent of dehydration, the primary objective of treatment is to replenish deficiencies in water and electrolytes. In cases of severe dehydration, it is recommended that patients be administered an intravenous bolus of isotonic fluid, such as saline or lactated Ringers, as a preventive measure against the development of hypovolemic shock. The administration of oral rehydration therapy has demonstrated a significant decrease in mortality rates associated with dehydrating diarrheal diseases, making it the preferred treatment option for children experiencing mild to moderate dehydration. Community healthcare providers have the ability to disseminate oral rehydration salts (ORS) and educate individuals on the process of preparing and administering the solution. The World Health Organization recommends a formulation that includes the following components: glucose, a sugar that aids in the absorption of sodium and water in the small intestine; sodium and potassium, to replenish electrolyte losses in the gastrointestinal tract; and citrate or bicarbonate, which aids in correcting the acidosis caused by diarrhea. The absorption of ORS solution occurs in the small intestine, even in cases of severe diarrhea. The current recommendation is to utilize a novel formulation with reduced osmolarity, consisting of 75 mEq/L of glucose and 75 mEq/L of sodium.

5.2.7. Antimicrobial Agents

The role of antimicrobials in the treatment of patients with secretory acute watery diarrhea is typically limited or secondary. Patients exhibiting symptoms and signs of infection with enteroinvasive organisms, such as fever, abdominal pain, toxicity, tenesmus, and frequent stools containing mucus and blood, should receive empiric treatment based on WHO protocols and local antimicrobial resistance patterns. The efficacy of fluoroquinolones against enteroinvasive bacteria, such as *Salmonella* and

Shigella spp., has been demonstrated, although there has been a noticeable rise in resistance. Infection of *Campylobacter* spp. prefer macrolides as their preferred drug. Infection. The treatment of giardiasis and amebiasis necessitates the administration of metronidazole or tinidazole.

5.2.8. Supplementary Treatment

Supplementing with zinc decreases the length and intensity of diarrhea and mortality in children with intestinal infection. However, there is no evidence to suggest that vitamin A has a similar effect. To mitigate the detrimental impact of diarrhea on nutrition, it is advisable to maintain feeding and enhance breastfeeding in infants. Patients should be promptly fed with energy-dense, low-osmolality foods in regular, small portions, and there should be an increase in feeding following the occurrence of diarrhea. Avoid using intestinal sedatives due to the decreased frequency of bowel movements, which leads to fluid stagnation in the gut lumen. This stagnation promotes the growth of organisms and maintains contact between the organisms and their toxins with the mucosa.

5.2.9. Prevention and Control

The provision of potable water and appropriate sewage disposal systems has been shown to decrease the prevalence of gastrointestinal infections. Tube wells are a method employed for the provision of potable water. The implementation of appropriate latrine infrastructure will contribute to the disruption of the fecal-oral transmission of gastrointestinal pathogens. Trained community members should provide health education on the significance of proper sanitary practices and breastfeeding. While these measures are expected to yield long-term effectiveness, achieving a short-term reduction in the prevalence of diarrheal diseases necessitates the implementation of more immediate interventions, such as vaccination. The effectiveness of rotavirus vaccination has been demonstrated in children residing in both developed and developing nations. During an outbreak in Mozambique in 2004, the efficacy of an oral cholera vaccine in preventing cases was demonstrated. Nevertheless, the widespread implementation of this approach has been limited due to its relatively brief duration of protection and challenges related to its availability.

The management of gastrointestinal infection epidemics involves identifying the origin(s) of the infection, detecting cases, and administering treatment, if needed, to prevent the spread of the disease. Handwashing and fly control are effective in preventing the transmission of enteric infection.

5.2.10. Traveler's Diarrhea

Individuals from developed nations who travel to tropical regions are susceptible to contracting traveler's diarrhea. Younger individuals, those taking proton pump inhibitors, and individuals who neglect personal hygiene precautions seem to have a higher risk. Enterotoxigenic *Escherichia coli* is the most prevalent type of pathogen. Both coli and enteroaggregative *Escherichia coli. Salmonella*, *Campylobacter*, *Shigella*, *Salmonella*, *Aeromonas*, *Plesiomonas*, and *Vibrio* spp. have been identified as additional bacteria. The predominant viral agents responsible for traveler's diarrhea are noroviruses and rotaviruses, while the predominant protozoan pathogens include *Giardia lamblia*, *Entamoeba histolytica*, and *Cryptosporidium hominis/ parvum*.

It is recommended that individuals traveling to regions with high endemicity be provided with typhoid and hepatitis A vaccinations. The administration of bismuth subsalicylate or probiotics has the potential to mitigate the risk of traveler's diarrhea. The efficacy of antibiotic prophylaxis in preventing traveler's diarrhea has been demonstrated, however, it is not recommended for the general population due to the potential negative consequences of antibiotics and the possibility of antibiotic resistance.

Antibiotic therapy effectively shortens the duration of symptoms in individuals who experience traveler's diarrhea, even in cases where a specific pathogen cannot be identified. The prevalence of *Campylobacter* spp. that are resistant to fluoroquinolones. The prevalent use of azithromycin is on the rise, indicating its potential as a viable alternative for managing traveler's diarrhea. Rifaximin represents an alternative, albeit not advisable, for patients afflicted with invasive disease. Patients should receive guidance on hydration and diet, in addition to a brief antibiotic treatment. Individuals without signs of invasive disease may find an antimotility agent advantageous.

5.2.11. Abdominal Pain

Peptic ulcer disease is frequently associated with upper abdominal pain, and the exacerbation of these symptoms may indicate the presence of a complication, such as perforation or penetration. Possible causes of upper abdominal symptoms accompanied by ulceration in the stomach or duodenum include infections such as tuberculosis, *Mycobacterium avium intracellulare*, cytomegalovirus, and herpes simplex virus. Other potential diagnoses include neoplasms, which can be either primary tumors or metastatic diseases, as well as infiltrative diseases. Acute pancreatitis is a prevalent etiology for acute upper abdominal pain, with gallstones and alcohol consumption being the primary causes globally. However, it is worth noting that infectious etiologies play a significant role in individuals with compromised immune systems. The clinical presentation of chronic pancreatitis includes symptoms such as abdominal pain, steatorrhea, and diabetes mellitus. The majority of cases worldwide are attributed to alcohol abuse. However, in certain regions of the tropics, tropical calcific pancreatitis is the most prevalent cause of chronic pancreatitis. This condition, which has an unknown cause, often affects children. Plain abdominal film may reveal pancreatic calcifications, while ultrasonography or computed tomography may reveal ductal dilatation. Biliary colic, acute cholecystitis, acute cholangitis, acute hepatitis, and liver abscess are conditions that can manifest as pain in the right upper quadrant. Pain in the left upper quadrant can potentially arise from splenic disorders, including splenomegaly, splenic abscess, or splenic infarction. When assessing the patient presenting with upper abdominal pain, it is crucial to take into account supradiaphragmatic etiologies, including pneumonia and myocardial infarction.

Several parasitic worms have the potential to induce nonspecific gastrointestinal symptoms, such as epigastric pain. Furthermore, parasitic infections affecting the biliary tract can result in acute pancreatitis. This is demonstrated by the migration of adult *Ascaris lumbricoides* worms from the jejunum to the papilla, causing blockages in the pancreatic and bile ducts.

The occurrence of pain in the right lower quadrant is frequently attributed to acute appendicitis. However, it is worth noting that an infection with *Yersinia* or *Campylobacter* can occasionally lead to intense pain that is erroneously diagnosed as appendicitis. It is imperative to take into account ectopic pregnancy, pelvic inflammatory disease, and adnexal pathologies in females experiencing acute lower abdominal pain.

One of the cardinal features of bowel obstruction is the presence of colicky abdominal pain. It can also be observed in children with intussusception. Peritonitis, stemming from perforated peptic ulcer, ileal perforation in typhoid fever, colonic perforation in amebic colitis, or rupture of a hydatid cyst, can lead to generalized abdominal pain and tenderness. Acute mesenteric ischemia is characterized by the presence of intense abdominal pain accompanied by minimal or absent tenderness. Aside from considering surgical emergencies, it is crucial to also consider the "medical" factors contributing to abdominal pain. Individuals diagnosed with sickle cell disease may experience acute episodes of pain as a result of vaso-occlusion, which can be challenging to differentiate from alternative etiologies of abdominal pain. Abdominal pain is a prevalent symptom observed in various infectious diseases, with malaria being particularly notable.

5.2.12. Abdominal Distension

Individuals diagnosed with ascites may present with symptoms such as abdominal pain, early satiety, or dyspnea as a result of diaphragm splinting. The examination of ascitic fluid serves two purposes in identifying the etiology of ascites. First, it aids in determining the presence of infection within the fluid. Spontaneous bacterial peritonitis is characterized by a polymorphonuclear leukocyte count exceeding 250 cells/mL, accompanied by a positive bacterial culture. Second, it aids in identifying the presence of underlying portal hypertension, which is indicated by a serum-ascites albumin gradient of 1.1 g/dL or higher. Cystic fibrosis and tuberculous peritonitis are prevalent etiologies. Chronic hepatic schistosomiasis frequently leads to the development of ascites in regions where it is prevalent. Ascites can be induced by malignancy through various mechanisms. In cases of peritoneal carcinomatosis, ascitic fluid cytology may yield positive results, whereas in cases of portal hypertension resulting from extensive liver metastases, it will yield negative results. In chylous ascites, the ascitic fluid appears cloudy due to the high levels of triglycerides; the most common causes in developing countries are infections leading to lymphatic obstruction, such as tuberculosis and filariasis. Tricuspid regurgitation, constrictive pericarditis, or any cause of right-sided heart failure can lead to cardiac ascites. Spontaneous bacterial peritonitis may complicate ascites due to cirrhosis; however, it is very rare in non-cirrhotic ascites, as these patients have a higher concentration of ascitic fluid opsonins. The classic presentation is with fever and abdominal pain and tenderness, but it may be asymptomatic or present with encephalopathy or renal failure.

A massive ovarian cyst can present with abdominal distension, but the central location of the swelling, presence of a fluid thrill, and absence of shifting dullness help to distinguish this from ascites.

Abdominal distension may be due to gas, either within or outside the bowel lumen. Extraluminal gas is seen in bowel perforation, which is a surgical emergency. Gaseous distension of the bowel may be due to mechanical obstruction or motility disorder. Bloating is a common symptom in lactose malabsorption, which is commonplace among Africans and Asians after childhood, and in irritable bowel syndrome.

5.2.13. Intestinal Obstruction

The cardinal features are colicky abdominal pain, vomiting, constipation, and abdominal distension. A bolus of worms can cause intraluminal obstruction in children with heavy Ascaris lumbricoides infestation; it may also serve as a lead point for intussusception and volvulus. Colorectal carcinoma is increasingly recognized in the tropics, but may not be evident until presentation with obstruction of the large bowel. The differential diagnosis includes inflammatory masses that can lead to intramural obstruction, such as: ileocecal tuberculosis, histoplasmosis, actinomycosis, amebiasis, schistosomiasis and angiostrongyliasis. Extramural obstruction is most commonly due to incarcerated hernia. Umbilical hernias are more common in African children, but usually the defects close spontaneously. Symptoms and signs of small bowel obstruction may also be seen in paralytic ileus, in which there is bowel dilatation without mechanical obstruction. This is a common complication of abdominal surgery, but may also occur in peritonitis or after trauma. Plain film or computed tomography of the abdomen in paralytic ileus shows gas in the colon and rectum, helping to differentiate it from small bowel obstruction in which the colon is decompressed. Treatment is supportive, consisting of fluid resuscitation, correction of electrolyte abnormalities (especially hypokalemia) and discontinuation of antikinetic drugs. Another motility disorder that may be misdiagnosed as mechanical obstruction is chronic intestinal pseudo-obstruction, which may occur in Chagas disease. Here, gross dilation of the colon (megacolon), most commonly involving the sigmoid colon, causes constipation; it may be complicated by toxic megacolon or volvulus.

5.3. Gastrointestinal Bleeding

Upper gastrointestinal bleeding, defined as bleeding emanating from a source proximal to the ligament of Treitz, presents with hematemesis and/or melena. It is most commonly due to bleeding peptic ulcer. In areas with a high prevalence of cirrhosis, bleeding from esophageal and gastric varices is common. Mallory–Weiss tears are mucosal lacerations at the gastroesophageal junction that are most commonly associated with repeated retching. Gastric and duodenal neoplasms can present with overt gastrointestinal bleeding, though occult blood loss is more common. Unusual causes of upper gastrointestinal bleeding include vascular abnormalities.

Hematochezia is most often due to colorectal sources but may be the first sign of a brisk upper gastrointestinal hemorrhage. Patients with infectious colitis present with bleeding in association with diarrhea, abdominal pain, and systemic upset. Gastrointestinal bleeding is a common complication of typhoid fever. Many causes of lower gastrointestinal bleeding that are common in the West – colonic diverticular bleeding, ischemic colitis, colorectal cancer, and hemorrhoids – are unusual in the tropics due to epidemiologic differences. Lymphoma and Kaposi sarcoma may affect any part of the gastrointestinal tract and are common causes of gastrointestinal bleeding in patients with AIDS.

The initial management of patients with acute gastrointestinal bleeding consists of fluid resuscitation and, if coagulopathy or thrombocytopenia is present, transfusion of blood products. Once patients are stabilized, endoscopy should be performed to diagnose and treat the source of bleeding. Cirrhotic patients with upper gastrointestinal bleeding are at risk for bacterial infections including spontaneous bacterial peritonitis; broad-spectrum antibiotics may reduce this risk.

5.4. Anatomic Differentials

5.4.1. Mouth

5.4.1.1. Dental Caries

Dental caries is a chronic disease in which the composition of the oral flora is altered as a result of chronic consumption of high-sugar substances. This leads to demineralization of the enamel, eventually causing a dental cavity. Dental caries is a major oral health problem worldwide, and the incidence is increasing in developing countries as people engage in Western dietary practices. Three factors are important in the prevention of caries: dietary counseling, oral hygiene, and fluoride supplementation.

5.4.1.2. Oral Cancer

Oral cancer should be suspected in any patient with a nonhealing ulcer or mass in the mouth.

As with all squamous cell carcinomas of the head and neck, the major risk factors are tobacco and alcohol use. Additional risk factors include viral infection (Epstein-Barr virus, which is strongly associated with nasopharyngeal carcinoma, human papillomavirus, and human immunodeficiency virus [HIV]) and betel-nut chewing, which is widespread in South and Southeast Asia.

5.4.1.3. Candidiasis

Oral infection with *Candida* ("thrush") is usually characterized by white plaques on the oral mucosa, though there is also an atrophic form that presents as erythema without plaques. It is a common finding in patients with HIV infection; other risk factors include treatment with antibiotics or steroids (both oral and inhaled). Treatment consists of a topical antifungal agent or, in patients with more severe disease, systemic therapy.

5.4.1.4. Herpes Simplex Virus Infection

Primary infection of the oral cavity with herpes simplex virus causes gingivostomatitis and pharyngitis. The lesions can be vesicular or ulcerative and may be associated with fever and cervical lymphadenopathy. Reactivation of the virus leads to vesicular lesions of the oral mucosa ("cold sores"). Treatment should be directed toward providing symptomatic relief; antiviral therapy may be helpful if primary infection is detected early or for patients with recurrent infection who can identify a characteristic precipitating factor or prodrome.

5.4.1.5. Cancrum Oris (Noma)

This is a gangrenous, polymicrobial infection affecting the orofacial tissues. It starts as a gingival ulceration, which, if left untreated, spreads rapidly through the soft and hard tissues of the mouth and face, breaching normal anatomic barriers and resulting in gross deformity. It is thought to occur after fecal–oral transmission in young children who are at risk due to a complex interplay between infection, malnutrition and immunocompromise – a combination that is common in impoverished areas of Africa, Asia and Latin America. The acute stage may present with unilateral facial pain and swelling, halitosis, oral discharge and systemic upset; management consists of broad-spectrum antibiotics and local wound care together with treatment of associated diseases and nutritional deficiencies. However, most patients are not brought to medical attention until the infection is well established – characterized by a necrotic center with a well-demarcated perimeter – at which time reconstructive surgery is required.

5.4.2. Esophagus

5.4.2.1. Esophagitis

The main presenting features are odynophagia, dysphagia, and retrosternal chest pain. While noninfectious conditions such as gastroesophageal reflux disease (GERD) and pill esophagitis are the most common causes in immunocompetent hosts, infections of the esophagus are common in the immunocompromised. In patients with HIV infection, the most common cause is esophageal candidiasis. While the presence of oropharyngeal candidiasis can be a clue to esophageal infection, its absence does not rule it out. Diagnosis can be made by endoscopy, which reveals white plaques on the esophageal mucosa; biopsy reveals the presence of budding yeasts. An alternative strategy is to undertake a therapeutic trial of a systemic antifungal agent; if the symptoms do not resolve within days, then further investigation is warranted. Cytomegalovirus esophagitis causes similar symptoms, but endoscopy reveals ulcerative lesions. Ulcers are also seen in herpes simplex virus esophagitis, but they tend to have heaped-up borders as opposed to the shallower lesions of cytomegalovirus; there may or may not be associated oropharyngeal lesions. It is important to note that a number of patients with HIV infection presenting with esophagitis may have simultaneous infection with more than one agent, whereas others will have no infection identified. The latter condition, named idiopathic esophageal ulcer, may respond to steroids.

5.4.2.2. Caustic Esophageal Injury

Caustic injuries to the esophagus may result from ingestion of acid or alkali. The main complaint is pain, and there may be signs of complications such as perforation, mediastinitis or peritonitis. Attempts at inducing emesis or neutralizing the ingested substance must be avoided, lest the injury be aggravated. Endoscopy may be helpful for risk stratification and guiding further management. Late complications include esophageal strictures, which cause dysphagia and necessitate dilation, and squamous cell carcinoma.

5.4.2.3. Esophageal Varices

Esophageal varices are relatively common in the tropics. The causes of portal hypertension can be classified as pre-hepatic, hepatic and post-hepatic. Pre-hepatic causes include the tropical splenomegaly syndrome and portal or splenic vein thrombosis. Hepatic causes may be classified as pre-sinusoidal, sinusoidal, and post-sinusoidal, exemplified by schistosomiasis, cirrhosis, and veno-occlusive disease, respectively. Budd–Chiari syndrome and cardiac causes (restrictive cardiomyopathy, congestive heart failure) are post-hepatic causes. Variceal bleeding carries a high mortality rate worldwide. Initial management consists of restoration of the circulating volume, with caution to avoid over-transfusion, the use of agents to reduce portal pressure (e.g., terlipressin or octreotide), and antibiotic prophylaxis. After stabilization, endoscopic variceal ligation is the ideal approach. For patients with refractory bleeding, balloon tamponade can be a temporizing measure while awaiting portosystemic shunting.

5.4.2.4. Megaesophagus

Marked dilation of the esophagus is the most common gastrointestinal manifestation of chronic Chagas disease and occurs due to a loss of neurons in the enteric nervous system. Dysphagia is the most prominent symptom, but patients may also complain of odynophagia and regurgitation; aspiration is a common complication. The condition cannot be reversed by antitrypanosomal agents, but symptomatic relief can be achieved through balloon dilations of the lower esophageal sphincter or through surgery.

5.4.2.5. Esophageal Cancer

Squamous cell carcinoma usually arises in the mid portion of the esophagus in patients with a history of tobacco and alcohol use or preexisting esophageal diseases. In contrast, adenocarcinoma affects the lower third of the esophagus in patients with Barrett's esophagus. Both types of cancer have a similar clinical presentation, with dysphagia and weight loss being the most common symptoms. Diagnosis is made at endoscopy with biopsy. Over half of patients present with incurable disease.

5.4.3. Stomach

A variety of gastroduodenal pathologies are related to infection with *Helicobacter pylori*. This Gram-negative, spiral-shaped bacterium adheres to the gastric epithelium and is able to survive in the acidic environment of the stomach due to a urease that converts urea into ammonia, which increases the pH of the immediate vicinity. It is spread by person-to-person (likely fecal–oral) transmission and is usually acquired at an earlier age in developing countries than in developed countries. It is found worldwide, though the prevalence is decreasing with improved sanitation and hygiene. Infection causes acute gastritis, which leads to chronic gastritis. Peptic ulcer disease is a common complication, while a small minority of patients with *H. pylori* infection go on to develop gastric adenocarcinoma or MALT (mucosa-associated lymphoid tissue) lymphoma.

5.4.3.1. Gastritis

Both inflammation of the stomach (gastritis) and damage to the gastric epithelium with minimal or no inflammation (gastropathy) may cause epigastric pain and nausea and vomiting, but they may be asymptomatic. The most common infectious cause of gastritis is *H. pylori* infection. A number of agents cause gastropathy, the most common being nonsteroidal anti-inflammatory drugs (NSAIDs), alcohol, and bile reflux.

5.4.3.2. Peptic Ulcer Disease

Population-based endoscopy studies have shown that the prevalence of peptic ulcer disease is almost 10% in the East, twice as high as in Western countries. Historically, duodenal ulcers were more common than gastric ulcers in the tropics – due to the higher prevalence of *H. pylori* and lower usage of NSAIDs – but this ratio is changing with time. While patients with peptic ulcer may be asymptomatic, the usual symptom is epigastric discomfort or pain, which may radiate to the back. The four major complications are hemorrhage, penetration, perforation, and gastric outlet obstruction. Bleeding peptic ulcer is a common cause of acute upper gastrointestinal hemorrhage; management consists of hemodynamic resuscitation, endoscopic therapy, and, for refractory cases, surgery. Treatment with a proton pump inhibitor reduces the risk of rebleeding after endoscopic hemostasis. The ulcer's penetration through the bowel wall induces severe pain; additional erosion leads to bowel perforation, resulting in peritonitis and requiring immediate laparotomy. Gastric outlet obstruction typically arises as a consequence of a persistent ulcer, resulting from the presence of chronic inflammation and fibrosis. Diagnostic testing for *H. pylori* should be conducted in all patients with peptic ulceration, either through endoscopy or noninvasive methods. While the eradication of *H. pylori* is a positive outcome, the treatment should involve the use of a proton pump inhibitor and two antibiotics, while considering the specific resistance patterns in the local area. Contrary to duodenal ulcers, which are seldom cancerous, gastric ulcers can have a malignant cause, thus requiring follow-up endoscopy to confirm resolution.

5.4.3.3. Gastric Neoplasms

Gastric cancer ranks as the second leading cause of cancer-related mortality on a global scale. The occurrence is rare in developed nations, but it is most prevalent in East Asia and certain regions of South America. Dietary factors and the prevalence of *H. pylori* may contribute to some of the geographic variation. The prevailing symptoms commonly observed include weight loss and abdominal pain, alongside additional manifestations such as dysphagia, early satiety, and iron deficiency anemia resulting from prolonged blood loss. A significant proportion of patients exhibit metastatic disease upon initial presentation, thereby rendering curative resection unfeasible.

Adenocarcinomas account for more than 90% of gastric cancers, while gastric MALT lymphomas constitute a minority. However, they are significant because early lesions can be treated with H. The exclusive use of *H. pylori* eradication therapy. Chemotherapy is necessary for cases of nonresponsive or recurrent disease.

5.4.4. The Small Bowel

A diverse range of pathological mechanisms leads to comparable histological abnormalities in the mucosal lining of the small intestine, leading to foreseeable clinical presentations. The initial occurrence involves the recruitment of lymphocytes into the epithelial layer, leading to the occurrence of intraepithelial lymphocytosis. Subsequently, there is an augmentation in the proliferation of crypt cells, leading to crypt hyperplasia. Subsequently, the depletion of villous cells results in progressive villous atrophy, ultimately culminating in the development of flat mucosa. Patients may experience symptoms such as diarrhea, steatorrhea, and weight loss as a result of mucosal malabsorption. Laboratory investigations have the potential to provide valuable insights into the scope of the malabsorption syndrome. Anemia can occur due to insufficiencies in iron, folate, and/or vitamin B12. In the case of vitamin B12, it suggests that the damage to the mucosal lining also affects the terminal ileum. The extension of the prothrombin time could potentially be attributed to a deficiency in vitamin K, which is classified as a fat-soluble vitamin, alongside vitamins A, D, and E. This deficiency is commonly observed in cases of fat malabsorption.

Causes of Malabsorption

- Infections
- Celiac disease
- Tropical sprue
- Bacterial overgrowth
- Crohn's disease
- Malignancies
- Immunoproliferative small intestinal disease
- Intestinal lymphoma
- Hypolactasia
- Pancreatitis
- Alcoholic pancreatitis
- Chronic calcific pancreatitis

Box 5.4

Vitamin D deficiency can lead to the development of osteomalacia or osteoporosis, as evidenced by the presence of hypophosphatemia, hypocalcemia, and elevated alkaline phosphatase levels. Parasitic infections, celiac disease, tropical sprue, bacterial overgrowth, and Crohn's disease are among the conditions that give rise to these histologic abnormalities and manifest with these clinical and laboratory characteristics (Box 5.4). Other disorders with distinct pathologic findings, such as intestinal lymphoma and amyloidosis, may exhibit comparable clinical manifestations. The fundamental tenets of managing disorders affecting the small intestinal mucosa encompass addressing the root cause of the condition and rectifying any potential deficiencies in essential nutrients. Additionally, adhering to a lactose-free and low-fat diet may yield advantageous outcomes.

5.4.4.1. Tropical Sprue

There have been reports of abnormalities in the small intestinal mucosa, leading to heightened intestinal permeability and reduced absorption, observed in individuals residing in and visiting specific tropical and subtropical nations. The disorder, known as tropical sprue or tropical enteropathy, is characterized by a chronic malabsorption syndrome. It can occur either after an episode of acute infectious diarrhea or develop gradually over time. In some cases, it can even develop years after leaving an area where the disease is common. The occurrence of this condition seems to be declining, primarily due to the growing acknowledgment of nontropical sprue, also known as celiac disease, and potentially also due to the rising utilization of antibiotics for individuals with acute diarrheal illnesses. The phenomenon under consideration is observed in the Indian subcontinent, Southeast Asia, and certain regions of the Caribbean. Nevertheless, it is not universally present in all tropical regions, as it is notably uncommon or nonexistent in Africa and other Caribbean areas, including Jamaica. The disease presentation in these areas exhibits significant heterogeneity, indicating that tropical sprue may encompass a range of related disorders. The cause of the disease is not yet known, but it is believed to be infectious based on the disease's epidemiology and its response to antibiotics. While several infectious agents have been suggested, there has been limited agreement among studies. Furthermore, the etiology of tropical sprue has been linked to folate deficiency, as evidenced by the high prevalence of folate deficiency in affected individuals and the observed histologic improvement following folic acid repletion. However, it is important to note that this theory, along with other theories such as malnutrition or excessive T-cell activity, are flawed due to the inability to establish a causal relationship. Tropical sprue exhibits clinical, laboratory, and endoscopic characteristics that closely resemble those of celiac disease. Although both conditions can exhibit patchy mucosal lesions, the villous atrophy in tropical sprue is generally less severe, with flat mucosa being rare. However, it is more widespread throughout the small intestine. The primary differentiating factors between tropical sprue and celiac disease include the lack of autoantibodies specific to celiac disease and the absence of clinical and histologic amelioration following a gluten-free dietary regimen. Therefore, tropical sprue can be considered a potential diagnosis, indicated by villous atrophy in a patient with malabsorption who resides or has previously resided in a region where the condition is prevalent. Antibiotics, typically tetracycline for 6 months, in conjunction with folic acid, can effectively treat the disease.

5.4.4.2. Celiac Disease

Celiac disease, also known as nontropical sprue or gluten-sensitive enteropathy, is a persistent inflammatory condition of the small intestine. It occurs when individuals with a genetic predisposition exhibit an abnormal immune reaction to wheat gluten and related proteins found in barley and rye. The condition, which was previously considered rare in tropical regions, has gained recognition due to the development of serologic tests that are both specific and sensitive. This recognition has extended to South Asians, Arabs residing in North Africa, and the Middle East. In previous instances, individuals residing in these regions exhibiting malabsorption and small intestinal villous atrophy, without any indications of parasitic infection or bacterial overgrowth, were likely subject to misdiagnosis as tropical sprue. The study of 259 Indian children attending a pediatric gastroenterology clinic in New Delhi provides evidence of the prevalence of celiac disease in a previously considered low-risk group. The findings reveal that more than 40% of the children were diagnosed with celiac disease. The condition typically manifests following the incorporation of gluten into the dietary intake of infants. However, it is widely acknowledged that adult-onset celiac disease can also occur in older individuals, including the elderly. It is worth noting that the prevalence of this condition is higher among females compared to males. With the growing acknowledgment of celiac disease, there has been an enhanced understanding of its diverse manifestations. While the typical disease is characterized by chronic diarrhea, abdominal distension, and failure to thrive or weight loss, a significant number of patients exhibit atypical disease, wherein extraintestinal symptoms such as delayed menarche in girls, neuropsychiatric symptoms, or osteomalacia are more prominent. Additionally, some individuals have silent or subclinical disease, displaying positive results on serologic testing and biopsy but lacking any symptoms. The serologic tests, namely IgA endomysial antibodies and IgA tissue transglutaminase antibodies, are highly effective in diagnosing celiac disease. These tests have a sensitivity of over 85% and a specificity of over 95%. Nevertheless, small bowel biopsy continues to be considered the preferred method due to several reasons. Firstly, in individuals who test positive for serologic markers, a biopsy serves to validate the diagnosis and rule out potential complications like lymphoma. Secondly, in patients who exhibit suggestive clinical characteristics but test negative for serologic markers, it is crucial to persist with the investigation, as around 10% of individuals with IgA-competent celiac disease are seronegative. In the past, the diagnosis was limited to individuals who exhibited villous atrophy upon biopsy. However, it is now acknowledged that patients with milder forms of mucosal damage, such as crypt hyperplasia or intraepithelial lymphocytosis alone, experience a mortality rate that is at least as high as that of individuals with severe villous atrophy. The current diagnostic criteria for celiac disease rely on a positive small bowel biopsy, which is characterized by the presence of intraepithelial lymphocytosis, crypt hyperplasia, and villous atrophy. Additionally, the patient's condition may improve clinically and/or histologically when gluten is eliminated from their diet. While serologic tests are not essential for diagnosing celiac disease, they can be beneficial in managing the condition. This is because a positive test result will become negative once the patient adheres to a rigorous gluten-free diet. The primary cause of nonresponsive celiac disease is typically the deliberate or unintentional consumption of gluten. If these factors are not considered, they may be attributed to concurrent conditions such as microscopic colitis (which is linked to celiac disease), refractory celiac disease, or enteropathy-associated T-cell lymphoma. Research in the field of epidemiology has demonstrated that individuals diagnosed with celiac disease exhibit a heightened susceptibility to both gastrointestinal and non-gastrointestinal malignancies.

5.4.4.3. Enteropathy with Protein Loss

The gastrointestinal tract may experience protein loss due to various factors, including: (1) erosive mucosal disease, characterized by the leakage of protein across damaged membranes; (2) non-erosive mucosal disease, characterized by altered epithelial permeability leading to protein loss; and/or (3) lymphatic disease, characterized by the leakage of lymph into the lumen. Intestinal infection is the primary etiology of non-erosive mucosal disease. Lymphatic dysfunction can arise from either obstruction, such as in the case of mesenteric tuberculosis, or impaired drainage, as observed in manifestations of portal hypertension or right-sided heart failure. The presence of hypoalbuminemia without protein malnutrition, proteinuria, or liver disease suggests the diagnosis. Treatment involves administering medium-chain triglycerides to provide nutritional support, in addition to correcting the underlying disorder.

5.4.4.4. Small Intestinal Disease with Immunoproliferative Syndrome

Immunoproliferative small intestinal disease (IPSID), also referred to as alpha heavy chain disease or Mediterranean lymphoma, is a type of MALT lymphoma. It is distinguished by the release of truncated immunoglobulin alpha heavy chains, lacking an accompanying light chain, by plasma cells that invade the bowel wall. Environmental factors, including one or more infectious agents, are believed to play a crucial role in the development of IPSID due to its distinctive epidemiology, which is limited to the Mediterranean, the Middle East, and Africa, as well as its association with inadequate sanitation and response to antibiotic therapy. Researchers have attempted to link this pathogen with IPSID by studying *H. pylori* and gastric MALT lymphomas. Despite the publication of one case report indicating an association, a subsequent case series has been unable to reproduce this finding. After identifying *Campylobacter jejuni* in a primary patient with IPSID, researchers analyzed six more patients and observed indications of *C. jejuni*. There is evidence to suggest that *C. jejuni* is present in four of these cases, indicating that this bacterium may play a role, at least partially, in eliciting the antigenic response in IPSID.

5.4.4.5. Pathology

The second, third, and fourth segments of the duodenum, as well as the proximal jejunum, experience the highest level of involvement.

However, there have been reports of ileal or complete involvement of the small bowel. Involvement of the stomach and colon is even more uncommon. The mucosa exhibits a noticeable increase in thickness, accompanied by infiltrations that give it a cobblestone-like appearance, as well as localized nodules or polypoid tumors. The typical vascular structure of the gastrointestinal tract is completely eliminated due to the extensive infiltration of plasma cells. The villi are reduced in length, while the crypts remain diminutive and are primarily concealed within the infiltrate.

5.4.4.6. Manifestations and Diagnosis of Clinical Conditions

The clinical presentation of the disease is marked by a pronounced malabsorption syndrome accompanied by symptoms such as diarrhea, abdominal pain, and weight loss. Palpable abdominal masses can be observed, whereas hepatosplenomegaly is indicative of an advanced stage of the disease. The laboratory results exhibit significant observations of hypoalbuminemia and hypogammaglobulinemia, which are indicative of protein-losing enteropathy. The presence of alpha heavy chains in the serum is indicative of the diagnosis, although it may not be present in a small number of patients. In the remaining cases, the biopsy specimens show positive immunohistochemical staining.

5.4.4.7. The Management and Prognosis

Bacterial therapy, specifically tetracycline with or without metronidazole for parasitic infections, has traditionally been used to treat early-stage IPSID. However, newer agents may also be effective in treating this condition. Chemotherapy may be necessary in cases of advanced disease. In instances of unresponsiveness, surgical intervention may be necessary to address the obstruction caused by bulky abdominal disease.

5.4.4.8. Pigbel's Enteritis Necroticans

The aforementioned condition is a necrotizing infection that can impact either the small or large intestine. It manifests subsequent to the consumption of food that contains the beta toxin produced by Clostridium perfringens. This condition primarily impacts individuals with chronic malnutrition who consume a meal rich in protein. It was initially identified in children and adults in Papua New Guinea following a pork feast, but has subsequently been reported in individuals from various regions of Asia and Africa. Decreased trypsin activity is a contributing factor to the infection, observed in cases of protein malnutrition and in individuals who consume foods with antitrypsin properties, such as sweet potatoes. The toxic substance induces tissue necrosis, primarily impacting the small intestine but occasionally extending to encompass the colon. The histologic analysis demonstrates a significant presence of inflammation and necrosis in the mucosa, accompanied by a substantial bacterial population on the affected surface. Abdominal pain and distension, bloody diarrhea, and shock are observed in the patients. The surgical removal of the affected portion of the bowel has the potential to be curative; however, the disease frequently results in mortality.

5.4.4.9. Intussusception

The term "intussusception" refers to the phenomenon of one segment of the bowel extending into another. Children account for 95% of cases, exhibiting the typical symptoms of colicky abdominal pain and vomiting, a right-sided abdominal mass (typically found at the ileocecal junction), and currant-jelly stool (resulting from the combination of blood and mucus). Non-operative treatment options for most cases include the use of air, saline, or barium enemas. The majority of cases are idiopathic, while the remaining cases can be attributed to various lesions in the intestine, such as Meckel's diverticulum, polyp, or vascular malformation, which can serve as precursors to intussusception. In contrast, adults diagnosed with intussusception typically exhibit an underlying disorder, with amebomas and schistosomal granulomas serving as the primary etiological factors, alongside benign and malignant neoplasms. Surgical resection is preferred over non-operative reduction due to the potential for underlying malignancies in adults with intussusception.

5.4.5. Colon

5.4.5.1. Appendicitis

Acute appendicitis is a prevalent etiology of acute abdominal pain, manifesting across various age groups. Appendiceal wall inflammation can give rise to ischemia, necrosis, and ultimately perforation, potentially leading to the development of a localized abscess or a more widespread peritonitis. The causative factor is the blockage of the appendix, typically caused by fecaliths or calculi. Nevertheless, the etiology of appendiceal obstruction exhibits age-related variations, wherein lymphoid hyperplasia is frequently observed in pediatric patients, and tumors are occasionally detected in adult individuals. Schistosome ova have been detected in the appendiceal wall of patients undergoing appendectomy in regions where schistosomiasis is prevalent. This indicates that certain parasitic infestations may play a role in the development of acute appendicitis. Irrespective of the underlying cause, the clinical manifestations of acute appendicitis exhibit similarities. The typical symptoms encompass pain that transitions from the periumbilical region to the right iliac fossa, fever, loss of appetite, and vomiting. However, diagnosing acute appendicitis may pose greater difficulties in pediatric and geriatric populations, as they may present with less distinct clinical features. The laboratory results exhibit a lack of specificity, although the presence of leukocytosis is typically observed. Ultrasonography or computed tomography can be used in regions where radiographic studies are available to confirm the diagnosis. However, it is important to note that surgical exploration should not be postponed if the clinical assessment strongly suggests the presence of acute appendicitis. In cases where patients exhibit symptoms shortly after their onset, the preferred course of treatment involves prompt appendectomy, accompanied by the administration of broad-spectrum antibiotics in cases of severe perforation. Conversely, patients experiencing symptoms for an extended period may be managed non-operatively with antibiotics. Acute gastroenteritis is a potential differential diagnosis for acute appendicitis, characterized by the presence of diarrhea as a prominent symptom and a more diffuse manifestation of abdominal pain. Conversely, gastroenteritis caused by *Yersinia* infection can manifest as mild diarrhea and abdominal pain in the right lower quadrant, leading to a misdiagnosis as appendicitis.

5.4.5.2. Tuberculosis of the Intestines

This condition has the potential to impact various segments of the gastrointestinal tract, with a particular emphasis on the ileocecal region. Furthermore, apart from the typical constitutional symptoms such as fever, night sweats, and weight loss, there may be indications of abdominal involvement, including distension caused by ascites, diarrhea resulting from malabsorption, obstruction due to stenosing disease, or the existence of an abdominal mass. Open pulmonary disease is present in less than 50% of patients diagnosed with intestinal tuberculosis. Laboratory examinations typically detect the presence of anemia and elevated levels of inflammatory markers, albeit lacking specificity. Tuberculin tests typically yield robust positive results in individuals who possess sufficient nourishment, while frequently yielding negative results in those afflicted with malnutrition or HIV infection. It is necessary to analyze sputum and gastric washings for the presence of tubercle bacilli. Radiographic contrast studies of the gastrointestinal tract reveal various alterations, such as the development of mucosal ulcers, the formation of strictures, the narrowing of segments, and the formation of fistulas. Colonoscopy can confirm the diagnosis by detecting acid-fast bacilli or caseating granulomas on a biopsy. However, it is important to note that these findings are not always present, and it can be challenging to differentiate other endoscopic findings from other colon diseases, particularly Crohn's disease. In certain cases, the diagnosis may be established solely through the utilization of laparoscopy or laparotomy, followed by microscopic examination and culture of biopsies. In cases where the available facilities for investigation are insufficient, it may be imperative to administer antituberculous medications to the patient based on a clinical diagnosis.

5.4.5.3. Inflammatory Bowel Disease (IBD)

The chronic inflammatory disorders of the bowel, namely Crohn's disease and ulcerative colitis, are believed to arise from the complex interaction of genetic factors, environmental factors, and the immune response of the host. Historically associated with Western societies, there is now a growing recognition that the prevalence of these diseases is on the rise in numerous developing nations. While it is widely acknowledged that the hygiene hypothesis may be an oversimplification of the underlying causes of these diseases, it is plausible that the altered Th1/Th2 balance, which arises from reduced childhood exposure to helminths, could contribute to the rising prevalence of these diseases in tropical countries experiencing demographic transition. Furthermore, it is probable that a significant portion of actual cases were previously misidentified as infectious colitis.

Celiac disease has the potential to affect various segments of the gastrointestinal tract, with a particular inclination towards the terminal ileum and cecum. Inflammatory lesions give rise to symptoms such as abdominal pain in the right lower quadrant, diarrhea, and weight loss. Ileocecal inflammatory lesions can be diagnosed through a differential approach, which encompasses various bacterial infections such as yersiniosis or actinomycosis, tuberculosis, histoplasmosis, parasitic infections like amebiasis, and helminthic infections such as strongyloidiasis. The examination of biopsy specimens at a microscopic level reveals the presence of transmural inflammation, lymphoid aggregates, and noncaseating granulomas. Distinguishing between Crohn's disease and intestinal tuberculosis can pose difficulties due to variations in clinical, endoscopic, and histologic characteristics. In regions where tuberculosis is prevalent, an empirical investigation is conducted to evaluate the efficacy of antituberculous medications. The management of Crohn's disease encompasses a combination of medical and surgical interventions. Medical interventions encompass the administration of broad-spectrum antibiotics and immunosuppressive agents. In cases where the disease is accompanied by complications such as strictures, fistulizing disease, or abscesses, surgical intervention becomes imperative.

Ulcerative colitis is characterized by inflammation at the rectum, which subsequently extends proximally. Proctosigmoidoscopy reveals reddened and raw mucosa. The results of the histologic examination indicate that the inflammation is confined to the submucosa. Furthermore, the lamina propria exhibits an inflammatory cell infiltrate, crypt abscesses display neutrophil accumulation, and the epithelium shows a depletion of goblet cells. Granulomas are not present. Ulcerative colitis is confined to the colon and rectum, unlike Crohn's disease where lesions can spread throughout the bowel. Therefore, if the disease does not respond to medical treatment, total colectomy is a curative procedure.

5.4.5.4. Megacolon

Individuals exhibiting symptoms of large bowel dilatation may present with symptoms such as abdominal pain, distension, and tenderness. Toxic megacolon has the potential to complicate various infectious colitis, such as *C. difficile*, and is a frequently encountered complication. Infection caused by *C. difficile* is observed in cases of fulminant colitis resulting from inflammatory bowel diseases. In rare instances, it may be attributed to drug-induced intestinal hypomotility. The abdominal examination reveals a notable presentation of abdominal distension accompanied by the absence of bowel sounds. The abdominal plain film reveals a significantly enlarged colon. Bacterial culture of stool should be conducted. The administration of *C. difficile* toxin and the detection of ova and parasites. Regardless of the cause, the recommended treatment is colectomy. Without surgical intervention, there is an unacceptable risk of bowel perforation and peritonitis.

On the other hand, certain individuals may exhibit large bowel dilatation without experiencing systemic toxicity. Constipation arises as a consequence of persistent intestinal pseudo-obstruction. The absence of ganglions in the enteric nervous plexus, as seen in Chagas disease, may be the cause.

5.4.5.5. Colon and Rectal Stenosis Lesions

Stenosing lesions of the bowel can arise due to various pathological conditions, including amebiasis, schistosomiasis, tuberculosis, and lymphogranuloma venereum, which primarily affects the rectum. Inflammatory strictures can also manifest in Crohn's disease or following an episode of diverticulitis, or they can be neoplastic. The cecum is the primary location for the development of amebomas, although any segment of the colon can be impacted. At times, there are instances where multiple amebomas develop in a single patient. The typical symptoms include chronic diarrhea accompanied by hematuria and localized abdominal pain, as well as the presence of one or more tender masses in the abdomen. The lesion is characterized by the presence of granulation tissue exhibiting regions of necrosis and fibroblast proliferation. Amebas are frequently challenging to locate; however, serologic tests yield positive results in more than 90% of instances. The implementation of targeted treatment leads to prompt resolution, obviating the need for surgical excision.

The presence of granulomatous lesions in the colon caused by schistosomiasis can lead to bowel constriction. Antischistosomal treatment can reverse early lesions. Surgical intervention may be necessary for the removal of infrequent fibrotic strictures.

5.4.6. Rectum and Anus

5.4.6.1. Proctitis

Rectal pain, tenesmus, and a mucopurulent rectal discharge are symptoms associated with inflammation of the rectum. Although the rectum can be affected by various infectious causes of colitis, isolated proctitis is predominantly a sexually transmitted infection (STI). It is typically observed in men who engage in unprotected anal intercourse with other men. The primary etiologies include gonorrhea, herpes simplex, lymphogranuloma venereum resulting from chlamydia infection (which is prevalent in Africa, South and Southeast Asia, and Central and South America), and syphilis. Proctitis can arise from noninfectious factors such as inflammatory bowel diseases, radiation exposure, ischemia, and neoplasia. The comprehensive diagnostic evaluation should encompass the examination of rectal swab cultures to detect gonorrhea, lymphogranuloma venereum, and herpes simplex virus, as well as blood samples for serologic testing of syphilis. Prior to the rectal examination, it is advisable to conduct STI testing, as certain lubricants possess bacteriostatic properties. Anoscopy may be contraindicated due to pain; if conducted, the mucosa exhibits signs of edema, redness, and fragility, accompanied by exudates or ulceration. In cases where proctitis is suspected to be caused by a sexually transmitted infection (STI), but the specific causative agent remains unidentified, it is recommended to initiate empiric antimicrobial therapy. The combination of ceftriaxone, doxycycline, and valacyclovir has demonstrated efficacy against the four primary etiological agents. It is crucial to identify and treat sexual partners, and it is important to provide counseling on barrier protection, as proctitis heightens the likelihood of HIV transmission.

5.4.6.2. Rectal Prolapse

Prolapse through the anus can occur in either the mucosa or all layers of the rectal wall. Typically, this is a secondary consequence of an underlying disorder. Diarrheal diseases, particularly shigellosis, parasitic infestations such as *Trichuris trichiura*, and malnutrition are frequently observed as underlying factors in children residing in tropical regions. Rectal prolapse is more prevalent in elderly women among adults, primarily caused by pelvic floor weakness resulting from vaginal delivery. The primary objective of treatment is to rectify the fundamental disorder, and in cases where repeated manual reductions are deemed necessary, surgical intervention may be employed.

5.4.6.3. Lesions in the Anus

Frequently encountered benign lesions in the vicinity of the anus encompassing ulcers and warts. Both can induce pruritus, hemorrhaging, and acute pain. Ulcers commonly arise as a result of infection with the herpes simplex virus, syphilis, or chancroid. Furthermore, individuals with HIV are particularly vulnerable to ulcers induced by cytomegalovirus, tuberculosis, and fungal infections. A subset of individuals diagnosed with HIV exhibit idiopathic anal ulcers, which are characterized by the absence of any identifiable infectious agents. *Condylomata acuminata*, commonly known as anal warts, are the result of infection with human papillomavirus, which is associated with sexual activity. It is important to differentiate between the exophytic, flesh-colored lesions and the flat lesions of condyloma lata, which are commonly observed in cases of secondary syphilis.

5.4.6.4. Anal Cancer

Squamous cell carcinoma, commonly known as cancer of the anal canal, constitutes a relatively minor fraction of gastrointestinal malignancies. Nevertheless, there has been a global rise in the occurrence of anal cancer, which can be attributed to the extensive prevalence of human papillomavirus infection. Patients who are co-infected with HIV may experience an elevated risk. Individuals exhibit symptoms of rectal bleeding or the presence of a mass at the anal verge. Chemoradiotherapy or surgery are the available treatment options.

5.5. Gastrointestinal Diseases in Patients with Human Immunodeficiency Virus (Acquired Immune Deficiency Syndrome (AIDS)

Acute HIV-1 infection manifests as a mononucleosis-like illness, characterized by generally mild gastrointestinal symptoms such as nausea, vomiting, and diarrhea. In certain instances, individuals may experience pancreatitis or hepatitis. Advanced HIV infection typically affects the gastrointestinal tract, primarily resulting in esophageal disease and chronic diarrhea (Box 5.5). Organ-specific diseases in individuals infected with HIV can typically be ascribed to one of three etiologies: inherent to the HIV infection, opportunistic infection, or the medications employed for HIV treatment or prevention of its complications. The causes differ based on the extent of immunosuppression.

Gastrointestinal Involvement in AIDS

- Dysphagia
- Candida esophagitis
- CMV esophagitis
- HSV esophagitis
- Idiopathic esophageal ulcer
- Diarrhea
- Opportunistic infections
  - CMV
  - Salmonellosis, campylobacteriosis
  - Tuberculosis, Mycobacterium avium-intracellulare infection
  - Cryptosporidium hominis/ parvum, Cyclospora cayetanensis, Isospora belli, Entamoeba
  - histolytica, Giardia lamblia, Strongyloides stercoralis
  - Microsporidiosis, cryptococcosis, coccidioidomycosis, histoplasmosis
- AIDS enteropathy
- Medications
- Lymphoma
- Malignancy - any location, due to
- Kaposi sarcoma
- Non-Hodgkin lymphoma

Box 5.5

Patients with AIDS frequently experience chronic diarrhea, which leads to substantial morbidity and mortality. Although the CD4 cell count remains unchanged, the underlying causes are comparable to those observed in individuals without HIV. As the infection progresses, there is an increase in the prevalence of parasitic, fungal, and viral infections. A considerable number of these pathogens can also be detected in individuals with AIDS who do not exhibit diarrhea, indicating the prevalence of asymptomatic infection. The workup should encompass the collection of stool specimens for bacterial culture, as well as examinations for ova and parasites. If the aforementioned methods fail to provide significant insights, the utilization of flexible sigmoidoscopy with biopsy could prove beneficial in the diagnostic process, particularly in the detection of cytomegalovirus infection. The appropriate course of action should focus on addressing the particular enteric pathogen that has been identified. In cases where certain infections, such as cryptosporidiosis and microsporidiosis, are the sole viable treatment options, commencement of antiretroviral therapy is recommended.

No enteric pathogens are found in a significant number of AIDS patients experiencing diarrhea. Villous atrophy and lymphocytic infiltration into the lamina propria are observed in small intestinal biopsy specimens obtained from these patients. The aforementioned idiopathic condition is referred to as AIDS enteropathy, which potentially signifies the mucosal reaction to atypical pathogens, such as HIV.

5.6. Summary

Diseases of the gastrointestinal (GI) system encompass a broad spectrum of conditions affecting the digestive tract, which includes the mouth, esophagus, stomach, small intestine, large intestine, and rectum, along with the liver, pancreas, and gallbladder. These conditions can range from mild to severe, impacting various functions of the digestive system and significantly affecting individuals' health and quality of life.

Common gastrointestinal disorders include GERD, peptic ulcer disease, irritable bowel syndrome (IBS), inflammatory bowel disease (IBD), which includes Crohn's disease and ulcerative colitis, gastrointestinal cancers, celiac disease, diverticulitis, and various infectious diseases like gastroenteritis. Symptoms of GI diseases are diverse, including abdominal pain, bloating, diarrhea, constipation, indigestion, vomiting, and weight loss or gain, reflecting the complex nature of these disorders.

The causes of gastrointestinal diseases are multifactorial, involving genetic predisposition, lifestyle factors such as diet and exercise, chronic stress, microbial infections, and environmental exposures. For example, GERD is often attributed to the reflux of stomach acid into the esophagus, whereas IBS and IBD are thought to result from a combination of genetic, immune, and environmental factors. Infectious gastroenteritis is caused by various pathogens, including viruses, bacteria, and parasites.

Diagnosis of GI diseases typically involves a combination of clinical evaluation, laboratory tests, imaging studies, and endoscopic procedures to visualize the interior of the digestive tract. Treatment strategies vary widely depending on the specific condition and can include dietary and lifestyle modifications, medications to manage symptoms or modify disease processes, and in some cases, surgical interventions.

Prevention of gastrointestinal diseases often focuses on lifestyle choices such as maintaining a healthy diet, regular exercise, minimizing stress, and avoiding known risk factors like tobacco and excessive alcohol use. Vaccinations and proper hygiene practices are also crucial in preventing infectious causes of GI diseases.

A Closer Look

Antimicrobial Agents

Antimicrobial agents are substances that inhibit or kill microorganisms, including bacteria, fungi, viruses, and parasites. They have revolutionized medicine, offering treatments for infections that were once life-threatening. These agents can be classified broadly into antibiotics (against bacteria), antifungals, antivirals, and antiparasitics.

Mechanisms of Action vary across antimicrobial classes. Antibiotics like penicillin and cephalosporins interfere with bacterial cell wall synthesis, while others, such as fluoroquinolones, target DNA replication. Antifungals, like azoles, typically inhibit cell membrane synthesis in fungi, while antivirals often disrupt viral replication or entry into host cells. Selecting the appropriate agent depends on identifying the infecting organism and understanding its vulnerabilities. Misuse or overuse, however, contributes significantly to the growing crisis of antimicrobial resistance (AMR), where microbes adapt to evade treatment.

Antimicrobial Resistance (AMR) is a pressing global health threat, driven by factors like excessive prescription, agricultural use, and suboptimal dosing. Resistant strains, such as MRSA (methicillin-resistant Staphylococcus aureus) and MDR-TB (multi-drug resistant tuberculosis), require alternative, often more toxic or expensive, therapies. Addressing AMR necessitates a multifaceted approach, including rigorous infection control practices, public health awareness, novel drug discovery, and policies to reduce antimicrobial misuse.

Recent Innovations in antimicrobial development focus on discovering new drug classes, repurposing existing drugs, and employing adjunct therapies to enhance efficacy. Nanotechnology is emerging in antimicrobial delivery, improving targeting and reducing side effects. Another promising area is phage therapy, where bacteriophages—viruses that infect bacteria—are used to target specific pathogens. Such advancements represent critical steps toward effective infection control in an era of rising resistance.

References

1. Almadi, M. A., Ghosh, S., & Aljebreen, A. M., (2009). Differentiating intestinal tuberculosis from Crohn's disease: a diagnostic challenge. *Am J Gastroenterol. 104,* 1003–1012.
2. Al-Saleem, T., Al-Mondhiry, H., (2005). Immunoproliferative small intestinal disease (IPSID), a model for mature B-cell neoplasms. *Blood. 105,* 2274–2280.
3. Anastassopoulos, K., Farraye, F. A., Knight, T., Colman, S., Cleveland, M. V., Pelham, R. W. (2016). A Comparative Study of Treatment-Emergent Adverse Events Following Use of Common Bowel Preparations Among a Colonoscopy Screening Population: Results from a Post-Marketing Observational Study. *Dig. Dis. Sci. 61,* 2993–3006.
4. Belsey, J., Epstein, O., & Heresbach, D., (2009). Systematic review: Adverse event reports for oral sodium phosphate and polyethylene glycol. *Aliment. Pharmacol. Ther. 29,* 15–28.
5. Bhatnagar, S., Gupta, S. D., & Mathur, M., (2005). Celiac disease with mild to moderate histologic changes is a common cause of chronic diarrhea in Indian children. *J Pediatr Gastroenterol Nutr. 41,* 204–209.
6. Bhattacharyya, A., Chattopadhyay, R., Mitra, S., & Crowe, S. E., (2014). Oxidative Stress: An Essential Factor in the Pathogenesis of Gastrointestinal Mucosal Diseases. *Physiol. Rev. 94,* 329–354.
7. Cello, J. P., & Day, L. W., (2009). Idiopathic AIDS enteropathy and treatment of gastrointestinal opportunistic pathogens. *Gastroenterology. 136,* 1952–1965.
8. Chan, A., Depew, W., & Vanner, S., (1997). Use of oral sodium phosphate colonic lavage solution by Canadian colonoscopists: Pitfalls and complications. *Can. J. Gastroenterol. Hepatol. 11,* 797486.
9. Davis, T. W., & Goldstone, S. E., (2009). Sexually transmitted infections as a cause of proctitis in men who have sex with men. *Dis Colon Rectum. 52,* 507–512.
10. de Silva, H. J., de Silva, N. R., de Silva, A. P., (2008). Emergence of inflammatory bowel disease "beyond the West": do prosperity and improved hygiene have a role? *Trans R Soc Trop Med Hyg. 102,* 857–860.
11. Driman, D. K., & Preiksaitis, H. G., (1998). Colorectal inflammation and increased cell proliferation associated with oral sodium phosphate bowel preparation solution. *Hum. Pathol. 29,* 972–978.
12. Enwonwu, C. O., Falkler, W. A., Jr, Phillips, R. S., (2006). Noma (cancrum oris). *Lancet. 368,* 147–156.
13. Fernández, J. F. J., Sainz, I.F.-U.; Ollo, B. Z., Dueñas, C. S., Guimera, M. M., González, A. E., Costas, J. J. V., (2018). Gastroduodenal lesions detected during small bowel capsule endoscopy: Incidence, diagnostic and therapeutic impact. *Rev. Esp. Enferm. Dig. 110,* 102–108.
14. Hagège, H., Laugier, R., Nahon, S., Coulom, P., Isnard-Bagnis, C., Albert-Marty, A., (2015). Real-life conditions of use of sodium phosphate tablets for colon cleansing before colonoscopy. *Endosc. Int. Open 3*, e346–e353.
15. Hill, D. R., & Ryan, E. T., (2008). Management of travelers' diarrhea. *BMJ. 337,* a1746.
16. Hogenauer, C., Langner, C., & Beubler, E., (2006). *Klebsiella oxytoca* as a causative organism of antibiotic-associated hemorrhagic colitis. *N Engl J Med. 355,* 2418–2426.

17. Hsu, M. H., Chang, I. W., & Tai, C. M., (2016). White Spots in the Rectum. *Gastroenterology, 151,* e15–e16.

18. Kosek, M., Bern, C., & Guerrant, R. L., (2003). The global burden of diarrhoeal disease, as estimated from studies published between 1992 and 2000. *Bull World Health Organ. 81,* 197–204.

19. Lecuit, M., Abachin, E., & Martin, A., (2004). Immunoproliferative small intestinal disease associated with *Campylobacter jejuni. N Engl J Med. 350,* 239–248.

20. Leong, R. W., (2009). Differences in peptic ulcer between the East and the West. *Gastroenterol Clin North Am. 38,* 363–379.

21. Lucas, M. E. S., Deen, J. L., von Seidlein, L., (2005). Effectiveness of mass oral cholera vaccination in Beira, Mozambique. *N Engl J Med. 352,* 757–767.

22. Ludvigsson, J. F., Montgomery, S. M., & Ekbom, A., (2009). Small-intestinal histopathology and mortality risk in celiac disease. *JAMA. 302,* 1171–1178.

23. Nam, S., Choi, I., Park, K., Ryu, K., Kim, B., Sohn, D., Nam, B., & Kim, C., (2010). Risk of hemorrhagic gastropathy associated with colonoscopy bowel preparation using oral sodium phosphate solution. *Endoscopy 42,* 109–113.

24. Pawlowski, S. W., Warren, C. A., & Guerrant, R., (2009). Diagnosis and treatment of acute or persistent diarrhea. *Gastroenterology. 136,* 1874–1886.

25. Plummer, M. P., Blaser, A. R., & Deane, A. M., (2014). Stress ulceration: Prevalence, pathology and association with adverse outcomes. *Crit. Care 18,* 213.

26. Ramakrishna, B. S., Venkataraman, S., & Mukhopadhya, A., (2006). Tropical malabsorption. *Postgrad Med, J., 82,* 779–787.

27. Rejchrt, S., Bureš, J., Široký, M., Kopáčová, M., Slezák, L., Langr, F. (2004). A prospective, observational study of colonic mucosal abnormalities associated with orally administered sodium phosphate for colon cleansing before colonoscopy. *Gastrointest. Endosc. 59,* 651–654.

28. Roy, S. K., Hossain, M. J., & Khatun, W., (2008). Zinc supplementation in children with cholera in Bangladesh: randomized controlled trial. *BMJ. 336,* 266–268.

29. Section on Pediatric Dentistry and Oral Health Preventive oral health intervention for pediatricians. (2008). *Pediatrics. 122,* 1387–1394.

30. Shah, N., DuPont, H. L., & Ramsey, D. J., (2009). Global etiology of travelers' diarrhea: systematic review from 1973 to the present. *Am J Trop Med Hyg. 80,* 609–614.

31. Steffen, R., (2005). Epidemiology of traveler's diarrhea. *Clin Infect Dis. 41*(Suppl 8), S536–S540.

32. Teixeira, A. R., Nitz, N., & Guimaro, M. C., (2006). Chagas disease. *Postgrad Med, J., 82,* 788–798.

33. Wallace, J. L., (2008). Prostaglandins, NSAIDs, and Gastric Mucosal Protection: Why Doesn't the Stomach Digest Itself? *Physiol. Rev. 88,* 1547–1565.

34. Watts, D. A., Lessells, A. M., Penman, I. D., & Ghosh, S., (2002). Endoscopic and histologic features of sodium phosphate bowel preparation-induced colonic ulceration: Case report and review. *Gastrointest. Endosc. 55,* 584–587.

35. Zwas, F. R., Cirillo, N. W., Ei-Serag, H. B., & Eisen, R. N., (1996). Colonic mucosal abnormalities associated with oral sodium phosphate solution. *Gastrointest. Endosc. 43,* 463–466.

Chapter 6

HEMATOLOGICAL DISORDERS

Contents

Introduction

Hematologic diseases encompass a wide spectrum of conditions that affect the blood and blood-forming organs, presenting a significant health burden worldwide. These diseases are characterized by their diverse nature, affecting millions of individuals with conditions that range from common to exceedingly rare. The American Society of Hematology emphasizes the complexity and breadth of hematologic diseases, noting that they not only include malignancies such as blood cell cancers but also a broad array of non-cancerous conditions.

Blood cell cancers, a critical subset of hematologic disorders, are perhaps the most recognized, encompassing leukemias, lymphomas, and myelomas. These malignancies represent a significant area of concern due to their impact on the body's ability to produce and regulate blood cells effectively. According to the National Cancer Institute, these cancers target the very foundation of the body's hematologic system, disrupting the normal production and function of white blood cells, red blood cells, and platelets.

Beyond these well-known cancers, hematologic diseases also include a myriad of genetic disorders, some of which are exceedingly rare. The National Institutes of Health highlights conditions such as hemophilia and thalassemia, which, though less common, pose substantial challenges to those affected. These genetic anomalies can lead to a wide range of symptoms, from mild to life-threatening, necessitating ongoing research and specialized care.

Anemia, another prevalent hematologic condition, is characterized by a deficiency in the number or quality of red blood cells, which are crucial for carrying oxygen throughout the body. The World Health Organization points out that anemia can result from various causes, including nutritional deficiencies, chronic diseases, infections, and inherited conditions, making it a global health concern with multifaceted implications.

Furthermore, hematologic diseases also intersect with other health conditions, such as HIV. The Centers for Disease Control and Prevention (CDC) report that individuals living with HIV may face an increased risk of certain blood-related conditions, including anemia and leukopenia, due to both the virus itself and the side effects of treatments.

Sickle cell disease represents another significant concern within the realm of hematologic disorders. This inherited condition, which alters the shape and functionality of red blood cells, can lead to severe pain, organ damage, and increased susceptibility to infections. The CDC underscores the importance of early diagnosis and comprehensive care in managing sickle cell disease and mitigating its impacts. Lastly, complications arising from medical treatments such as chemotherapy or blood transfusions further complicate the landscape of hematologic diseases. The American Cancer Society discusses how treatments intended to combat cancers and other conditions can inadvertently affect the blood and its components, leading to additional health challenges that require careful management.

Thus, the spectrum of hematologic diseases is broad, affecting millions with conditions ranging from blood cell cancers to rare genetic disorders, anemia, and complications related to other illnesses like HIV, sickle cell disease, and the aftereffects of treatments such as chemotherapy or transfusions. This diversity underscores the need for ongoing research, patient education, and advancements in treatment to address the complex needs of those affected by these disorders.

Orientation and Directional Terms

Term	Definition	Illustration
Anemia	A condition in which there is a deficiency of red blood cells or hemoglobin, leading to fatigue and weakness due to reduced oxygen delivery to tissues.	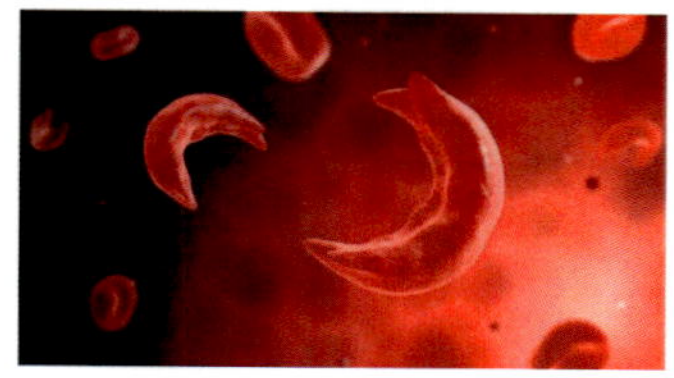
Immunohistochemistry	A laboratory technique used to detect specific antigens in cells of a tissue section using labeled antibodies, commonly used in diagnosing diseases.	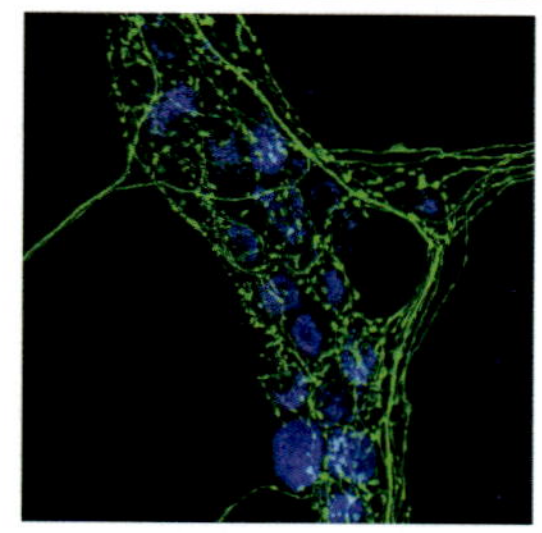
Immunophenotyping	A laboratory technique that uses antibodies to identify cells based on the proteins they express on their surface. It's used to diagnose diseases like leukemia and lymphoma, and is also used in basic research.	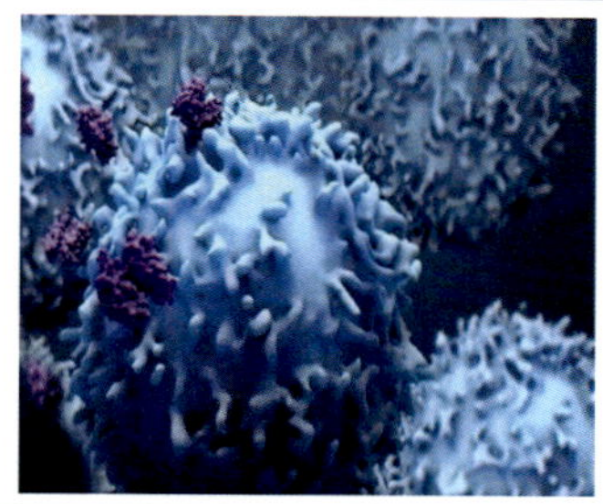
Anti-Phospholipid Antibody Testing	A test to detect antibodies that mistakenly target phospholipids, associated with clotting disorders and autoimmune diseases.	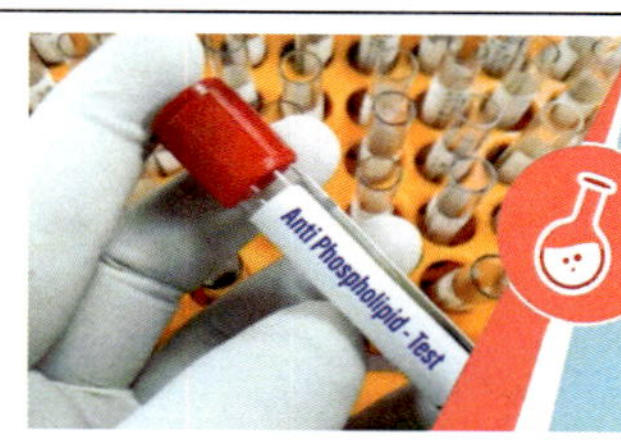
Hematological disorders	Hematologic diseases are disorders which primarily affect the blood and blood-forming organs. Hematologic diseases include rare genetic disorders, anemia, HIV, sickle cell disease and complications from chemotherapy or transfusions.	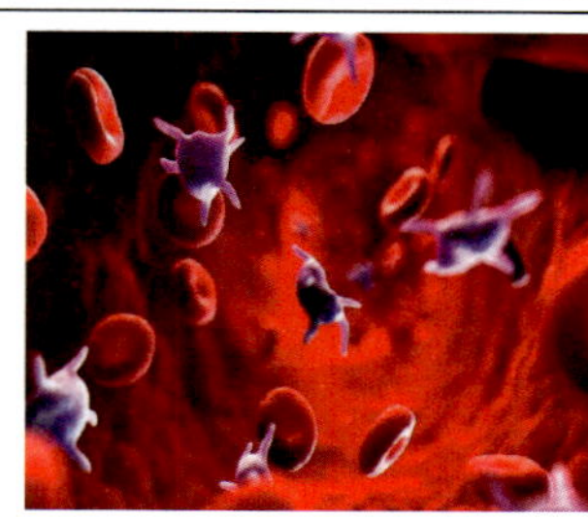

6.1. Anemia: General Approach

Definition:

- **Functional definition**: A significant reduction in red cell mass and a corresponding decrease in the 0_2 carrying capacity of the blood.
- **Laboratory definition**: A reduction of the Hemoglobin concentration, red cell mass or hematocrite, to below normal levels.
- In women of childbearing age, their blood values are 10% lower than men. Therefore, anemia may be defined as an HCT of <10% below the mean values for age, sex, and altitude
- Hgb or Hematocrite could be falsely elevated (plasma volume), e.g., hemorrhage, burns, vigorous diuresis, dehydration, all leading to *Hemoconcentration*
- Hgb or Hct may be falsely low (plasma volume), leading to *Hemodilution*, e.g., Splenomegaly, congestive heart failure (CHF), cirrhosis, pregnancy

Epidemiology:

- In Ethiopia, a study conducted by Zein Ahmed Zein in Gondar, rural population indicated a prevalence rate of anemia to be very high (40.5%), and anemia was the fourth leading cause of hospitalization and hospital deaths in 1982 in Gondar.
- Another study done in Black Lion Hospital in 1987 G.C. showed that anemia is the 3rd cause of hematology admissions.
- Analysis of admissions to hospitals in Ethiopia showed that anemia accounted for 0.5–4% of all admissions and 25% of hematological diseases-related admissions.
- Iron deficiency anemia is the most common type of anemia globally, mainly in developing countries like Ethiopia.
- Sickle cell disease and thalassemias are not reported in Ethiopia but are common in other African countries. Hereditary hemolytic anemias aren't common in our country.

Clinical Approach to Patients with Anemia: Anemia is a manifestation of an underlying pathological condition. It results from:

- Under production;
- Increased destruction/hemolysis;
- Blood loss /bleeding;
- Multifactorial: a combination of these.

History: Accurate history provides information crucial to the diagnosis of the underlying cause.

- Nutritional /dietary history;
- Underlying diseases;
- Blood loss: GI or Genito urinary blood loss;
- Family history of anemia;
- Exposure to drugs/toxins, e.g., methyldopa;

- Geographical location;
- Pregnancy.

Symptoms:

- Depend on the rapidity of development of anemia, the age of the patients, and the presence of an underlying disease. They are often non-specific.
- Fatigue, dizziness, dyspnea, palpitation, syncope, exercise and cold intolerance, angina,
- Tinnitus, vertigo, throbbing headache,
- Anorexia, indigestion, nausea, bowel irregularity (due to shunting of blood from the splanchnic bed)
- Irritability, difficulty in concentration, worsened dementia and.
- Impotence or decreased libido
- Intermittent claudication.

Physical Examination: A comprehensive examination with emphasis on the following findings should be made.

- Skin and mucous membrane: look for pallor, icterus, bleeding sites, leg ulcer
- Spooning of fingernails in iron deficiency anemia
- Atrophy of the tongue, sore tongue (glossitis), angular stomatitis, which may be seen in iron deficiency anemia.
- Abdomen: splenomegaly, hepatomegaly, evidence of gallstone.
- Pelvic and rectal examination: to look for possible sites of bleeding.
- Bone tenderness and Lymphadenopathy to rule our hematologic malignancies and
- Neurological: gait, reflexes, vibration, and position sense, which may help to look for neurologic changes associated with Vit B_{12} deficiency.
- Fundoscopy: retinal hemorrhage
- Cardiovascular system; modest tachycardia, wide pulse pressure hyperdynamic precordium, flow murmur. In severe forms of chronic anemia patients may develop CHF with S3 gallops.

Laboratory Study:

i. **Complete Blood Count:** Hgb, Hct, ESR, Platelet count, WBC with differential.

ii. **Red Blood Cell Indices:**

- Mean Ccorpuscular volume (MCV): Hct/RBC: normal value is 80–95 fl.
- Mean corpuscular hemoglobin (MCH): Hgb/RBC: 27–32 pg.
- Mean corpuscular hemoglobin (MCHC): Hgb/Hct 32–36%.

iii. **Examination of the Peripheral Blood Smear:** Examine the cellular morphology, shape, size, color, abnormality of other cells.

Red Cell Morphology:

- Normochromic normocytic RBCs are seen in normal individuals and in anemia of chronic diseases
- Anisopoikilocytes: Variation in size and shape may be seen in iron deficiency anemia
- Hypochromic microcytic anemia: is seen in iron deficiency anemia, anemia of chronic diseases, thalassemia and sideroblastic anemia (SBA)
- Macrocytic RBCs: Macro-ovalocytes with hyper segmented neutrophils indicate

Megaloblastic anemia and myelodysplasia.

- Schistocytes (fragmented RBC/helmentcells): Microangiopathies, DIC, vasculitis, prosthetic heart valve

Classification of Anemia:

i. Pathophyisiologic Classifications (Based on the Underlying Disease):

a. Anemia Associated with Impaired RBC Production:

- Aplastic anemia
- Iron deficiency
- Myelodysplastic syndrome.
- Megaloblastic anemia
- Anemia of CRF
- Anemia of chronic diseases
- Drug related

b. Anemia Associated with Increased RBC Loss or Destruction:

- **Bleeding**
- **Hereditary Hemolytic Anemia:**
  - o Hemoglobinopathies, sickle cell disease, Thalassemia
  - o Primary disorder of RBCs
  - o RBC erythropathies (G6 PDH, PK deficiency)
- **Acquired Hemolytic Anemia:**
  - o Autoimmune
  - o Drug induced hemolytic anemia
  - o Microangiopathies (e.g., DIC)
  - o Traumatic

ii. Morphological Classification:

a. Hypochromic Microcytic Anemia:

- Inherited: Thalassema, sideroblastic anemia;
- Acquired: IDA, Anemia of chronic diseases.

b. Macrocytic Anemia: (MCV > 100 fl)

- With megaloblastic marrow: megaloblastic anemia;
- With normoblastic marrow: Hemolysis, acute bleeding.

c. Normchromic Normocytic:

- Anemia of chronic disease;
- Early iron deficiency anemia;
- Aplastic anemia;
- Anemia of CRF.

Adaptation to Chronic Anemia: The main consequence of anemia is tissue hypoxia.

Compensatory Mechanisms:

i. Intrinsic Red Cell Adjustments (Adaptations):

- Modulation of O_2 affinity by increased generation of 2,3-diphosphoglycerate in erythrocytes.
- It bounds to Hgb, causing a rightward shift in O_2^- Hgb dissolution curve.

This allows more O_2 to be unloaded from the RBC at any given blood O_2 tension.

ii. Cardiovascular Adjustment:

- Increase in cardiac output occurs at Hgb level of 7–8 gm%: the increase in cardiac output coupled with modest tachycardia creates a hyperdynamic state and hence systolic ejection murmur
- Peripheral vascular resistance decreases, thereby facilitating tissue perfusion; clinically this is evidenced by wide pulse pressure.

iii. Local Changes in Tissue Perfusion: Redistribution of blood flow to vital organs at the expense of reduced blood flow to less vital organs.

iv. Reduction of mixed venous O_2 tension to increases the arterio-venous O_2 difference. Individuals tend to survive at extremely low hemoglobin levels (even as low as 3 gm %) due to these compensatory mechanisms.

Ø **Therapeutic Considerations and Indications:** In the management of anemic patients carefully remember the following points:

- Identify and correct the cause of anemia.
- Administration of Hematinines such as Iron, Vit B_{12} or folate without correct diagnosis of the cause of anemia is an unacceptable practice in the treatment of anemia.
- Therapeutic modalities include iron, folate, Vit. B_{12}, pyridoxine (B_6) blood transfusion, steroids (in hemolytic anemia) splenectomy, erythropoietin, bone marrow transplant (aplastic anemia), and androgens.
- Carefully weigh the risks of blood transfusion over its advantages. When to transfuse blood in chronic anemia:
  - o Anemia severe enough to cause congestive heart failure;
  - o Hypoxic manifestations: Irritability, unconsciousness, angina;
  - o Surgical or gynecologic patient awaiting surgery.

NB: No threshold of Hct/Hgb that mandates transfusion; the decision to administer blood must be based on the functional status and symptomatology of the patient.

- Consider the risk of blood transfusion;
- Adhere to blood component transfusion (packed RBC, FFP, cryoprecipitate, platelets);
- Consider whole blood only when there is volume loss due to hemorrhage.

i. Microcytic Anemias:

a. **Iron Deficiency Anemia (IDA):** Learning objectives: at the end of this topic, the student will be able to:

- Understand iron metabolism;
- Describe the characteristic features of IDA;
- List the various causes of IDA;
- Know the clinical manifestations and common specific laboratory findings of IDA;
- List some of the differential diagnosis of IDA;
- Understand the management of IDA;
- Identify possible reasons for inadequate response to therapy and indications for parenteral iron administration;
- List the possible causes of anemia of chronic diseases with their features, pathogenesis, and principles of therapy.

Definition: Iron deficiency anemia occurs when body iron stores become inadequate for the needs of normal RBC production (erythropoiesis).

It's characterized by:

- Hypochromia and microcytosis of the circulating erythrocytes (RBCs);
- Low plasma iron and ferretine concentration;
- A transferrin saturation of < 15% (normally ~ 35%);
- Iron deficiency anemia is a manifestation of diseases, not by itself a complete diagnosis;
- It is the most common cause of anemia worldwide.

Iron Metabolism:

- Daily 10–30mg iron ingested, 5–10% absorbed to balance precisely the amount lost (1 mg) under physiologic condition
- Amount absorbed can increase up to *five-fold* if body iron store is depleted or erythropoiesis is accelerated.
- Absorbed as hem and non-hem iron in the duodenum and proximal jejunum

Iron Absorption:

- Is facilitated by: Stomach acidity, ascorbic acid, citrates, while
- Is limited/reduced by: Phosphates,

oxalates, TTC, tannates (tea) and pyrates (plant food)

Transferrin is the transport protein that carries iron in the plasma and ECF. Sequences of events in the development of IDA

- Mobilization and depletion of iron stores;
- Decreased plasma Fe^{2+} and ferretin concentration;
- Iron deficient erythropoiesis;
- Iron deficiency anemia – hypo-chromic microcytic cells.

Etiologies of Iron deficiency Anemia:

1. Chronic Blood Loss:
- Uterine
- Gastrointestinal, e.g., esophageal varices; hiatal hernia; peptic ulcer disease; aspirin ingestion; Carcinoma of the stomach, ceacum, colon or rectum; *hook worm infestation*; colitis; piles; diverticulosis; etc.
- Rarely hematuria, hemoglobulinuria, pulmonary hemosiderosis, self inflicted blood loss
- Disorders of hemeostasis, intravascular hemolysis

2. Increased Demands:
- Prematurity in newborns;
- Rapid growth (as in adolescent) growth spurt;
- Pregnancy.

3. **Mal Absorption of Iron:** Gastrectomy, celiac disease.
4. **Poor Diet:** A contributory factor in many countries but rarely the sole cause

Clinical Manifestation:

- Is insidious in onset and progressive in course;
- Patients often present with nonspecific symptoms mentioned above with/without some specific symptoms.

Specific Symptoms:

- Pica: craving for unusual food substance (amylophagia, geophagia, pagophagia).
- Increased GI absorption of lead – lead poisoning.
- Koilonychia – spooning of the finger nails.
- Plummer–Vinson/Peterson – Kelly syndrome: characterized by IDA, koilonychia, and dysphagia due to post cricoid esophageal web).

Laboratory Findings:

1. Peripheral Blood Morphology and RBC Indices:
- ↓MCV, ↓MCH, ↓MCHC, and hypochromic microcytic RBCs with occasional target cells and pencil-shaped poikilocytes;
- ↓ Reticulocyte count;
- Dimorphic peripheral films (mixed normal RBCs and microcytic hypochromic RBCs);
- Combined iron and folate /B_{12} deficiency;
- On those with recent iron therapy;
- Those with recent blood transfusion.

2. Serum Iron and Total Iron-Binding Capacity (TIBC):
- ↓ serum iron and TIBC (hence IBC is < 10% saturated). This is in contrast to other forms (e.g., ACD).

3. Serum ferritine is decreased.
4. **Free Erythrocyte Protoporphyrine (FEP): Non-Specific:** It increased during the early phase of iron deficiency anemia, lead poisoning, sideroblastic anemia, and erythropoietic porphyria.

5. **Bone Marrow Iron:** Complete absence of iron from stores (macrophages) and absence of siderotic iron granules from developing erythroblasts
6. Investigation to Establish the Underlying Cause:

- Stool for occult blood;
- CXR to exclude pulmonary hemosiderosis;
- U/A for hematuria or hemosiderinuria;
- Pelvic–gynecologic studies;
- Cr^- labeling of RBCs with 5-day collection of stools;
- Upper and lower GI radiologic and Endoscopic studies;
- Bronchoscopy.

Differential Diagnosis of Hypochromic, Microcytic Anemia:

1. With ↓ body iron stores - IDA:
2. **With Normal Body or Body Iron Store:**

- Impaired iron metabolism: Anemia of chronic diseases (ACD);
- Disorder of globin synthesis: Thalassemia;
- Disorders of hem synthesis: sideroblastic anemia;
- Both impaired iron metabolism and defective globin synthesis: lead poisoning.

Treatment of Iron Deficiency Anemia:

1. Identify the underlying cause and treat it.
2. Correct anemia and replenish stores by oral iron:

- Ferous sulfate 300 mg (60 mg elemental iron) 3x/day for 4–6 months
- Absorption increased by giving between meals, but side effects are less if given with meals.

Common Side Effects: GI upset, nausea, dyspepsia, constipation /diarrhea. If the side effects are not tolerable, reduce the dose or change brand, e.g., to ferrous gluconate or ferrous lactate syrup.

- Response to treatment: An expected daily rise of hemoglobin by 0.1–0.2 gm /dL in
- Follow-up: Reticulocytosis will start at 3–4 days and peak on the 10th day of initiation of treatment.
- An increase in Hgb concentration of at least 2 gm/dL after 3 weeks of therapy is considered as a good response.
- Treatment should be continued for about 3 months after resolution of anemia to replenish the iron store.

1. Inadequate Response may Imply:
    - Continuing hemorrhage;
    - non compliance to therapy;
    - Wrong diagnosis;
    - Mixed deficiency - associated folate or vit B_{12} deficiency;
    - Another cause for anemia, e.g., malignancy, inflammation;
    - Malabsorption - rare cause;
    - Use of slow-release preparations.
2. **Parentral Iron:** Indications:
    - Oral Iron intolerance despite modification in dosage regimen;
    - Malabsorption;
    - Inability or unwillingness to take orally.
    - Iron-dextran complex or iron sorbitol citrate can be used Intra-muscularly or intra-venous route.

Dose (ml) = 0.0442 (desired Hgb - Observed Hgb.) X weight (kg) + (0.26 x weight kg)

3. **Anemia of Chronic Diseases (ACD):** It occurs in association

with a variety of chronic inflammatory and malignant diseases.

4. Etiologies:

i. Chronic Inflammatory Diseases:

a. Infections: E.g., pulmonary abscess, TB, Osteomyelitis, pneumonia, bacterial endocarditis

b Non-infectious: E.g., Rheumatoid arthritis, SLE (systemic lupus erythematous) and other connective tissue diseases, sarcoidosis, Crohn's disease

ii. Malignant Diseases: E.g., carcinoma, lymphoma, sarcoma

Characteristic Features are:

- NCNC or mildly hypochromic indices and red cell morphology;
- Mild and non progressive anemia (Hgb rarely < 9.0 g/dL): Severity being related to severity of underlying disease;
- Both serum iron and TIBC are reduced;
- Serum ferritine is normal or raised; and
- Bone marrow storage iron is normal but erythroblast iron is reduced.

Pathogenesis is related to release of cytokines which mediate

- Decreased release of iron from macrophages to plasma;
- reduced RBC life span (80 days) in effective erythropoiesis;
- Inadequate erythropoietin response to anemia.

Treatment of anemia of chronic diseases:

- Correction of underlying disease;
- Erythropoietin (40–80% success rate);
- Correction of reversible contributors (iron, folate, cobalamine supplements if necessary).

Sideroblastic Anemia:

- Refractory anemia with hypochromia with marrow iron;
- Many pathological ring sideroblasts are found in the bone marrow;
- Is caused by defect in hem synthesis.

Classification:

- Hereditary (sex linked recessive trait);
- Acquired;
- Primary: Myelodysplasia;
- Secondary:
  - o Malignant diseases of the marrow;
  - o Drugs, e.g., cycloserin alcohol, lead;
  - o Others: hemolytic anemia, megaloblastic anemia, malabsorption.
  - o 15% of marrow erythroblasts are ring sideroblasts in hereditary and 1^0 acquired forms.
- **Lead Poisoning:**
  - o Inhibits both hem and globin synthesis.
  - o Interferes with breakdown of RNA by inhibiting the enzyme pyrimidine-5 nucleotidase Þ accumulation of denatured RNA in red cells giving rise to basophilic stippling.
  - o Hypo chromic/Hemolytic anemia with bone marrow ring sideroblasts.
  - o Free erythrocyte protoporphyrin is raised.
- **Management:**
  - o Pyridoxine, folic acid therapy: may bring some response;
  - o Repeated transfusion is ultimate choice.

6.2. Diagnostic Techniques for Hematological Disorders

The following section provides a description of the advancements in diagnostic techniques used to evaluate hematologic disorders, as presented in Box 6.1. One notable advancement has occurred in the field of genetic testing, which was in its early stages of development in 1990. Furthermore, there have been notable advancements in the utilization of antibodies for laboratory analysis, resulting in significant implications for various diagnostic procedures. Laboratories are authorized to conduct the chosen tests in accordance with the Clinical Laboratory Improvement Amendments (CLIA), as specified in the standard requirements. CLIA is a federal initiative designed to oversee and govern laboratory testing procedures. It mandates that clinical laboratories obtain certification from the Centers for Medicare and Medicaid Services (FDA) prior to accepting human samples for diagnostic testing (FDA, 2021).

Box 6.1 selected new or improved hematologic diagnostic techniques since 1990.

Assesses Molecular or Physiologic Functions: Genetic testing:

i. Phenotype Characterization:
   - Immunophenotyping: Immunohistochemistry and flow cytometry.
   - Other flow cytometry tests: Eosin-5-maleimide test for hereditary spherocytosis, and glycosylphosphatidyl-inositol (GPI)-anchored proteins in paroxysmal nocturnal hemoglobinuria.
   - Fluorescence in situ hybridization (FISH).

ii. Functional Assays:
   - Viscoelastic testing: Thromboelastography and rotational thromboelastometry.
   - Platelet function testing: Platelet function analysis and platelet aggregometry.
   - Anti-phospholipid antibody testing.

6.2.1. Genetic Testing

Genetic testing has become extensively accessible for clinical diagnostic purposes. It assists clinicians in providing genetic counseling to families, monitoring patients who are affected, and determining appropriate treatment options. In the last three decades, researchers have successfully identified genetic variants that are linked to numerous hematologic diseases. The committee examines a number of genetic variants in the following sections.

The responses to the items in the statement of task are as follows:

- Genetic testing is employed for the purpose of identifying hereditary variations in an individual's DNA, thereby aiding in the diagnosis of an inherited genetic disorder, including but not limited to hemoglobinopathy, Diamond-Blackfan anemia, Fanconi anemia, and various other hematologic disorders that are inherited. Genetic testing is employed for the identification of somatic genetic variants acquired in cancer, thereby facilitating the diagnosis process, determining the most suitable therapeutic interventions to address these genetic alterations, and monitoring the effectiveness of therapy through the detection of minimal residual disease.
- The progress made in molecular and genetic diagnostics has enhanced the identification of inherited and somatic diseases, including the aforementioned hematological diseases.

- There exist a multitude of instances of hematologic diseases in which genetic testing is employed as an integral component of the established standard of care. Several illustrative examples are provided herein. Germline genetic variants, such as those found in hemoglobin genes, are frequently observed in patients. Hemoglobinopathies represent the prevailing single-gene disorders on a global scale, manifesting in more than 330,000 births each year. These diseases can be caused by mutations in either the alpha globin or beta globin genes (Traeger-Synodinos & Harteveld, 2014). DNA sequencing analysis can be conducted to confirm or elucidate the precise genetic variant and establish a conclusive diagnosis of the alpha or beta globin genes.

  Hematological disorders can be diagnosed through gene panel tests, which aim to identify hereditary factors contributing to neutropenia (reduced neutrophil count), thrombocytopenia (decreased platelet count), and hemolytic anemia (decreased red blood cell count). Children who may have Diamond-Blackfan anemia should undergo genetic testing by sequencing a set of ribosomal genes that have been identified as potential causes of this condition. Patients who exhibit pancytopenia, characterized by low levels of white blood cells, hemoglobin, and platelets, often undergo genetic testing to differentiate between idiopathic aplastic anemia and inherited bone marrow failure syndromes. This differentiation is crucial as the treatment approaches for these conditions may vary.

  Genetic testing for somatic (acquired) genetic variants is a customary component of the diagnostic process for numerous malignancies. Its purpose is to aid in the identification of the specific cancer type, offer prognostic insights, and contribute to informed treatment choices. An illustration of this can be seen in the inclusion of FMS-like tyrosine kinase 3 mutations within a comprehensive cancer-risk genetic panel for acute myelogenous leukemia.
- The widespread availability of genetic testing in clinical practice occurred approximately in 2014 (Ee et al., 2015).
- The committee lacks knowledge regarding any disparities pertaining to these techniques, except for the widely recognized disparities observed in the field of healthcare. Individuals belonging to ethnic minority groups and those with low socioeconomic status, who face challenges in accessing healthcare services, would consequently experience limited availability of these approaches.
- The latest gene sequencing techniques exhibit enhanced speed and, in certain instances, possess the capability to identify genetic alterations that were previously undetectable using previous methods.
- None of the aforementioned methods evaluate impairments in functioning. These tools possess utility solely in the context of diagnosis and disease monitoring.
- These tests can only be conducted by laboratories that have been approved by CLIA. The interpretation of the test should be conducted by a qualified clinician, such as the patient's clinical provider, genetic counselor, or laboratory medicine provider who is

responsible for signing the test report.

- The widespread adoption of genetic testing techniques is minimally hindered, provided that tissue or DNA samples can be transported to specialized laboratories.
- DNA sequencing tests conducted in CLIA-approved laboratories are highly precise in detecting sequence variants, provided that the tissue sample used is optimal. The level of accuracy, typically exceeding 99% (Yin et al., 2021), is contingent upon factors such as the origin of the tissue, potential DNA contamination from other cellular entities, and the extent of sequencing coverage for the particular test.

6.2.1.1. Characterization of Phenotypes

6.2.1.1.1. Immunophenotyping

Immunophenotyping is a commonly employed technique in the field of cell classification and diagnosis. It involves the utilization of antibodies that specifically target antigens found in particular tissues and cells. This method enables the identification of both normal and malignant cell types, as well as the determination of the organ from which they originate (Magaki et al., 2019). Laboratories can identify specific proteins expressed on the surface or inside cells of a patient's blood or tissue sample by utilizing the specific binding of an antibody to its target antigen. Immunohistochemistry is a technique employed for the analysis of cells within tissue sections on microscope slides, enabling the examination of cells within the framework of adjacent histologic tissues. Flow cytometry is a technique that involves the examination of antibodies that are bound to cells in a liquid suspension. This method enables the simultaneous analysis of multiple markers on each individual cell.

6.2.2. Immunohistochemistry

Immunohistochemistry (IHC) is a robust methodology employed to investigate the interaction between an antibody and antigen, with the aim of identifying and determining the precise location of particular antigens within cells present in tissue sections observed on microscope slides. In contrast to flow cytometry, immunohistochemistry (IHC) enables the visualization of cells of interest within the broader tissue context, thereby offering valuable diagnostic insights. The specific immuno-phenotype identified through immunohistochemistry (IHC) is crucial for diagnosing lymphoma and other forms of cancer, and it is increasingly offering predictive and prognostic insights. Furthermore, the determination of a patient's eligibility for immunotherapy treatments is contingent upon the expression of specific antigens. As an illustration, immunotherapy for lymphoma and other cancer types involves the utilization of antibodies targeting programmed death-ligand 1 (PD-L1), CD19, and CD30 (Cho, 2022). Prior to administering an immunotherapy treatment, it is imperative to confirm the expression of these proteins by the cancer, as cancers lacking the target antigen would not exhibit a response.

The responses to the items in the statement of task are as follows:

- Immunohistochemistry (IHC) is a diagnostic technique applicable to a diverse range of lymphomas and solid tumors. It serves the purpose of providing a more precise characterization of hematologic cancer cells (Herold & Mitra, 2022). Additionally, it can aid in bolstering clinical diagnosis.
- Immunohistochemistry (IHC) has been extended to evaluate predictive and prognostic biomarkers in various types of cancer. Each year, this technique consistently makes progress by

identifying new biomarkers and developing antibodies to detect them in tissues (Magaki et al., 2019).

- The methodology is employed for the evaluation of predictive and prognostic biomarkers in various malignancies, encompassing those associated with the breast, gastrointestinal tract, lung, hematolymphoid, and central nervous system.
- The clinical application of immunohistochemistry (IHC) dates back to the early 2000s.
- The committee lacks knowledge regarding any disparities pertaining to these techniques, with the exception of the widely recognized disparities observed in the field of healthcare. Individuals belonging to ethnic minority groups and those with low socioeconomic status, who face challenges in accessing healthcare services, would consequently experience limited availability of these approaches.
- Previous methodologies employed cell and tissue staining techniques in conjunction with light microscopy to investigate cellular morphology for diagnostic purposes. Immunohistochemistry (IHC) is an advanced technique that enhances the analysis of protein expression, enabling more precise identification of cell phenotypes that were previously undetectable.
- These methods do not evaluate impairments in performance. They are exclusively utilized for the purposes of diagnosis and disease monitoring.
- These tests can only be conducted by laboratories that have been approved by CLIA. The College of American Pathologists has established guidelines for the standardization and analytic validation of immunohistochemical tests (Magaki et al., 2019). In order to ensure accurate interpretation by a trained pathologist, it is necessary to employ suitable controls during the administration of these tests (Magaki et al., 2020).
- The widespread use of this technique is minimally hindered, provided that tissue samples can be transported to specialized laboratories.
- In the context of CLIA-approved laboratories, the reliability of IHC tests is significantly enhanced when conducted in conjunction with the appropriate control samples.

6.2.3. Flow Cytometry

Flow cytometry leverages the capacity of an antibody to selectively bind to its designated antigen. Here, patient cells are combined with cocktails of antibodies, each labeled with a distinct fluorescent compound. The suspension of individual cells is subsequently evaluated using a flow cytometer to identify the cells that emit distinct fluorescent wavelengths. The intensity of the fluorescence is then correlated with the degree of protein expression. Protein expression patterns are employed for the purpose of identifying and classifying the cells that have been labeled. As an illustration, this technique is employed to quantify CD4+ T cell populations and other lymphocyte subgroups in the investigation of distinct immunodeficiency disorders and immune-related ailments. According to Weir & Borowitz (2001), flow cytometry is employed to diagnose distinct sub-types of leukemia.

The responses to the items in the statement of task are as follows:

- Flow cytometry is a diagnostic technique that can be employed to further characterize hematologic cancer cells and diagnose a diverse range of leukemias and immunodeficiency disorders (Herold & Mitra, 2022). Additionally, it can be utilized to monitor minimal residual disease in the bone marrow of individuals with leukemia.

- The field of flow cytometry is witnessing a continuous expansion in the range of predictive and prognostic biomarkers employed for various malignancies. Each year, this technique consistently makes progress by identifying new biomarkers and developing antibodies to detect them in tissues (Magaki et al., 2019).
- This approach does not evaluate impairments in performance and is solely employed for diagnostic objectives.
- Flow cytometry has been utilized in clinical settings since the 1980s (Picot et al., 2012).
- The committee lacks knowledge regarding any disparities pertaining to this technique, with the exception of the widely recognized disparities observed in the field of healthcare. Individuals belonging to ethnic minority groups and those with low socioeconomic status, who face challenges in accessing healthcare services, would consequently experience limited availability of these approaches.
- Previous methodologies employed cell and tissue staining techniques in conjunction with light microscopy to investigate cellular morphology for diagnostic purposes. Flow cytometry enhances the aforementioned technique by analyzing the expression of particular proteins, thereby providing a more precise assessment of cell characteristics, some of which were previously undetectable before the introduction of this method.
- These methods do not evaluate impairments in performance. They are exclusively utilized for the purposes of diagnosis and disease monitoring.
- These tests can only be conducted by laboratories that have been approved by CLIA. The College of American Pathologists has established guidelines for the standardization and analytic validation of flow cytometry tests (Magaki et al., 2019). To ensure accurate interpretation by a trained pathologist, it is necessary to employ suitable controls during the administration of these tests (Magaki et al., 2020).
- The widespread adoption of this technique is minimally hindered, provided that tissue samples can be transported to specialized laboratories.
- Flow cytometry tests exhibit high reliability when conducted in a laboratory that has been approved by CLIA, and when the appropriate control samples are run concurrently.

6.2.4. Other Flow Cytometry Tests

6.2.4.1. Hereditary Spherocytosis Test Using Eosin-5-Maleimide

Hereditary spherocytosis (HS) exhibits clinical heterogeneity and is distinguished by the presence of mild to moderate hemolysis, which arises from abnormalities in the proteins of the red cell membrane. Hemolytic anemia, jaundice, and splenomegaly are the distinctive symptoms of HS. Hemolytic anemia refers to the destruction of red blood cells in the spleen and their subsequent removal from the bloodstream. Splenomegaly is characterized by a yellowish tone to the skin. Symptoms may manifest during infancy; however, it is worth noting that certain individuals with HS may exhibit no symptoms or experience mild symptoms, leading to a delayed diagnosis. Confirmation of the diagnosis is established through blood tests. Splenectomy, the surgical removal of the spleen, is advised for patients with severe anemia caused by HS, as it effectively treats hemolytic anemia. Additional interventions for patients experiencing severe hemolysis encompass folate supplementation and blood transfusions.

The presence of hemolytic, aplastic, and megaloblastic crises is also observed in individuals with HS. Hemolytic crises frequently arise because of a viral infection that induces heightened erythropoiesis of erythrocytes. Hemolytic crises are generally mild, although blood transfusions may be necessary. Hemolytic crises are more prevalent and less frequent compared to aplastic crises, which are also induced by viral infections, specifically parovirus B19.

The responses to the items in the statement of task are as follows:

- The diagnostic procedure for HS involves the utilization of the eosin-5-maleimide (EMA) test.
- In the past, prior to the introduction of the EMA test, the diagnosis of HS was established through the utilization of osmotic fragility testing. The osmotic fragility test is a method used to evaluate the ability of red blood cells to withstand hemolysis. This is achieved by treating the cells with different concentrations of sodium chloride solution, which induces osmotic stress. The test exhibits a high level of accuracy; nevertheless, the administration process is arduous and relies on the proficiency of the individuals responsible for its execution. The sensitivity of the test in detecting abnormalities is contingent upon the presence of a minimum of 2% spherocytes within the red blood cells. Therefore, in cases of less severe or unusual types of HS, the test may not detect any abnormalities (Chari & Prasad, 2018). The osmotic fragility testing and the EMA binding test have a strong agreement, but the EMA binding test has shown greater sensitivity and specificity in detecting HS (Chari & Prasad, 2018). The EMA test utilizes flow cytometry technology to analyze proteins present in the membrane of red blood cells, with a primary focus on band 3 protein. The EMA test is highly sensitive in detecting a significant decrease in the amount of band 3 protein in red blood cells in patients with HS.
- This test provides a more precise assessment of the impairments mentioned earlier.
- The test became widely available in nearby 2015 (Christensen et al., 2015).
- The committee lacks knowledge regarding any disparities pertaining to this technique, except for the widely recognized disparities observed in the field of healthcare. Individuals belonging to ethnic minority groups and those with low socioeconomic status, who face challenges in accessing healthcare services, would consequently experience limited availability of this approach. Underresourced facilities may lack access to a flow cytometer (Chari & Prasad, 2018).
- In contrast to the osmotic fragility tests that were previously employed, the EMA test offers several advantages in the diagnosis of HS. These include its simplicity, cost-effectiveness, high reproducibility, and reduced labor intensity (Chari & Prasad, 2018).
- This method does not evaluate

impairments in performance. It is exclusively utilized for the diagnosis and disease monitoring.

- Regarding prerequisites, the EMA test must be conducted by a laboratory that has been approved by CLIA.
- The widespread adoption of this technique is minimally hindered, provided that blood samples can be transported to specialized laboratories.
- According to a study comparing the sensitivity and specificity of HS screening tests, the EMA-binding test was found to be the most effective screening test. However, it is important to note that false negatives may still occur. It is recommended to exercise caution in clinical correlation (Mothi et al., 2021).

6.2.5. Proteins Attached to Glycosylphosphatidylinositol in Cases of Paroxysmal Nocturnal Hemoglobinuria

Paroxysmal nocturnal hemoglobinuria (PNH) is an uncommon medical condition characterized by an acquired disorder of hematopoietic stem cells. This disorder is characterized by a deficiency of GPI-anchored surface proteins in the affected stem cell clones. PNH is clinically distinguished by the presence of bone marrow failure, thrombosis, and chronic hemolytic anemia.

The diverse range of clinical manifestations and unpredictable progression of the disease pose difficulties in diagnosing and treating patients. Nevertheless, significant progress has been achieved over the past 15 years in comprehending the molecular and cellular biology of PNH, as well as in identifying the specific molecular abnormality that causes the PNH abnormality (Richards et al., 2000).

The genotypic lesion in PNH has been elucidated through the application of molecular biology techniques, whereas the phenotypic abnormalities in PNH have been effectively characterized through the utilization of monoclonal antibodies and flow cytometry. Flow cytometry has been widely recognized as a dependable diagnostic method for PNH and for quantifying the presence of the PNH clone in different hematopoietic cell lineages since 1985.

As previously mentioned, there exists a significant level of heterogeneity in the expression patterns and levels of GPI-linked proteins across different cell types, potentially indicating heterogeneity in lineage. When diagnosing PNH using flow cytometry, it is important to consider the various expression patterns of GPI-linked proteins. A comprehensive understanding of the cellular distribution of GPI-linked antigens and their expression during various stages of hematopoietic cell differentiation is crucial for interpreting results in PNH (Richards et al., 2000).

The responses to the items in the statement of task are as follows:

- GPI-linked protein analysis is commonly employed for diagnosing PNH.
- Flow cytometry, which analyzes GPI-linked proteins on red blood cells and granulocytes, offers a targeted and highly sensitive screening method for the diagnosis and monitoring of PNH clones. The diagnosis was previously established using the sucrose lysis test or the acidified serum test (Ham test), both of which are characterized by lower accuracy and increased time requirements.
- Flow cytometry is a more precise method for diagnosing PNH and quantifying the presence of the PNH clone in different hematopoietic cell

lineages, as mentioned earlier.

- The analysis of GPI-linked proteins has been feasible since 1985.
- The committee lacks knowledge regarding any disparities pertaining to this technique, except for the widely recognized disparities observed in the field of healthcare. Individuals belonging to ethnic minority groups and those with low socioeconomic status, who face challenges in accessing healthcare services, would consequently experience limited availability of these approaches.
- In the past, the diagnosis of PNH relied on the sucrose lysis test and acidified serum lysis, commonly known as the Ham test. However, these diagnostic methods have become outdated and have been replaced by flow cytometry, which is now used to detect GPI-linked proteins (CD55 and CD59) on the surface of blood cells.
- These methods are exclusively employed for the purposes of diagnosis and disease monitoring, and do not offer insights into the extent of impairments in functioning.
- Flow cytometry is the preferred method for diagnosing and monitoring PNH, and it must be conducted by a laboratory that has been approved by CLIA.
- The widespread adoption of this technique is minimally hindered, if blood samples can be transported to specialized laboratories.
- Regarding the acknowledged constraints associated with the analysis of GPI-linked proteins, it has been observed that recent transfusions have the potential to diminish the sensitivity of this assay and impede its precision (Mayo Clinic, 2023).

6.2.6. Fluorescence In Situ Hybridization

The cytogenetic technique known as FISH was developed during the early 1980s. FISH employs fluorescent DNA probes to selectively target distinct chromosomal sites within the nucleus, resulting in the generation of colored signals that can be detected through the utilization of a fluorescent microscope. FISH has assumed a progressively significant function in the identification of distinct biomarkers and genetic translocations within solid and hematologic neoplasms. The integration of conventional microscopic cytogenetic analysis with molecular techniques has played a crucial role in the advancement of personalized medicine. The applications of FISH have expanded beyond its initial development in the 1980s to encompass a wider range of genetic diseases, hematologic malignancies, and solid tumors (Hu et al., 2014). FISH applications have made significant progress in identifying new chromosomal rearrangements, amplifications, and deletions that are linked to the development of different types of cancer, including both hematopoietic and non-hematopoietic malignancies (Hu et al., 2014).

The responses to the items in the statement of task are as follows:

- FISH is employed for the purpose of both primary identification and regular identification of chromosomal rearrangements, amplifications, and deletions that are linked to the development of diverse hematopoietic and non-hematopoietic malignancies. The BCR-ABL fusion protein is recognized as a key factor in the development of chronic myelogenous leukemia. It arises from a chromosomal translocation t(9:22), which can be easily identified using FISH. The utilization of FISH for the identification of this translocation is crucial for the surveillance of disease status, as it exhibits greater sensitivity compared to conventional chromosomal karyotyping.

- The FISH technique does not necessitate the cultivation of cells and can be employed to promptly assess fresh or paraffin-embedded interphase nuclei (Hu et al., 2014).
- According to Hu et al. (2014), FISH is employed for the identification of various types of malignancies, including multiple myeloma, myelodysplastic syndrome, as well as hematopoietic and non-hematopoietic malignancies such as lung cancer, prostate cancer, breast cancer, and melanoma.
- The utilization of FISH as a clinical test gained significant popularity in the late 1980s, following its initial development in the early 1980s (Hu et al., 2014).
- The committee lacks knowledge regarding any disparities pertaining to these techniques, except for widely recognized disparities in healthcare. Individuals belonging to ethnic minority groups and those with low socioeconomic status, who face challenges in accessing healthcare services, would consequently experience limited availability of these approaches.
- According to Sabath (2004), FISH analysis has the capability to analyze a larger number of cells compared to standard cytogenetics, enabling the detection of even small populations of neoplastic cells. According to Huber et al. (2018), FISH is widely regarded as the most reliable cytogenetic technique for identifying diseased or malignant cells that exhibit chromosomal rearrangements or gene aberrations.
- These methods do not evaluate performance impairments. These devices are exclusively employed for the diagnosis and disease monitoring.
- FISH must be conducted by a laboratory that has been approved by CLIA.
- The widespread adoption of this technique is minimally hindered, provided that tissue samples can be transported to specialized laboratories.
- When conducted in a CLIA-approved laboratory with the appropriate control samples run simultaneously, this test is highly dependable. Nevertheless, the efficacy of a FISH test in identifying a specific genetic anomaly is contingent upon the configuration of the DNA probe employed in said test. Only genetic aberrations that are already known are identified, provided that the specific probe is accessible and it is unlikely that other genetic abnormalities would be detected, according to Bishop (2010).

6.2.7. Functional Assays

6.2.7.1. Viscoelastic Hemostatic Assays (VHAs)

VHAs, such as thromboelastografy (TEG) and rotational thromboelastometry (ROTEM), are diagnostic tests that provide a quantitative assessment of the formation and dissolution of blood clots in whole blood. Significant hemorrhaging is a grave medical complication that can arise from external trauma, surgical intervention, invasive procedures, or an underlying medical condition such as the rupture of an aneurysm or a peptic ulcer. Various congenital disorders, such as von Willebrand disease or hemophilia A or B, are linked to a deficiency in the coagulation factory. These disorders can result in substantial bleeding, even in cases of minor injuries. In addition, the administration of prescribed anticoagulants and anti-platelet agents has the potential to induce a coagulopathic condition, which can result in the occurrence of excessive bleeding in relation to trauma or medical interventions. Moreover, significant acute hemorrhage can result in coagulopathy as a consequence of diminished levels of coagulation factors. According to Shaydakov et al. (2022), individuals experiencing or anticipated significant bleeding would derive advantages from a precise evaluation of the operational condition of the hemostatic system, enabling healthcare professionals to deliver the most effective treatment. An additional medical condition linked to atypical blood coagulation is venous thromboembolism. A number of frequently employed blood tests are utilized to evaluate blood coagulation, encompassing prothrombin time, international normalized ratio, activated partial thromboplastin time, platelet count, fibrinogen concentration, and D-dimer. According to Shaydakov et al. (2022), these tests serve the purpose of clinically diagnosing coagulopathy, monitoring the effectiveness of anticoagulation therapy, and aiding in the management of bleeding episodes.

The responses to the items in the statement of task are as follows:

- VHAs are valuable for diagnosing coagulopathy or prothrombotic condition. In the fields of cardiovascular surgery, liver transplantation, trauma care, and for patients undergoing continuous dialysis or cardiac extracorporeal membrane oxygenation, TEG and ROTEM are commonly employed. According to Morcom (2018), the tests are employed in individuals experiencing post-partum hemorrhage, gastrointestinal bleeding, and severe epistaxis, as well as in specific post-operative patients. The ROTEM test has been employed as a point-of-care assessment tool to enhance the efficacy of hemostatic resuscitation in individuals with trauma. ROTEM parameters are utilized in trauma to inform treatment decisions. According to Veigas et al. (2016), ROTEM offers insights into platelet function and fibrinogen reserve.
- VHAs have been advocated as a superior alternative to conventional coagulation tests in the treatment of trauma patients. This is primarily attributed to their ability to provide rapid results and offer a comprehensive assessment of clot formation and thrombolysis.
- VHAs are effective in accurately evaluating specific impairments such as coagulopathy and prothrombotic state. Additionally, they are useful in predicting the need for massive transfusion and providing guidance for transfusions (Veigas et al., 2016).
- The TEG technology was created in 1948. Since then, TEG has developed into a widely utilized noninvasive test that accurately quantifies the whole blood's capacity to create and dissolve a blood clot. According to Shaydakov et al. (2022), the utility of TEG was observed in liver transplant patients during the 1980s, and subsequently demonstrated in cardiac surgery during the 1990s.
- The committee is not cognizant of any documented disparities pertaining to these techniques, apart from the widely recognized disparities observed in the realm of healthcare. Individuals belonging to ethnic minority groups and those with low socioeconomic status, who face challenges in accessing healthcare services, would consequently experience limited availability of these approaches.
- The utilization of previously established

techniques in combination with viscoelastic assays, such as TEG and ROTEM, has not been supplanted by these alternative methods. Viscoelastic assays yield faster results compared to conventional coagulopathy tests like prothrombin time and partial prothrombin time. Therefore, TEG and ROTEM are particularly valuable when prompt laboratory results are required for treatment determinations.

- These methods do not evaluate performance impairments. These devices are exclusively employed for the diagnosis and disease monitoring.
- These tests must be conducted by a laboratory that has been approved by CLIA.
- The administration of these tests occurs at the location and may not be universally accessible across all institutions, despite the widespread adoption of both TEG and ROTEM in clinical settings.
- As long as the test is conducted by a CLIA-certified laboratory, there are no established constraints.

6.2.8. Platelet Function Analysis (PFA-100)

PFA-100 employs a microprocessor-controlled instrument/cartridge system (PFA-100TM) specifically developed for the evaluation of primary hemostasis related to platelets in regularly collected whole blood samples. Platelet dysfunction has been identified as a potential etiological factor for bleeding diathesis, particularly in patients who are critically ill and at risk of experiencing life-threatening hemorrhages. Furthermore, the aforementioned test is employed for the purpose of detecting platelet dysfunction induced by acetylsalicyclic acid (Mammen et al., 1998).

The responses to the items in the statement of task are as follows:

- Platelet function analysis is employed to assist in diagnosing platelet dysfunction or to assess the risk of bleeding before surgery in patients experiencing bleeding symptoms.
- PFA-100 offers several advantages, including its minimal blood volume requirement, compatibility with non-skilled personnel, and its rapid and automated nature.
- The PFA-100 is employed as a screening tool due to its rapidity in obtaining results. In cases where the test yields abnormal results, it is necessary to conduct formal platelet aggregation studies by a proficient laboratory medicine technician to validate the diagnosis.
- Efforts have been undertaken since the early 1970s to identify a device capable of providing a comprehensive assessment of platelet-related primary hemostasis on a global scale.
- The committee lacks knowledge regarding any disparities pertaining to this technique, with the exception of the widely recognized disparities observed in the field of healthcare. Individuals belonging to ethnic minority groups and those with low socioeconomic status, who face challenges in accessing healthcare services, would consequently experience limited availability of these approaches.
- Adenosine diphosphate (ADP) or epinephrine can induce platelet aggregation, which is assessed by the PFA-100 test. On the other hand, formal investigations on platelet aggregation encompass the analysis of various substances that stimulate platelets, as well as the evaluation of platelet

reactions to varying concentrations of said substances.

- These methods do not evaluate impairments in performance. These devices are exclusively employed for the diagnosis and disease monitoring.
- PFA-100 should be conducted by a laboratory that has been approved by CLIA.
- The widespread adoption of this technique is minimally hindered, provided that blood samples can be transported to specialized laboratories.
- The PFA-100 has a restricted scope in evaluating specific platelet agonists, namely epinephrine and ADP, and is thus commonly employed as a screening test. Light transmission aggregometry is typically employed in formal platelet aggregation studies to validate a positive outcome obtained from the PFA-100 test, particularly when there is suspicion of a congenital platelet disorder such as Bernard Soulier syndrome or Glanzmann's thrombasthenia. A comprehensive range of platelet agonists, such as ADP, arachidonic acid, collagen, epinephrine, and high- and low-dose ristocetin, among others, is assessed using light transmission aggregometry.

6.2.9. Anti-Phospholipid Antibody Testing

Individuals with autoimmune diseases commonly exhibit the presence of anti-phospholipid antibodies (APLAs), which are auto-antibodies responsible for initiating the formation of anomalous blood clots. The production of antiphospholipid antibodies typically occurs as part of a typical immune response, wherein the immune system produces an antibody targeting phospholipids present in the cellular membrane of endothelial cells that line blood vessels. Clots typically develop as a result of damage to endothelial cells. Nevertheless, upon binding to the phospholipids present on endothelial cells, these antibodies have the ability to initiate the creation of an anomalous clot even in the absence of any harm.

The identification of antiphospholipid syndrome is contingent upon the identification of circulating antiphospholipid antibodies (APLAs) in conjunction with other clinical presentations. APLA testing is conducted in cases where patients have experienced the formation of blood clots or exhibit an abnormally extended partial thromboplastin time. Testing plays a crucial role in elucidating the underlying factors contributing to recurrent miscarriages, as well as aiding in the diagnosis and assessment of autoimmune disorders. APLAs, also known as lupus anticoagulants, are frequently observed in individuals diagnosed with systemic lupus erythematosus. However, it is important to note that this nomenclature is misleading, as APLAs can also be detected in non-lupus individuals and exhibit pro-thrombotic properties rather than anticoagulant effects.

Antiphospholipid antibodies are frequently present in individuals who experience recurrent venous thromboembolism or other abnormal clotting, repeated miscarriages, or autoimmune diseases like systemic lupus erythematosus and multiple sclerosis (MS). In certain instances, individuals diagnosed with cancer may also possess antibodies that diminish in intensity following cancer treatment. There exists a correlation between the presence of antiphospholipid antibodies and an elevated susceptibility to clotting, as well as an increased likelihood of experiencing recurrent miscarriages, premature labor, and pre-eclampsia. Individuals with autoimmune diseases (such as lupus, rheumatoid arthritis, and systemic sclerosis), infections (such as HIV, mononucleosis, and rubella), and cancers (such as solid tumors, leukemias, and lymphomas) as well as those who have used specific drugs (such as procainamide, phenothiazines, and oral contraceptives) have been found to have one or more antiphospholipid antibodies (Labcorp, 2022).

The responses to the items in the statement of task are as follows:

- Diagnostic tests are employed for individuals presenting with atypical thrombi, recurrent miscarriages, or autoimmune disorders such as systemic lupus erythematosus, rheumatoid arthritis, or systemic sclerosis.
- Devreese et al. (2020) have reported advancements in the standardization of tests and guidelines pertaining to lupus anticoagulant testing, as well as immunological assays related to anticardiolipin and antibeta2-glycoprotein1 antibodies.
- The present examination does not assess impairments in cognitive or physical abilities but rather assists in the identification of antiphospholipid syndrome in individuals presenting with atypical thrombi, recurrent miscarriages, or autoimmune disorders.
- The anticardiolipin antibody test, classified as an antiphospholipid antibody test, has gained significant popularity in the diagnostic process for individuals diagnosed with antiphospholipid syndrome since the mid-1980s (Pierangeli, 2006).
- The committee lacks knowledge regarding any disparities pertaining to these techniques, with the exception of the widely recognized disparities observed in the field of healthcare. Individuals belonging to ethnic minority groups and those with low socioeconomic status, who face challenges in accessing healthcare services, would consequently experience limited availability of these approaches.
- Over the past 27 years, there have been numerous publications of consensus guidelines and proposals for testing antiphospholipid antibodies. These efforts have significantly enhanced the standardization of testing, resulting in improved test accuracy (Devreese et al., 2020).
- These methods do not evaluate impairments in performance. These devices are exclusively employed for the diagnosis and disease monitoring.
- Plasma-based clotting assays are employed to identify lupus anticoagulants, while enzyme immunoassays are utilized to identify solid-phase antibodies. These antibodies encompass anticardiolipin antibodies, antibodies to β2-glycoprotein 1 (β2GP1), and various other antibodies. To ascertain the existence of antiphospholipid syndrome, it is necessary to conduct tests for both lupus anticoagulants and immunoassays targeting anticardiolipin and β2GP1 antibodies (Labcorp, 2022). These tests must be conducted by a laboratory that has been approved by CLIA.
- The widespread adoption of this technique is minimally hindered, provided that blood samples can be transported to specialized laboratories.
- The administration of anticoagulant therapies has the potential to yield inaccurate positive outcomes for lupus anticoagulants (Labcorp, 2022).

It is anticipated that in the forthcoming years, advancements in genetic sequencing tests will persist in enhancing the diagnosis and evaluation of hematological disorders. As the number of genetic syndromes increases, the diagnostic accuracy of these tests will further improve. Furthermore, there will be ongoing advancements in technology that enable the execution of sequencing tests at a faster pace and with reduced sample sizes. Presently, there is ongoing development of tests aimed at sequencing cell-free DNA in the bloodstream, to monitor the presence of genetic mutations in cancer cells across various anatomical regions. Presently, cell-free DNA tests are being employed within the realm of research, with the anticipation that they will revolutionize the field of diagnosis and disease monitoring, thereby augmenting the quality of clinical care provided to patients in the forthcoming years.

6.3. Summary

Hematological disorders encompass a wide range of conditions affecting the blood and its components, including red blood cells, white blood cells, platelets, and the bone marrow — the body's site for blood cell production. These disorders can be broadly classified into three main categories: anemias, clotting disorders, and cancers of the blood.

Anemias, one of the most common hematological disorders, occur when there's a deficiency of red blood cells or hemoglobin in the blood, leading to reduced oxygen transport to the body's tissues. This can result from nutritional deficiencies (like iron, vitamin B12, or folate), inherited conditions (such as sickle cell anemia or thalassemias), or other factors like chronic diseases or bone marrow failure.

Clotting disorders, or coagulopathies, involve problems with blood clot formation. Hemophilia and von Willebrand disease are examples of inherited clotting disorders, characterized by prolonged bleeding or excessive bleeding, even from minor injuries. On the other end of the spectrum are conditions that lead to excessive clotting, such as DVT and pulmonary embolism, which can be life-threatening if not treated promptly.

Blood cancers, including leukemia, lymphoma, and myeloma, arise from the abnormal growth and proliferation of different types of blood cells. These cancers can have a significant impact on the body's ability to fight infection, carry oxygen, and control bleeding. Treatment varies widely depending on the type of cancer and may include chemotherapy, radiation therapy, and bone marrow transplantation.

Diagnosis of hematological disorders involves a range of tests, including complete blood counts (CBC), blood smears, bone marrow biopsies, and genetic testing. Treatment depends on the specific condition and its severity but may involve dietary supplements, medications to stimulate blood cell production or prevent clotting, chemotherapy, or bone marrow transplantation. Advances in medical research continue to improve the understanding and management of these complex disorders, offering hope for better outcomes and quality of life for affected individuals.

A Closer Look

Functional Assays

Functional assays are laboratory techniques designed to measure biological activity, cell function, or the efficacy of compounds in a given system. These assays are crucial for drug discovery, diagnostics, and understanding disease mechanisms, as they provide insights into how biological entities like cells, enzymes, or receptors perform under various conditions.

Cell-Based Assays assess cellular responses to stimuli or drugs, revealing insights into cell viability, proliferation, cytotoxicity, and apoptosis. These assays are pivotal in cancer research and immunology, where responses to treatments like chemotherapy or immune checkpoint inhibitors need precise evaluation. Techniques like the MTT assay, which measures metabolic activity, help in assessing cell viability, while flow cytometry allows researchers to examine specific cell markers and understand cell populations in complex tissues.

Enzyme Activity Assays focus on evaluating enzymatic reactions, often used in drug discovery to screen for enzyme inhibitors or activators. These assays are especially relevant for diseases like hypertension, where drugs targeting enzymes (e.g., ACE inhibitors) play a key role. The assays are performed by measuring product formation, substrate depletion, or changes in absorbance or fluorescence, enabling a quantitative analysis of enzyme function in real time.

Reporter Assays use genetic markers or fluorescent tags to assess gene expression, protein interactions, or cellular responses to certain stimuli. Common in genetic and molecular biology research, reporter assays allow the visualization of complex processes, such as signal transduction pathways, which are essential in cancer biology and regenerative medicine.

Technological Advancements in functional assays continue to drive innovation in biomedical research. High-throughput screening and automation enable rapid testing of thousands of compounds, accelerating drug discovery. Additionally, microfluidics and lab-on-a-chip technologies provide miniaturized environments for cell-based assays, conserving resources and allowing more precise control over experimental conditions. Functional assays thus remain invaluable in bridging the gap between theoretical research and clinical application, offering the tools necessary to develop effective diagnostics and treatments.

References

1. Kuwajima, M., & Iijima, K. (1996). Recent advances in laboratory approaches to hematologic disorders. PubMed. Retrieved from https://pubmed.ncbi.nlm.nih.gov/8816057.
2. Crezee, I. (2013). Chapter 20. Hematology: Blood and blood disorders. In Z. (Ed.), Hematology: Blood and blood disorders. Retrieved from https://dx.doi.org/10.1075/Z.181.20HEM.
3. Belyaeva, E. (2023). Hematology: General questions. Scientific Journal of Hematology, 8(4), 2-13. https://doi.org/10.12737/2409-3750-2023-8-4-2-13.
4. Choudhry, V. (2013). Editorial: Advances in diagnosis of hematological disorders. Indian Journal of Medical Research, 138(5), 751-752. https://doi.org/10.1007/s12098-013-1146-0.
5. Kuwajima, M., & Iijima, K. (1996). Recent advances in laboratory approaches to hematologic disorders. PubMed. Retrieved from https://pubmed.ncbi.nlm.nih.gov/8816057.
6. Crezee, I. (2013). Chapter 20. Hematology: Blood and blood disorders. In Z. (Ed.), Hematology: Blood and blood disorders. Retrieved from https://dx.doi.org/10.1075/Z.181.20HEM.
7. Belyaeva, E. (2023). Hematology: General questions. Scientific Journal of Hematology, 8(4), 2-13. https://doi.org/10.12737/2409-3750-2023-8-4-2-13.
8. Choudhry, V. (2013). Editorial: Advances in diagnosis of hematological disorders. Indian Journal of Medical Research, 138(5), 751-752. https://doi.org/10.1007/s12098-013-1146-0.

Chapter 7

METABOLIC SYNDROME

Contents

Introduction

Metabolic syndrome (MetS) is characterized by a collection of metabolic irregularities, encompassing hypertension, central obesity, insulin resistance, and atherogenic dyslipidemia. This condition is closely linked to an elevated susceptibility to the development of diabetes, as well as atherosclerotic and nonatherosclerotic cardiovascular disease (CVD). MetS pathogenesis encompasses a combination of genetic and acquired factors that collectively contribute to the ultimate pathway of inflammation that ultimately results in CVD. MetS has garnered considerable significance in recent times as a result of the rapid and substantial rise in global obesity rates. Prompt identification is crucial for implementing lifestyle and risk factor adjustments. This chapter provides a comprehensive examination of the epidemiology and pathogenesis of MetS, elucidates the involvement of inflammation in MetS, and presents a summary of current natural therapies for MetS.

Orientation and Directional Terms

Term	Definition	Illustration
Metabolic Syndrome	A cluster of conditions including high blood pressure, high blood sugar, excess body fat around the waist, and abnormal cholesterol levels that increase the risk of heart disease, stroke, and diabetes.	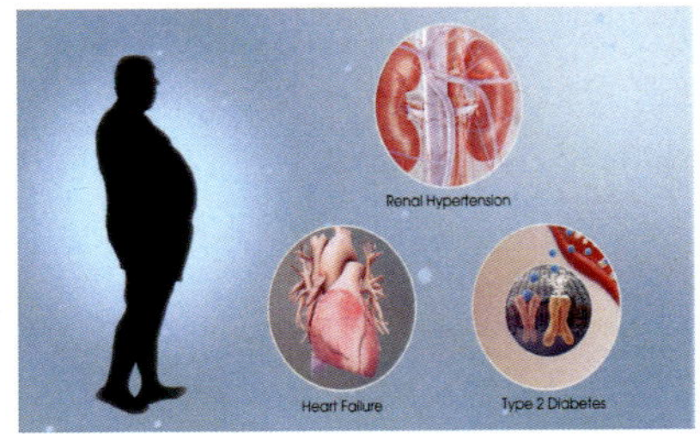
Insulin Resistance	A condition in which the body's cells do not respond effectively to insulin, leading to elevated blood glucose levels, commonly associated with type 2 diabetes.	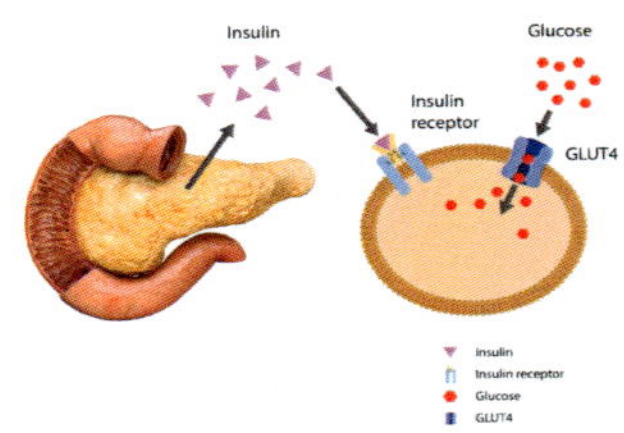
Obesity	A condition characterized by excessive body fat that increases the risk of health problems, often measured by body mass index (BMI).	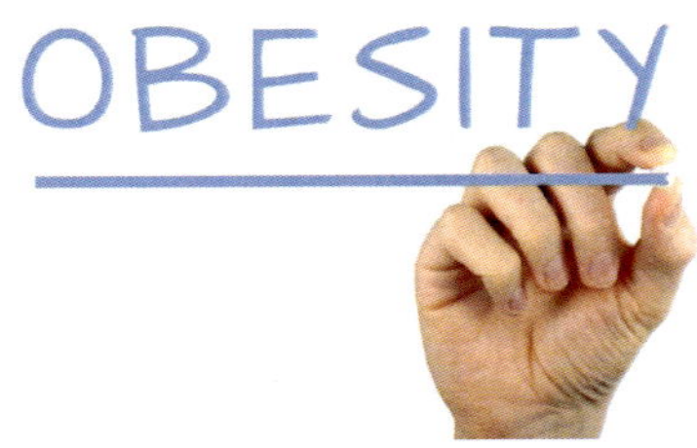
Pharmacotherapy	The use of drugs to treat diseases, which can include medications targeting metabolic pathways for chronic conditions.	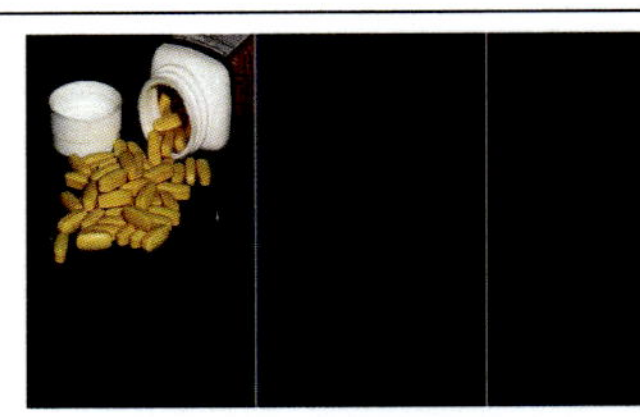
Nutraceuticals	Foods or food-derived products with health benefits beyond basic nutrition, often used to prevent or treat disease.	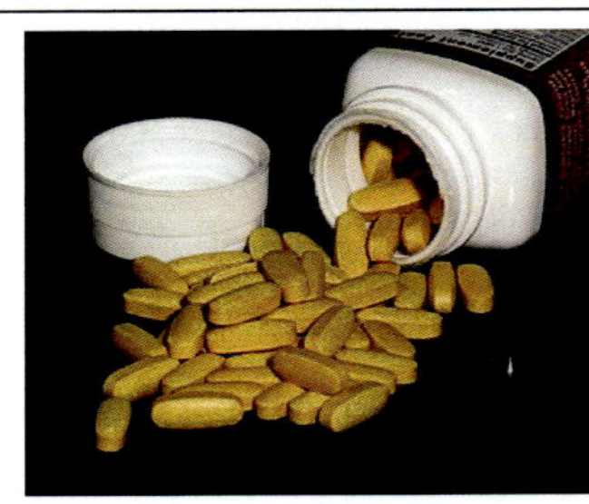

7.1. Overview

The objective of this chapter is to present a comprehensive examination of the pathophysiology underlying MetS and elucidate the interconnections among its various constituents. Due to the extensive nature of this topic, not all facets will be addressed. In this chapter, a bibliographic reference is provided for each topic to facilitate further investigation. This study constitutes a non-systematic literature review conducted using the databases PubMed and Google.

In a Portuguese population, an epidemiological study conducted by Armindo Sousa Ribeiro et al (2018) revealed that 23.8% of the population has MS. The prevalence of MS is higher among 24 males who do not smoke, do not consume significant amounts of alcohol, lead a sedentary lifestyle, have a high body mass index (BMI), and its prevalence increases with age. Different cardiovascular risk factors (CVRFs) play varying roles in the MetS.

CVDs are the primary contributors to mortality and morbidity in Western societies, affecting individuals of all genders. This phenomenon carries significant social and economic implications.

CVDs are the leading cause of death globally. According to the 2010 Global Burden of Disease Study, CVD is responsible for approximately 15.6 million deaths annually globally, accounting for 29.6% of all deaths. Despite efforts to decrease the mortality rate in Europe caused by CVD, it continues to be the primary cause of death, accounting for over 4 million deaths annually, which represents 45% of all recorded deaths in Europe. Among CVDs, coronary heart disease (CHD) continues to be the leading cause of mortality in both males and females, accounting for 19% and 20% respectively.

7.2. The Relationship Between Metabolic Syndrome and Cardiovascular Risk Factors (CVRF)

7.2.1. Definition

Multiple definitions of MS exist. MS encompasses a collection of pathophysiological factors that contribute to an elevated susceptibility to the development of type 2 diabetes mellitus (DM) and CVD. Currently, efforts have been undertaken to establish a unified set of criteria in order to achieve a consensus on the diagnosis.

The diagnostic criteria or components of MS have been proposed by the World Health Organization (WHO), International Diabetes Federation (IDF), National Cholesterol Education Program Adult Treatment Panel III (NCEP-ATP III), and the American Association of Clinical Endocrinologists (AACE) (Table 7.1).

The resolution of differences between definitions of MS and the unification of criteria were deliberated upon by representatives from the International Defense Forces (IDF) and the American Heart Association/National Heart, Lung, and Blood Institute (AHA/NHLBI)-ATP III Guidelines in 2009. The unification of criteria, also known as harmonizing theMetS, is widely employed in numerous international works and publications to define MS.

Table 7.1. *The Metabolic Syndrome Encompasses Various Components, as Defined by the National Cholesterol Education Program Adult Treatment Panel III (ATP III), the WHO), the AACE, and the IDF*

	ATP III	WHO	AACE	IDF
Triglycerides ≥ 150 mg/dl	X	X	X	X
HDL <40 mg/dl in men and <50 mg/dl in women	X	X	X	X
Blood pressure > 130/85 mmHg	X	X	X	X
Insulin Resistance (IR)		X		
Fasting glucose >100 mg/dl	X		X	X
Glucose 2h: 140 mg/dl			X	
Abdominal Obesity	X			X
High body mass index		X	X	
Microalbuminuri a		X		
Risk factors and or diagnosis	3 plus IR	More than 2	Clinical Criteria	Abdominal Obesity

Source: https://www.intechopen.com/.

This definition necessitates the presence of three out of the following five criteria:

- The presence of fasting blood glucose levels exceeding 100 mg/dl or the administration of antidiabetic therapy involving insulin or oral antidiabetic medications.
- An increase in systolic blood pressure below 130 mmHg or diastolic blood pressure below 85 mmHg, or the administration of antihypertensive medication.
- The cholesterol levels of high-density lipoprotein (HDL) are typically below 40 mg/dl in men and 50 mg/dL in women.
- When triglyceride levels are below 150 mg/dL or when specific lipid-lowering agents are being used
- The abdominal circumference is 102 cm for men and 88 cm for women.

The implementation of the concept of MS was executed in a sequential fashion. The clinical significance of this is immense as it can detect patients at a high risk of developing CVD and/or diabetes mellitus (DM), enabling a proactive intervention.

The concept that CVRF exhibits a propensity for aggregation facilitates an earlier identification of MS, thereby enabling the prompt implementation of therapeutic interventions, whether pharmacological or non-pharmacological.

7.2.2. Historical Development

The fascination with the MS is not a recent phenomenon. The terminology has undergone changes over time.

Approximately 260 years ago, prior to the characterization of MS, Morgagni, an Italian anatomist and physician, established a correlation between visceral obesity, arterial hypertension (AHT), atherosclerosis, hyperuricemia, and recurrent occurrences of sleep apnea. During the mid-20th century, French physicist Vague initially established the correlation between android obesity and the heightened occurrence of diabetes mellitus (DM) and CVD. Avogaro and Crepaldi coined the term "plurimetabolic syndrome" in the 1960s to describe the coexistence of obesity, acute hypertension (AHT), and diabetes mellitus (DM). The researchers confirmed that these abnormalities were prevalent within the population and were associated with an elevated risk of cardiovascular complications. Around 10 years later, Haller established a connection between this group of risk factors and atherosclerosis.

In 1980, Vague proposed that adipose tissue in isolation had minimal impact on the development of diabetes mellitus in individuals who were obese. The existing body of knowledge indicates that central or android obesity is a contributing factor to the development of diabetes mellitus (DM) and atherosclerosis, and it has an impact on insulin secretion, in contrast to gynoid obesity. The phenomenon in question was referred to as syndrome X by Reaven in 1988. It encompasses a combination of hyperglycemia, insulin resistance, obesity, dyslipidemia, and hypertension. Reaven (year) proposed that the primary pathophysiological characteristics of syndrome X were insulin resistance and the subsequent elevation of blood insulin levels. This, in turn, was identified as a risk factor for CVD.

The term "insulin resistance syndrome" was coined by Ferrannini et al. in 1991. In 1993, Van Gaal coined the term MS to encompass all comorbidities linked to visceral obesity, and this terminology is currently in use.

The understanding of MS has undergone substantial development over the past decade, leading to the emergence of various clinical definitions proposed by different scientific societies. In a broad sense, MS is commonly characterized as the accumulation of multiple cardiovascular risk factors (CVRF) within a single individual. The fundamental components utilized in the categorization and assessment of MS encompass obesity, deviations in glycemic metabolism, iatrogenic dyslipidemia, and hypertension.

The WHO established the definition of the MetS in 1998. The National Cholesterol Education Program-Adult Treatment Panel III (NCEP-ATP III) introduced a revised definition of MS in 2001. Under this revised definition, glycemia is no longer regarded as a crucial factor, but rather as one of the diagnostic components of MS.

Following the validation of evidence establishing a correlation between central obesity and cardiovascular risk, there has been a growing inclination to assign greater importance to this diagnostic factor in the context of MS. In 2004, the IDF established a revised definition of MS, which emphasizes the importance of central obesity, as determined by the abdominal circumference, for accurate diagnosis. The implementation of this particular definition resulted in a notable rise in the occurrence of MS within a significant portion of the examined populations, with a particular emphasis on the elderly demographic.

In 2005, the American Heart Association/ National Heart, Lung, and Blood Institute (AHA/NHLBI) conducted a reassessment of the criteria and upheld the criteria established by the NCEP-ATP III. This decision was based on the rationale that the NCEP-ATP III criteria do not highlight a singular cause for MS and are more straightforward to implement. The cutoff point of fasting blood glucose was adjusted from 110 to 100 mg/dl, as recommended by the American Diabetes Association (ADA) for diagnosing diabetes mellitus (DM). Nevertheless, the initial Brazilian Guideline for the Diagnosis of Treatment of Multiple Sclerosis, published in 2005, employs the diagnostic criteria outlined in the NCEP-ATP III, published in 2001. Within the IDF criteria, the abdominal circumference component assumes a crucial role, as a smaller waist circumference is indicative of a higher prevalence of MS compared to the ATP III definition. Nevertheless, there is a correlation between increased abdominal circumference in older individuals and decreased body mass index (BMI) compared to younger adults.

7.2.3. The Incidence of Metabolic Syndrome

The occurrence of MS exhibits regional disparities, wherein diagnosis is influenced by factors such as age, race, sex, and classification.

The DARIOS study conducts a comprehensive analysis of 11 studies involving a total of 24,670 Spanish individuals between the ages of 35 and 74. The analysis adheres to the criteria outlined in the IDF/NHLBI/AHA-2009 study. The findings reveal a prevalence rate of 32% in men and 29% in women.

The prevalence rate of the West of Scotland Coronary Prevention Study (WOSCOPS), which is among the largest in Europe, is reported to be 26.2%.

The NHANES III, conducted in the USA, revealed that 7% of individuals aged 20 to 29, 42% of individuals aged 60 to 69, and 44% of individuals aged over 70 had MS. The overall prevalence of MS among the 8,814 adults who participated in the study was 23.7%. The findings of this study indicate a positive correlation between age and incidence, particularly after the age of 40. Furthermore, there were notable differences observed based on ethnicity, with Hispanics exhibiting the highest prevalence of 31.9% compared to Caucasians (23.8%) and African-Americans (21.6%). A comparable prevalence was observed in both genders, albeit with a higher incidence in Caucasian males and African-American and Hispanic females.

According to the findings of the Diabetes Epidemiology Collaborative Analysis of Diagnostic Criteria in Europe (DECODE) study conducted in Europe in 2004, the prevalence of MS was reported to be 15.7% among males and 14.2% among females. Epidemiological investigations pertaining to MS have indicated a substantial prevalence of MS within Western societies, which is progressively escalating as a consequence of the rising rates of obesity, particularly among younger cohorts.

There is a scarcity of research on the occurrence of MS in Portugal. In 2004, an epidemiological investigation was conducted in Porto, revealing a prevalence of MS at 23.9%. Notably, the prevalence was higher among females (27%) compared to males (19.1%).

The VALSIM study, conducted in 2008, aimed to investigate the prevalence of MetS and its associated cardiovascular complications among the adult population in Portugal. The study focused on primary care settings in continental Portugal, Azores, and Madeira. A total of 719 family doctors took part in this study. The research was conducted from April 2006 to November 2007. A cohort of 16,856 individuals, ranging in age from 18 to 96, were assessed, with mean ages of 58.1 ± 15.1 years. The study revealed a significant occurrence of MS in adults, impacting 27.5% of the analyzed population. The prevalence was higher in females (28.7%) compared to males (26%). The findings of this study indicate a positive correlation between age, body mass index, and abdominal perimeter with the prevalence of MS. This study additionally provided evidence of the correlation between metabolic risk factors, such as MS, and the incidence of cardiac events, stroke, and diabetes mellitus (DM). There was observed regional variation in the prevalence of MS, with higher rates observed in Alentejo (30.99%), Madeira (29.38%), Central Region (28.79%), and North Region (28.17%). Conversely, Algarve (24.42%), Lisbon and Tagus Valley (25.71%), and Azores (26.05%) exhibited lower prevalence rates.

7.3. Insulin Resistance and Metabolic Syndrome

The precise etiology of MS remains incompletely elucidated; however, the prevailing hypothesis posits that insulin resistance plays a pivotal role, thus leading to the designation of MS as insulin resistance syndrome. Insulin resistance can be described as a dysfunction in the peripheral action of insulin, leading to an elevated level of insulin in the bloodstream, which is necessary for the maintenance of normal blood glucose levels. Central obesity and the excessive release of free fatty acids from adipose tissue are identified as predisposing factors for insulin resistance. The determination of the increase in glycogenesis and gluconeogenesis, increased triglyceride production, and the secretion of very low-density lipoproteins (VLDL) is contingent upon the presence of free fatty acids within the liver.

Insulin is a hormone that inhibits the breakdown of fats. It is synthesized in pancreatic beta cells and is released into the bloodstream after binding to its receptor, initiating its metabolic effects. The insulin receptor is a glycoprotein that is located across the cell membrane. It consists of four subunits that are connected by disulfide bridges. These subunits include two extracellular alpha subunits that contain the domain responsible for binding insulin, and two β subunits that contain an extracellular domain, a transmembrane domain, and an intracellular domain. Insulin binds to both the α and β subunits, and the activation of tyrosine kinase in the β subunit is the initial step in the action of insulin on glucose metabolism. The process of tyrosine kinase activation and subsequent phosphorylation of the β subunit of the insulin receptor initiates the phosphorylation reaction of multiple tyrosine residues within a group of proteins known as insulin receptor substrate (IRS). These proteins, namely IRS-1, IRS-2, IRS-3, and IRS-4, are responsible for the most precise signaling cascade mediated by insulin. Additional forms of the protein include growth factor receptor-bound protein 2 (GRB2)-associated binding protein 1 (Gab-1), Shc, and p62.

The four IRS proteins exhibit several structural similarities, with a notable similarity being the presence of the phosphotyrosine-binding domain (PTB). This domain serves as the recognition sequence for asparagine-proline glutamic phosphotyrosine acid (NPEpY), which is situated in the juxta membrane region of the β receptor of insulin. This entity plays a role in the interaction between insulin receptor (IRS) proteins and the COOH-terminal domain of the proteins, enabling them to bind to the SH2 domains. The four IRS proteins exhibit variations in tissue distribution, in addition to their shared characteristics. The SH2 domain is comprised of a total of 100 amino acids and serves as the binding site for phosphotyrosine. Proteins containing the SH2 domain are crucial for transmitting the insulin signal and performing its functions.

The initial substrate that was identified was the IRS-1 gene, which is situated on chromosome 2q36–37. IRS-1 plays a crucial role in various functions of insulin, including the stimulation of nitric oxide (NO) synthetase, the activation of the iN+ pump, and the relaxation of blood vessels through the activation of protein kinases by mitogens (MAP kinase).

The IRS-2 gene is located on the 13q34 chromosome. The structural and functional similarities between the IRS-2 and IRS-1 proteins are notable, with the primary distinction residing in the specific region encompassing amino acids 591 and 789 within the IRS-2 protein. IRS-2 is predominantly located in the cellular cytosol, in contrast to IRS-1.

The expression of IRS-3 in human cells is not observed. The protein IRS-4 is composed of a total of 1,257 amino acids and is situated within the cellular membrane of diverse organs where it is expressed. The initial identification of this phenomenon occurred in embryonic kidney cells. The gene known as IRS-4 is located on the X chromosome.

The relaxation of blood vessels is induced by insulin, which achieves this by stimulating the production of nitric oxide (NO) in the endothelial cells of blood vessels. Additionally, insulin reduces the intracellular calcium concentration in muscle and smooth muscle cells by decreasing the sensitization of the light chains of calcium (Ca^{2+})-myosin. The activation of the phosphatidylinositol 3-kinase/protein kinase B (PI3K/Akt) signaling pathway and the stimulation of glucose transport in skeletal muscle and vascular adipose tissue are responsible for these effects. Insulin resistance leads to an elevation in lipolysis, resulting in a higher production of fatty acids. This, in turn, enhances the inhibition of insulin's lipolytic effect, leading to an increase in lipolysis.

Insulin resistance refers to the impaired capacity of skeletal muscle and adipose tissue to uptake glucose, as well as the liver's inability to suppress gluconeogenesis in response to elevated insulin levels.

There is a growing body of evidence supporting the existence of causal relationships between insulin resistance and hypertension. There remain numerous uncertainties regarding the underlying mechanisms that establish a connection between the two conditions. However, apart from the shared genetic predisposition between insulin resistance and AHT, there exist several alternative mechanisms that may elucidate this phenomenon.

AHT can be treated by targeting the renin-angiotensin-aldosterone system (RAAS). Alterations in the RAAS play a significant role in insulin resistance, and the shared molecular mechanisms of insulin resistance and androgenetic thiase (AHT) remain poorly comprehended.

The RAAS is known to have a significant impact on MS. Angiotensinogen, a protein with a molecular weight of 58 kDa, is primarily synthesized in the liver during normal physiological processes. However, it can also be synthesized in lesser quantities in adipocytes, mesangial cells, and epithelial cells of the proximal contoured tubule, as well as in the brain, specifically neurons and glial cells. The enzymatic activity of renin in the glomerular juxta cells of the kidney leads to the cleavage of angiotensinogen at the amino-terminal acid of 10 NH2, resulting in the formation of angiotensin I. Angiotensin I is a peptide that lacks biological activity and undergoes hydroxylation through the action of the enzyme angiotensin converter, resulting in the formation of an octapeptide known as angiotensin II.

The RAAS exhibits autocrine and paracrine mechanisms in multiple tissues, with particular prominence observed in skeletal muscle, smooth muscle of blood vessels, kidneys, heart, and pancreas. The transmembrane protein known as the angiotensin (AT) II receptor is classified as a member of the receptor family that is associated with the G protein. This receptor family is further divided into two types: type I (AT1) and type II (AT2). The AT1 receptor genes were successfully cloned in 1992, while the AT2 receptor genes were cloned in 1994. The interaction between angiotensin II and the AT1 receptor results in the phosphorylation of multiple proteins, including IRS-1 and IRS-2. This process establishes the P110/PI3K subunit as the shared activation mechanism within the insulin signaling pathway. Insulin resistance arises from the suppression of insulin by inhibiting the processes involved in glucose transportation and vasodilation.

Skeletal muscle plays a significant role in the pathogenesis of insulin resistance, a condition that accounts for approximately 75–95% of glucose metabolism. Skeletal muscle is the largest tissue in the body that is sensitive to insulin and serves as the primary location for the utilization of glucose stimulated by insulin. The metabolic dysregulation linked to obesity and physical inactivity is primarily caused by skeletal muscle resistance to insulin. This resistance plays a crucial role in the development of MS. Various mechanisms may contribute to the reduced signaling and action of insulin in skeletal muscle. These mechanisms include the expansion of adipose tissue and the increase in inflammatory adipokines, heightened activity of the RAAS, decreased mitochondrial oxidative capacity of muscle mitochondria, heightened accumulation of intramuscular lipids, and elevated levels of reactive oxygen species (ROS).

Inducing the formation of oxygen free radicals through the enzyme nicotinamide adenine dinucleotide phosphate (NADPH) oxidase, angiotensin II exerts prooxidant and pro-inflammatory effects that regulate various physiological processes, including apoptosis, inflammation, cell growth, fibrosis, and insulin sensitivity. ROS are generated through the electron transport chain within the mitochondria, and their levels tend to rise in circumstances necessitating the oxidation of substrates, such as glucose. Transcript factors, including factor nuclear kappa B (NF-KB) protein-1 and hypoxia-inducible factor-1 (HIF-1), are activated by various ROS. These transcription factors play a crucial role in the development of insulin resistance in skeletal muscle.

Hyperinsulinemia can modify certain elements of the RAAS, such as pro-fibrotic stimulants and pro-inflammatory actions facilitated by angiotensin II, which can contribute to the development of CVD.

Obesity has emerged as a global epidemic, prompting a significant number of scientific publications in recent times. Consequently, novel frameworks were being developed, while the previous obstacles remain unresolved. Obesity is a persistent medical condition that has emerged as a significant concern in numerous developed nations, primarily attributed to its heightened prevalence, correlation with diverse ailments, and substantial economic ramifications. The body has developed various regulatory mechanisms to maintain the energy reserves of body fat during periods of negative energy balance. The aforementioned regulation is accomplished through the equilibrium of glucose absorption in the intestines, glucose production in the liver, and glucose absorption and metabolism in peripheral tissues. The regulation of blood glucose is facilitated by insulin through its ability to stimulate glucose uptake in both muscle and liver tissues, while simultaneously inhibiting hepatic gluconeogenesis. Despite the initial alteration in insulin tolerance, blood glucose levels remain within normal range due to the capacity of pancreatic β cells to enhance insulin secretion, thereby mitigating pre-existing insulin resistance. The overabundance of nutrients leads to the enlargement of adipocytes, which in turn contributes to the emergence of several chronic health conditions, including type 2 diabetes mellitus, insulin resistance, impaired glucose tolerance, and dyslipidemia. These conditions ultimately contribute to the development of CVDs. There exists compelling evidence indicating that cellular hypoxia plays a significant role in the pathophysiology of adipocytes and potentially contributes to the dysfunction observed in obesity, thereby influencing metabolic changes.

According to the WHO, obesity is characterized as an atypical or excessive buildup of adipose tissue, which can lead to disruptions in an individual's overall health. In comparison to females, males exhibit a higher propensity for the accumulation of intra-abdominal adipose tissue. Men, on average, possess twice the quantity of visceral fat compared to women and exhibit a greater incidence of metabolic disorders linked to obesity and MS.

Obesity is linked to an increased prevalence of type 2 diabetes mellitus, insulin resistance, atrial hypertension, dyslipidemia, certain forms of cancer, and CVD. The deposition of fat tissue occurs in two primary compartments, namely the subcutaneous and central or visceral regions. Obesity can be categorized into two main types: central obesity and peripheral obesity. Central obesity is distinguished by the excessive growth and enlargement of adipocytes surrounding the internal organs within the abdomen, and is linked to an increased likelihood of developing MS.

Excessive nutrient intake leads to adipocyte hypertrophy, which in turn promotes the development of insulin resistance and glucose intolerance. The triglycerides found in adipose tissue serve as the primary energy reservoir within the human body. Consequently, adipose tissue functions as a highly efficient energy storage mechanism, enabling the survival of organisms during periods of famine.

Recent research has indicated that low oxygen levels in fat tissue can significantly impact the cellular processes of chronic inflammation, infiltration of macrophages, decrease in adiponectin levels, increase in leptin levels, apoptosis of adipocytes, and dysfunction of the endoplasmic reticulum and mitochondria in obese white adipose tissue.

Hypoxia has been observed to impede the process of pre-adipocyte differentiation while concurrently promoting the release of leptin and vascular endothelial growth factor (VEGF) in fully developed adipocytes.

Several genes, including HIF-1γ (hypoxia-inducible factor 1°), vascular endothelial growth factor VEGF, glucose transporter-1 (GLUT-1), heme oxygenase-1, and pyruvate dehydrogenase kinase 1, regulate the effects of hypoxia. The study revealed that, in the presence of hypoxia in adipose tissue, the expression of all genes exhibited an increase, with the exception of VEGF messenger ribonucleic acid (mRNA).

Adipose tissue can be classified into two distinct types, namely white adipose tissue and brown adipose tissue, each serving unique physiological roles. The primary role of brown adipose tissue is to generate thermal energy. Our comprehension and perception of white adipose tissue have undergone substantial transformations over the past 15 years. Presently, white adipose tissue is regarded as both a storage site for energy in the form of triglycerides and the primary organ responsible for secreting and regulating hormones in the organism. White adipose tissue is responsible for the synthesis and release of diverse proteins. The proteins in question were originally classified as adipocytokines. Presently, the term "adipokines" is widely accepted to refer to the group of proteins that are produced and released by adipose tissue, as not all proteins are classified as cytokines.

In conjunction with adipokines and fatty acids, adipose tissue is responsible for the synthesis of various lipid compounds, including steroid hormones, prostaglandins and prostanoids, cholesterol, and retinol. It is important to note that adipocytes do not synthesize cholesterol and retinol, but rather store and release them.

The hormone leptin, which is synthesized by white adipose tissue, was first identified by Friedman et al. in 1994. The hormone known as leptin, or OB protein, is a 16 kilodaltons hormone that is synthesized from a protein with a molecular weight of 18 kilodaltons. The process of cleavage results in the synthesis of leptin protein. Numerous tissues, such as the white and brown adipose tissue, stomach, placenta, mammary gland, ovarian follicles, and various others, exhibit the expression of leptin. The expression of this protein is predominantly observed in adipose tissue, although it is also present in lesser quantities within the brain and cerebrospinal fluid.

The hormone leptin exerts its effects in both the central nervous system, specifically the hypothalamus, and the peripheral organs. This finding has facilitated our understanding that adipose tissue serves not only as a site for energy storage but also functions as an endocrine organ. Adipokines, including tumor necrosis factor alpha (TNF-κ), interleukin (IL)-β, and IL-6, are produced by white adipose tissue and are known to have inflammatory properties. Obesity is associated with an elevation in the production of inflammatory interleukins, which play a role in the pathogenesis of insulin resistance and the MetS. Adipokines play diverse roles, particularly in regulating energy balance (e.g., leptin) and insulin sensitivity, glucose metabolism (e.g., adiponectin), inflammation (e.g., TNF-κ), immunity (e.g., adipsin), lipid metabolism (e.g., cholesterol ester transfer protein), blood pressure control (e.g., angiotensinogen), hemostasis (e.g., plasminogen activation inhibitor-1), and angiogenesis (e.g., vascular epidermal growth factor).

7.3.1. The Connection Between Low Oxygen Levels and Poor Insulin Resistance

Inflammation plays a significant role in both obesity and type 2 diabetes mellitus (DM), as it contributes to the development of insulin resistance by impeding the activity of IRS-1 and IRS-2 in the insulin signaling pathway.

Obesity is distinguished by a persistent state of inflammation accompanied by elevated levels of inflammatory markers, such as haptoglobin, IL-6, C-reactive protein (CRP), plasminogen activator inhibitor-1 (PAI-1), and TNF-α. Chronic hyperinsulinemia and insulin resistance are caused by high levels of cytokines, such as TNF-α, IL-6, and IL-1β, produced by adipose tissue, and low levels of specific adiponectins.

During periods characterized by positive energy balance, there is an observed augmentation in the accumulation of white adipose tissue, which serves the purpose of storing surplus triglycerides. As a result, the adipose tissue experiences hypoxia as a consequence of reduced vascularization. The precise contributions of hypoxia to obesity and insulin resistance in adipose tissue remain uncertain. The regulatory responses facilitated by HIF-1 are contingent upon the extent and duration of its influence.

Hypoxia-induced factor 1 (HIF-1) is a heterodimeric transcription factor that is comprised of two subunits: the β subunit, which has a molecular weight of 120 kDa, and the β subunit, which has a molecular weight ranging from 91 to 94 kDa. The transcriptional activity of HIF-1 is determined by the α subunit (HIF-1γ), and its upregulation is observed in response to hypoxia. The HIF-1 subunit, also known as an aryl hydrocarbon receptor nuclear translocator (tRNA), is consistently expressed. HIF-1κ undergoes hydroxylation at proline and asparaginyl residues under normoxic conditions, facilitated by the enzyme prolylhydroxylase (PHD). This process enhances the binding of HIF-1κ to a ubiquitin ligase complex. HIF-1 mediates proteosomal degradation in this process. The inhibition of hydroxylation and activation of HIF-1 target genes occurs under hypoxic conditions.

The activation of HIF-1α induces fibrosis in adipose tissue, leading to an augmented infiltration of macrophages into the tissue. This infiltration subsequently facilitates a more pronounced escalation in inflammation, accompanied by a concurrent reduction in insulin sensitivity. VEGF is a gene that HIF-1 targets. VEGF facilitates angiogenesis, an essential mechanism for the differentiation of adipocytes and the proliferation of adipose tissue.

7.4. Obesity and Metabolic Syndrome

A layer of cells known as the endothelium forms the inner surface of the blood vessel. Endothelial dysfunction refers to the disruption of the secretion of vasodilatory stimuli, including nitric oxide (NO) and prostacyclin (PGI2), as well as vasoconstrictive stimuli, such as endothelin-1 (ET-1) and angiotensin II. Insulin resistance can be induced by changes in vascular endothelial function within adipose tissue. Insulin resistance is associated with an elevated rate of free fatty acid release from adipose tissue, thereby contributing to the development of diabetic dyslipidemia. The levels of HDL-cholesterol, low-density lipoprotein (LDL) cholesterol, and free fatty acids decreased, while they increased. The activation of the inflammatory response leads to the recruitment of monocytes and lymphocytes to the endothelial cells, resulting in an augmented supply of glucose and free fatty acids to the cells. Consequently, an excessive generation of oxygen free radicals occurs, leading to an elevation in metabolic and hemodynamic deterioration. Intramitochondrial enzymatic oxy-reduction leads to an elevation in free radicals and nitrites, thereby facilitating apoptosis and compromising vascular endothelial function. This modification leads to impaired insulin metabolism, resulting in increased insulin resistance.

The correlation between insulin resistance and hypertension in individuals with obesity. The sole etiology of AHT in 78% of males and 65% of females is obesity. There is a growing body of evidence supporting the causal link between insulin resistance and AHT. In normal physiological conditions, insulin, and insulin growth factor-1 (IGF-1) promote the widening of blood vessels by stimulating the synthesis of nitric oxide (NO) and decreasing the level of calcium within the smooth muscle cells of blood vessels. The sensitization of myosin-Ca^{2+} light chains is also enhanced. The activation of the PI3K enzyme and the Akt protein mediates these actions. The activation of the PI3K/Akt pathway triggers vascular relaxation, which is facilitated by the production of nitric oxide (NO) by endothelial cells. This process involves the phosphorylation of endothelial NO synthetase.

Individuals diagnosed with acute hypertension (AHT) exhibit elevated levels of fasting and postprandial insulin when compared to non-hypertensive individuals with an equivalent body mass index. Secondary AHT does not occur, but essential AHT does. This phenomenon can be attributed, at least in part, to the influence of insulin on muscle tissue, which serves as the primary site for glucose utilization induced by insulin.

A correlation exists between blood pressure and the skeletal muscle's proportion of type II fibers, which exhibit lower insulin sensitivity compared to type I fibers. In typical physiological circumstances, a correlation exists between the availability of insulin mediated by glucose and the subsequent augmentation of blood flow in response to insulin. The observed decrease in this response is observed in individuals who are obese and have insulin resistance, indicating a resistance to the action of insulin in relation to the production of vascular nitric oxide (NO). The rapid growth of adipose tissue in a hypoxic environment at an early stage poses challenges, leading to the creation of conditions that promote an upregulation of HIF-1α expression.

There exists empirical evidence indicating that individuals with insulin resistance and hyperinsulinemia are more susceptible to the onset of acute hepatitis (AHT) as a result of cellular irregularities in insulin signaling pathways. These abnormalities are closely linked to metabolic and hemodynamic changes. Metabolic abnormalities have been found to be associated with hypertension, which can be attributed to pathophysiological mechanisms involving the sympathetic-adrenergic system, cellular cation imbalance, heightened inflammation, oxidative stress, and the RAAS.

The role of RAAS in insulin resistance is significant, as it exhibits greater activity in visceral adipose tissue relative to peripheral adipose tissue. The presence of insulin resistance in individuals who are obese is partially linked to the antagonistic effects of angiotensin II (AT II). This leads to a reduction in nitric oxide (NO) production accompanied by an increase in vasoconstriction and a decrease in glucocorticoid receptor 4 (GLUT-4) in skeletal muscle. Additionally, it reduces the uptake of glucose and decreases vasodilation in tissues. In typical circumstances, the RAAS serves as a regulatory mechanism for blood pressure. The heightened activity of the RAAS results in an augmented synthesis of adrenocorticotropic hormone (ATII), thereby inducing activation of the sympathetic nervous system, insulin resistance, sodium retention, and augmented intravascular volume. Additionally, it is implicated in the development of kidney disease, hypertension, insulin resistance, and left ventricular hypertrophy.

Insulin resistance and hypertension are frequently associated with a shared genetic predisposition. Individuals with insulin resistance and AHT have been found to have genetic abnormalities, specifically mutations on chromosome 7q. This chromosome also contains other genes that play a crucial role in regulating blood sugar levels, blood pressure, and obesity.

Hyperinsulinemia has the potential to directly induce the reabsorption of sodium and water within the renal system, resulting in an augmentation of extracellular volume and subsequently leading to acute kidney injury (AHT).

The stimulation of the sympathetic nervous system (SNS) through the elevation of norepinephrine concentration is an additional mechanism through which insulin can induce hypertension. The observed rise in pulse and blood pressure can be attributed to the direct impact on sodium reabsorption in the kidney, peripheral vasoconstriction, and heightened cardiac output.

7.5. Management of Metabolic Syndrome

MetS is linked to a higher likelihood of developing both atherosclerotic and nonatherosclerotic CVD. The ongoing debate revolves around whether the risk is a cumulative result of its individual components or if the clustering of these components leads to a synergistic risk. Motillo and colleagues' recent meta-analysis revealed that MetS is associated with a twofold increase in the risk of CVD outcomes and a 1.5-fold increase in all-cause mortality. The management of MetS entails a two-pronged strategy that integrates lifestyle modifications and pharmacological interventions with the aim of reducing CVD.

7.5.1. Lifestyle Modification

As previously mentioned, MetS arises due to an imbalance between caloric intake and metabolic demands. The implementation of lifestyle modifications is crucial in effectively managing the underlying risk factors. The implementation of weight reduction and the maintenance of an optimal body weight are crucial strategies for both prevention and management. The objective of weight reduction is to achieve a decrease of 7–10% in initial body weight within a timeframe of 6–12 months, while also reducing caloric consumption by 500–1,000 calories per day. Dietary modification has the potential to regulate various components of MetS. For instance, reducing the consumption of saturated fats, trans fats, cholesterol, sodium, and simple sugars has been shown to be beneficial in managing dyslipidemia, hyperglycemia, and hypertension. Diets characterized by high or low fat content have been found to worsen atherogenic dyslipidemia. Therefore, it is generally advised to consume 25–35% of one's daily caloric intake in the form of fat. The prudent utilization of bariatric surgery has demonstrated advantages in individuals with severe obesity. Weight loss contributes to enhancement in all aspects of physical activity. Physical activity enhances the intake of calories, facilitating weight reduction and decreasing the risk of CVD. Engaging in moderate-intensity exercise for approximately 30–60 minutes and making deliberate changes to a sedentary lifestyle can be advantageous for managing MetS.

7.5.2. Pharmacotherapy

In addition to altering the fundamental risk factors, pharmacotherapy is an alternative approach for preventing CVD. Prominent pharmacological interventions encompass the administration of statins for the management of dyslipidemia, the utilization of antiplatelet drugs to mitigate prothrombotic risk, and the implementation of insulin sensitizers to reduce the likelihood of developing diabetes. There is currently no singular pharmacological intervention for MetS, and the existing pharmacotherapy and accompanying comorbidities require the extended administration of multiple medications. This poses a significant challenge for patients, as it leads to polypharmacy and diminished adherence. Consequently, there is an increasing fascination with utilizing naturally existing substances to reduce the likelihood and advancement of MetS, although their impact on long-term cardiovascular results and long-term adherence remains uncertain.

7.5.3. Nutraceuticals in the Management of Metabolic Syndrome

Nutraceuticals refer to dietary supplements that offer health benefits in addition to their fundamental nutritional value. A range of natural compounds obtained from plant extracts, spices, herbs, and essential oils have been shown to possess significant advantages in the treatment of individuals diagnosed with MetS (Table 7.2). Due to the ongoing investigation into the potential benefits of these nutraceuticals, it is not advisable to consider them as substitutes for the pharmacotherapies presently employed in the treatment of MetS.

Table 7.2. *Nutraceuticals in Metabolic Syndrome*

Source	Active Ingredient	Actions
Turmeric (*Curcuma longa*)	Curcumin	Anti-inflammatory, antioxidant ↑ Insulin sensitivity ↓ Obesity ↓ Leptin and ↑ Adiponectin
Garlic (*Allium sativum*)	Allicin	Anti-inflammatory Antioxidant ↑ Insulin sensitivity ↓ Total cholesterol and triglycerides ↑ Adiponectin levels
Cinnamon (*Cinnamomum verum*)	Polyphenols	Antithrombotic Anti-inflammatory ↑ Insulin sensitivity Improves fasting blood glucose, blood pressure, and body composition
Rhizoma coptidis	Berberine	↑ Insulin sensitivity ↓ Body weight ↓ Triglycerides ↓ Systolic blood pressure
Neem (*Azadirachta indica*)	Neem oil	↑ Insulin secretion ↓ Postprandial hyperglycemia
Bergamot orange (*Citrus bergamia*)	Bergamot essential oil	Anti-inflammatory and antioxidant effects ↓ Lectin-like oxidized low-density lipoprotein receptor-1 expression ↓ Reactive oxygen species formation
Cumin (*Cuminum cyaminum*)	Cuminaldehyde	↓ Lipid levels ↓ Blood glucose levels

Fenugreek (*Trigonella foenum*)	Saponins, galactomannan	↓ Body weight ↓ Triglycerides and total cholesterol ↑ Insulin sensitivity ↓ Postprandial blood glucose
Cardamom (*Elettaria cardamomum*)	Terpenine, cineol	↓ Systolic blood pressure ↓ Platelet aggregation
Ginger (*Zingiber officinale*)	Gingerols, shogaols, parasols	Anti-inflammatory ↓ Cyclooxygenase-2, ↓ 5-lipoxygenase ↓ Systolic blood pressure
Grapes (*Vitus vinifera*)	Resveratrol, 3,5,4′-trihydroxy-*trans*-stilbene	↓ Adipogenesis ↑ Lipolysis ↓ Insulin resistance ↓ Body mass index
Onions (*Allium cepa*)	Quercetin	Anti-inflammatory Antioxidant ↓ Adipogenesis ↑ Lipolysis ↓ Blood glucose ↓ cholesterol levels
Fish oils (omega fatty acids)	Polyunsaturated fatty acids	↓ Lipogenesis ↑ Fatty acid oxidation Regulate peroxisome proliferator-activated receptor gamma
Broccoli (*Brassica oleracea*)	Sulforaphrane	Activates nuclear factor erythroid 2-related factor 2 Antioxidant Anti-inflammatory

Here, we outline the nutraceuticals that have been researched and have demonstrated certain advantages in MetS.

7.5.3.1. Curcumin

Curcumin is a compound derived from the spice turmeric (*Curcuma longa*), which is widely utilized in the regions of south-east Asia. Differentuloylmethane, the active constituent, is recognized for its anti-inflammatory and antioxidative characteristics. Curcumin has demonstrated the ability to inhibit the activation of NF-kB, thereby attenuating the inflammatory cascade through the downregulation of pro-inflammatory cytokine expression. Additionally, it downregulates the expression of TNF-κ and suppresses the expression of plasminogen activator inhibitor type-1, which is implicated in the promotion of thrombosis. In addition to its effects on obesity, curcumin has been observed to inhibit the Wnt/β-catenin pathway and induce activation of peroxisome proliferator-activated receptor gamma in hepatic stellate cells. Curcumin has the ability to disrupt leptin signaling, leading to an increase in the expression of adiponectin. The detrimental impact on obesity and the advantageous impact on insulin sensitization, along with the mitigation of inflammatory pathways, are advantageous outcomes in individuals with MetS.

7.5.3.2. Garlic

Allium sativum, commonly known as garlic, possesses medicinal properties due to its antioxidant and antithrombotic effects. The study conducted by Padiya et al. revealed that the consumption of raw garlic enhances insulin sensitivity in rats fed fructose, suggesting potential analogous effects in human subjects. Reinhart et al. conducted a meta-analysis comprising 29 randomized placebo-controlled trials to examine the impact of garlic consumption on lipid profiles. The findings of this study indicate that the intake of garlic is associated with a reduction in total cholesterol and triglyceride levels. In a separate investigation, Gomez-Arbelaez et al. conducted a study to examine the impact of aged garlic extract on adiponectin levels among individuals diagnosed with MetS. The application of aged garlic extract over a period of 12 weeks demonstrated a positive impact on adiponectin levels. The garlic derivatives contain organosulfur compounds that contribute to its anti-inflammatory effect. Garlic exhibits a promising potential as a natural therapy for MetS owing to its thiol groups, which possess antioxidant properties that aid in combating inflammation mediated by ROS.

7.5.3.3. Cinnamon

Cinnamon (Cinnamomum verum), obtained from the bark of a tree, is commonly employed as a spice and flavor enhancer in traditional medicinal practices of China and India. Cinnamon extracts and polyphenols possess various advantageous properties in the context of MetS, including antithrombotic, insulin-sensitizing, lipid-lowering, anti-inflammatory, and antioxidant effects. The insulin-like activity of cinnamon polyphenols has been observed in various studies, which have documented enhancements in glycemic control and lipid levels. Ziegenfuss et al. conducted a randomized placebo-controlled trial to establish the efficacy of an aqueous extract of cinnamon in ameliorating fasting blood glucose levels, blood pressure, and body composition among individuals diagnosed with MetS. The complete understanding of the mechanistic pathways involved in this process remains elusive. Nevertheless, certain investigations conducted on mouse models suggest that cinnamon extracts possess the ability to modulate the expression of adipocyte genes, thereby enhancing glucose transport (specifically GLUT 4) and insulin signaling.

7.5.3.4. Berberine

The alkaloid berberine, derived from the plant *Rhizoma coptidis*, is utilized in China due to its antimicrobial properties and recognized for its antidiabetic effects. Research conducted on animals with insulin resistance has demonstrated that the administration of berberine leads to enhancements in body weight, triglyceride levels, and insulin sensitivity. Berberine functions by increasing the expression of genes related to energy utilization and decreasing the expression of genes related to lipogenesis. Similar to metformin and thiazolidinediones, it exhibits an insulin-sensitizing effect through the activation of adenosine monophosphate-associated protein kinase in adipocytes. Research conducted on individuals with MetS has documented a decrease in waist circumference, triglyceride levels, and systolic blood pressure, particularly among females.

Azadirachta indica, commonly referred to as neem or nim tree, is recognized for its medicinal properties. The administration of neem extract has been found to be linked to an enhanced glucose tolerance through the reduction of glucosidase activity in the intestines and pancreas, thereby contributing to the amelioration of postprandial hyperglycemia. Previous studies have also reported an elevation in glucose-6-phosphate dehydrogenase activity, leading to an increase in glucose utilization. In addition, Neem extracts have been found to facilitate the regeneration of pancreatic beta cells, thereby enhancing the secretion of insulin.

7.5.3.5. Bergamot Oil

Bergamot essential oil is a citrus sap obtained from *Citrus bergamia*, and possesses properties that can combat cancer, inflammation, microorganisms, and anxiety. The antioxidant properties of bergamot oil are particularly noteworthy in the context of MetS. The study conducted by Mollace et al. investigated the impact of the antioxidant constituent found in bergamot oil on the expression of LOX-1 and the generation of free radicals in the context of carotid injury in rats. The study found that balloon injury was linked to the proliferation of smooth muscle cells, the formation of neointima, the generation of ROS, and an increase in the expression of LOX-1. The administration of bergamot essential oil prior to treatment in these rats resulted in a reduction in neointima formation, LOX-1 expression, and free-radical generation, thereby mitigating the extent of stenosis. Additional natural compounds, including procyanins, 6-shogoal procyanins, and flavonoids, have been linked to antioxidant properties that could potentially offer advantages in the treatment of MetS.

7.5.3.6. Resveratrol

Resveratrol, also known as 3,5,4′-trihydroxystilbene, is a polyphenol that can be found in various plants, including grapes and nuts, as well as in its derivatives like wine. The sirtuin pathway is activated by this substance, thereby governing various cellular processes associated with metabolism, oxidation, and the process of aging. It positively impacts cellular energy balance by reducing adipogenesis and promoting lipolysis through various mechanisms. Additionally, it inhibits cyclooxygenase, leading to an antioxidant effect. Resveratrol's efficacy in MetS has been investigated in both animal models and human subjects. Promising outcomes have been observed in clinical investigations conducted on individuals diagnosed with insulin resistance and nonalcoholic fatty liver disease. Indeed, the utilization of resveratrol has demonstrated efficacy in enhancing insulin sensitivity, glucose tolerance, as well as overall weight and body mass index among individuals diagnosed with MetS.

7.5.3.7. Quercetin

Quercetin, a flavonoid derived from plants, is present in various vegetables and fruits, including onions, berries, and tea. It has been documented to possess anti-inflammatory and antioxidant metabolic properties. Quercetin exerts its effects through mitochondrial pathways that are implicated in adipokinesis and lipolysis, which are key factors in the progression of obesity. Rivera et al. conducted a study to investigate the impact of quercetin on Zucker rats with obesity. The present study observed that rats administered with quercetin exhibited reduced blood pressure, decreased cholesterol levels, and diminished insulin resistance in comparison to rats that did not receive this treatment. An anti-inflammatory effect in the visceral adipose tissue was observed with higher doses of quercetin. The metabolic implications of quercetin use in humans, particularly in men with an apolipoprotein E genotype, were investigated by Pfeuffer et al. The findings of their study revealed that quercetin has a positive impact on metabolic parameters, including waist circumference, postprandial blood glucose, and lipids. However, it was also observed that quercetin led to an elevation in inflammatory markers, such as TNF-κ.

7.5.3.8. Omega Fatty Acids

The protective role of omega-3 long-chain polyunsaturated fatty acids (PUFAs) in diseases related to MetS has been the subject of extensive investigation in various epidemiological studies [47]. Two particular PUFAs, namely eicosapentaenoic acid and DHA, which are highly prevalent in fish oils, have garnered significant interest, resulting in substantial societal recommendations for prevention. Studies have demonstrated that 48 PUFAs can hinder the production of fats and trigger the breakdown of fats in the liver and adipose tissue. This is achieved by controlling important transcription factors, such as the peroxisome proliferator-activated receptors and sterol regulatory element binding protein [49–52]. Although PUFAs have shown positive effects on different aspects of MetS, there is currently a lack of long-term evidence supporting their effectiveness in preventing hard cardiovascular endpoints. Nevertheless, the presence of robust pathophysiological correlates for the underlying mechanisms is promising and warrants additional investigation.

7.5.3.9. Sulforaphane

Sulforaphane, a phytochemical derived from Brassica vegetables like broccoli, has recently demonstrated promising potential in the treatment of MetS owing to its antioxidant and anti-inflammatory characteristics. Sulforaphane stimulates the activation of nuclear factor erythroid 2-related factor 2, which is a transcription factor involved in antioxidant activity. Multiple animal studies have shown that sulforaphane has a protective effect against several disorders, including hypertension, hyperlipidemia, and diabetes, which are all important aspects of MetS [52–54].

7.6. Summary

MetS is a widespread and well-documented cause of both atherosclerotic and nonatherosclerotic CVD. There are notable disparities in the diagnostic criteria and definition of MetS, indicating a shift in the comprehension of this condition over time. The primary pathophysiological drivers for MetS appear to be a combination of different stimuli that ultimately lead to a state of chronic inflammation. Current treatments for different aspects of MetS are constrained by a range of factors. The limited number of medications that have demonstrated significant efficacy in achieving long-term outcomes poses a challenge in selecting an appropriate therapeutic approach. Furthermore, the chronic nature of the constituents of MetS necessitates the extended and frequently indefinite utilization of diverse pharmaceuticals, such as statins. This results in a heightened prevalence of adverse effects associated with drug usage and a lack of adherence from patients. Within this framework, the advancement of easily accessible nutraceuticals with minimal adverse effects may hold potential in the creation of innovative treatments.

A Closer Look

Pharmacotherapy

Pharmacotherapy, the use of medications to manage and treat disease, is a cornerstone of modern medicine that addresses a wide range of health conditions through targeted drug interventions. This field is integral to the broader discipline of pharmacology and involves understanding drug mechanisms, therapeutic effects, side effects, and optimal dosing. Pharmacotherapy's primary goal is to restore and maintain health, either by alleviating symptoms or, in some cases, curing diseases. The development of a pharmacotherapy plan is a complex, patient-centered process that takes into account individual needs, existing health conditions, and other medications a patient might be taking.

The advancement of pharmacotherapy has dramatically reshaped healthcare over the past century. Breakthroughs in pharmacotherapy include the discovery of antibiotics, which revolutionized the treatment of infections, and the development of insulin for diabetes management. More recent innovations involve medications targeting complex diseases like cancer, cardiovascular disease, and mental health disorders. The sophistication of these drugs, such as monoclonal antibodies and gene therapies, has introduced a new era of precision medicine, where treatments are tailored based on genetic and biomarker information.

Pharmacotherapy's scope is extensive, covering medications for chronic conditions like hypertension and diabetes, acute conditions like infections, and severe conditions like cancer. Each type of drug class—antibiotics, analgesics, anticoagulants, antidepressants, and others—operates through specific mechanisms that influence body systems in different ways. For instance, antibiotics target bacterial infections by interfering with bacterial cell wall synthesis or protein production, while antidepressants aim to balance neurotransmitters in the brain to alleviate mood disorders. However, despite these benefits, drug therapy is not without risks. Side effects and adverse drug reactions are prevalent concerns, especially with polypharmacy, where multiple drugs are used concurrently. Managing these risks involves careful monitoring and adjustments to minimize potential negative outcomes.

Pharmacotherapy also faces several ethical and economic challenges. One ethical concern is the accessibility of life-saving drugs, particularly for underprivileged populations. In terms of economics, high drug prices can hinder patient access, leading to disparities in treatment outcomes. The development of pharmacotherapy is costly, with research and clinical trials for a single drug potentially costing billions and taking many years to reach approval. This process is rigorously monitored by regulatory bodies such as the Food and Drug Administration (FDA) in the U.S. and the European Medicines Agency (EMA) in Europe to ensure the efficacy and safety of medications.

A critical element in the future of pharmacotherapy lies in pharmacogenomics, the study of how genes affect an individual's response to drugs. By understanding genetic factors that influence drug metabolism, clinicians can better predict which patients will benefit from a specific medication and at what dose. This has already seen practical application in areas like oncology, where personalized medicine has improved outcomes. Despite these advancements, challenges remain, such as managing side effects, patient adherence, and understanding complex drug interactions. Pharmacotherapy will continue to evolve as new drugs are discovered, and existing ones are refined, ultimately aiming to provide safer, more effective treatments for a wide range of conditions.

References

1. Aggarwal, B. B., (2010). Targeting inflammation-induced obesity and metabolic diseases by curcumin and other nutraceuticals. *Annu Rev Nutr 30,* 173–199.
2. Bastard, J. P., Jardel, C., Bruckert, E., et al., (2000). Elevated levels of interleukin 6 are reduced in serum and subcutaneous adipose tissue of obese women after weight loss. *J Clin Endocrinol Metab 85*(9), 3338–3342.
3. Beltrán-Sánchez, H., Harhay, M. O., Harhay, M. M., et al., (2013). Prevalence and trends of metabolic syndrome in the adult, U. S., population, 1999–2010. *J Am Coll Cardiol 62*(8), 697–703.
4. Bhat, M., Kothiwale, S. K., Tirmale, A. R., et al., (2009). Antidiabetic properties of Azardiracta indica and Bougainvillea spectabilis: in vivo studies in murine diabetes model. *Evid Based Complement Alternat Med 2011,* 561625.
5. Boden, G., & Shulman, G. I., (2002). Free fatty acids in obesity and type 2 diabetes: defining their role in the development of insulin resistance and beta-cell dysfunction. *Eur J Clin Invest 32*(Suppl. 3), 14–23.
6. Bremer, A. A., (2014). Resveratrol use in metabolic syndrome. *Metab Syndr Relat Disord 12*(10), 493–495.
7. Cao, H., Graves, D. J., & Anderson, R. A., (2010). Cinnamon extract regulates glucose transporter and insulin-signaling gene expression in mouse adipocytes. *Phytomedicine 17*(13), 1027–1032.
8. Chen, S., Zhao, X., Ran, L., et al., (2015). Resveratrol improves insulin resistance, glucose and lipid metabolism in patients with non-alcoholic fatty liver disease: a randomized controlled trial. *Dig Liver Dis 47*(3), 226–232.
9. Dai, Y., Mercanti, F., Dai, D., et al., (2013). LOX-1, a bridge between GLP-1R and mitochondrial ROS generation in human vascular smooth muscle cells. *Biochem Biophys Res Commun 437*(1), 62–66.
10. de Souza, C. G., Sattler, J. A., De Assis, A. M., et al., (2012). Metabolic effects of sulforaphane oral treatment in streptozotocin-diabetic rats. *J Med Food 15*(9), 795–801.
11. Flachs, P., Horakova, O., Brauner, P., et al., (2005). Polyunsaturated fatty acids of marine origin upregulate mitochondrial biogenesis and induce beta-oxidation in white fat. *Diabetologia 48,* 2365–2375.
12. Ford, E. S., Giles, W. H., & Dietz, W. H., (2002). Prevalence of the metabolic syndrome among US adults: findings from the third National Health and Nutrition Examination Survey. *JAMA 287*(3), 356–359.
13. Fried, S. K., Bunkin, D. A., & Greenberg, A. S., (1998). Omental and subcutaneous adipose tissues of obese subjects release interleukin-6: depot difference and regulation by glucocorticoid. *J Clin Endocrinol Metab 83*(3), 847–850.
14. Gillies, P. J., Bhatia, S. K., Belcher, L. A., et al., (2012). Regulation of inflammatory and lipid metabolism genes by eicosapentaenoic acid-rich oil. *J Lipid Res 53,* 1679–1689.
15. Gobal, F., Deshmukh, A., Shah, S., et al., (2011). Triad of metabolic syndrome, chronic kidney disease, and coronary heart disease with a focus on microalbuminuria: death by overeating. *J Am Coll Cardiol 57*(23), 2303–2308.

16. Gomez-Arbelaez, D., Lahera, V., Oubina, P., et al., (2013). Aged garlic extract improves adiponectin levels in subjects with metabolic syndrome: a double-blind, placebo-controlled, randomized, crossover study. *Mediators Inflamm 2013,* 285795.

17. Grundy, S. M., Hansen, B., Smith, S. C., Jr, et al., (2004). American Heart Association, National Heart, Lung, and Blood Institute, American Diabetes Association. Clinical management of metabolic syndrome: report of the American Heart Association/National Heart, Lung, and Blood Institute/American Diabetes Association conference on scientific issues related to management. *Arterioscler Thromb Vasc Biol 24*(2), e19–e24.

18. Grundy, S. M., (2008). Metabolic syndrome pandemic. *Arterioscler Thromb Vasc Biol 28*(4), 629–636.

19. Guo, W., Xie, W., Lei, T., et al., (2005). Eicosapentaenoic acid, but not oleic acid, stimulates beta-oxidation in adipocytes. *Lipids 40,* 815–821.

20. Hotamisligil, G. S., Murray, D. L., Choy, L. N., et al., (1994). Tumor necrosis factor alpha inhibits signaling from the insulin receptor. *Proc Natl Acad Sci USA, 91*(11), 4854–4858.

21. Juhan-Vague, I., Alessi, M. C., Mavri, A., et al., (2003). Plasminogen activator inhibitor-1, inflammation, obesity, insulin resistance and vascular risk. *J Thromb Haemost 1*(7), 1575–1579.

22. Lee, Y. S., Kim, W. S., Kim, K. H., et al., (2006). Berberine, a natural plant product, activates AMP-activated protein kinase with beneficial metabolic effects in diabetic and insulin-resistant states. *Diabetes 55*(8), 2256–2264.

23. Leiherer, A., Stoemmer, K., Muendlein, A., et al., (2016). Quercetin impacts expression of metabolism- and obesity-associated genes in SGBS adipocytes. *Nutrients 8*(5), 10.3390/nu8050282.

24. Lewis, G. F., & Steiner, G., (1996). Acute effects of insulin in the control of VLDL production in humans. Implications for the insulin-resistant state. *Diabetes Care 19*(4), 390–393.

25. Lichtenstein, A. H., Appel, L. J., Brands, M., et al., (2006). Diet and lifestyle recommendations revision 2006: a scientific statement from the American Heart Association Nutrition Committee. *Circulation 114*, 82–96.

26. Lindsay, R. S., Funahashi, T., Hanson, R. L., et al., (2002). Adiponectin and development of type 2 diabetes in the Pima Indian population. *Lancet 360*(9326), 57–58.

27. Matsuzawa, Y., Funahashi, T., & Nakamura, T., (2011). The concept of metabolic syndrome: contribution of visceral fat accumulation and its molecular mechanism. *J Atheroscler Thromb 18*(8), 629–639.

28. Mehta, P. K., & Griendling, K. K., (2007). Angiotensin II cell signaling: physiological and pathological effects in the cardiovascular system. *Am J Physiol Cell Physiol 292*(1), C82–C97.

29. Mendez-del Villar, M., Gonzalez-Ortiz, M., Martinez-Abundis, E., et al., (2014). Effect of resveratrol administration on metabolic syndrome, insulin sensitivity, and insulin secretion. *Metab Syndr Relat Disord 12*(10), 497–501.

30. Miller, J. M., Kaylor, M. B., Johannsson, M., et al., (2014). Prevalence of metabolic syndrome and individual criterion in US adolescents: 2001–2010 National Health and Nutrition Examination Survey. *Metab Syndr Relat Disord 12*(10), 527–532.

31. Mollace, V., Ragusa, S., Sacco, I., et al., (2008). The protective effect of bergamot oil extract

on lecitine-like oxyLDL receptor-1 expression in balloon injury-related neointima formation. *J Cardiovasc Pharmacol Ther 13*(2), 120–129.

32. Mottillo, S., Filion, K. B., Genest, J., et al., (2010). The metabolic syndrome and cardiovascular risk a systematic review and meta-analysis. *J Am Coll Cardiol 56*(14), 1113–1132.
33. Ouchi, N., Ohishi, M., Kihara, S., et al., (2003). Association of hypoadiponectinemia with impaired vasoreactivity. *Hypertension 42*(3), 231–234.
34. Padiya, R., Khatua, T. N., Bagul, P. K., et al., (2011). Garlic improves insulin sensitivity and associated metabolic syndromes in fructose fed rats. *Nutr Metab (Lond) 8,* 53, 7075-8-53.
35. Pant, S., Deshmukh, A., Gurumurthy, G. S., et al., (2014). Inflammation and atherosclerosis – revisited. *J Cardiovasc Pharmacol Ther 19*(2), 170–178.
36. Pendurthi, U. R., & Rao, L. V., (2000). Suppression of transcription factor Egr-1 by curcumin. *Thromb Res 97*(4), 179–189.
37. Perez-Rubio, K. G., Gonzalez-Ortiz, M., Martinez-Abundis, E., et al., (2013). Effect of berberine administration on metabolic syndrome, insulin sensitivity, and insulin secretion. *Metab Syndr Relat Disord 11*(5), 366–369.
38. Pfeuffer, M., Auinger, A., Bley, U., et al., (2013). Effect of quercetin on traits of the metabolic syndrome, endothelial function and inflammation in men with different APOE isoforms. *Nutr Metab Cardiovasc Dis 23*(5), 403–409.
39. Pischon, T., Girman, C. J., Hotamisligil, G. S., et al., (2004). Plasma adiponectin levels and risk of myocardial infarction in men. *JAMA 291*(14), 1730–1737.
40. Reinhart, K. M., Talati, R., White, C. M., et al., (2009). The impact of garlic on lipid parameters: a systematic review and meta-analysis. *Nutr Res Rev 22*(1), 39–48.
41. Rivera, L., Moron, R., Sanchez, M., et al., (2008). Quercetin ameliorates metabolic syndrome and improves the inflammatory status in obese Zucker rats. *Obesity (Silver Spring) 16*(9), 2081–2087.
42. Singh, S., & Aggarwal, B. B., (1995). Activation of transcription factor NF-kappa B is suppressed by curcumin (diferuloylmethane) [corrected]. *J Biol Chem 270*(42), 24995–25000.
43. Song, M.-Y., Kim, E.-K., Moon, W.-S., et al., (2009). Sulforaphane protects against cytokine- and streptozotocin-induced β-cell damage by suppressing the NF-κB pathway. *Toxicol Appl Pharmacol 235*(1), 57–67.
44. Tooke, J. E., & Hannemann, M. M., (2000). Adverse endothelial function and the insulin resistance syndrome. *J Intern Med 247*(4), 425–431.
45. Tripathy, D., Mohanty, P., Dhindsa, S., et al., (2003). Elevation of free fatty acids induces inflammation and impairs vascular reactivity in healthy subjects. *Diabetes 52*(12), 2882–2887.
46. Tsigos, C., Kyrou, I., Chala, E., et al., (1999). Circulating tumor necrosis factor alpha concentrations are higher in abdominal versus peripheral obesity. *Metabolism 48*(10), 1332–1335.
47. Vanecková, I., Maletínská, L., Behuliak, M., et al., (2014). Obesity-related hypertension: possible pathophysiological mechanisms. *J Endocrinol 223*(3), R63–R78.

Chapter 8

AGING AND NEUROLOGICAL DISORDERS

Contents

Introduction

Neurological disorders exert a significant impact on global health. According to the latest estimates, the neurological disorders such as Alzheimer's and other dementias, Parkinson's disease, multiple sclerosis, epilepsy, and headache disorders (specifically migraine, tension-type headache [TTH], and medication-overuse headache [MOH]) that were examined in the Global Burden of Disease (GBD) Study account for approximately 3% of the global burden of disease. Despite appearing to be a relatively modest proportion, dementia, epilepsy, migraine, and stroke are among the leading contributors to disability-adjusted life years (DALYs) within the top 50 causes (Murray et al., 2012).

According to Murray et al. (2012), migraine and epilepsy account for approximately 33% and 25% of the overall neurological burden, respectively. Additionally, dementia and Parkinson's disease are among the top 15 conditions that have experienced significant increases in burden over the past decade. In 2010, neurological disorders accounted for 5.5% of years lived with disability (YLDs), which is equivalent to 42.9 million YLDs. Migraine, epilepsy, and dementia were identified as some of the leading causes of YLDs, ranking among the top 25. According to Vos et al. (2012), migraine is the most prevalent neurological disorder, accounting for over 50% of neurological young learning disabilities (YLDs) or 2.9% of global YLDs. Epilepsy, on the other hand, represents 1.1% of global YLDs.

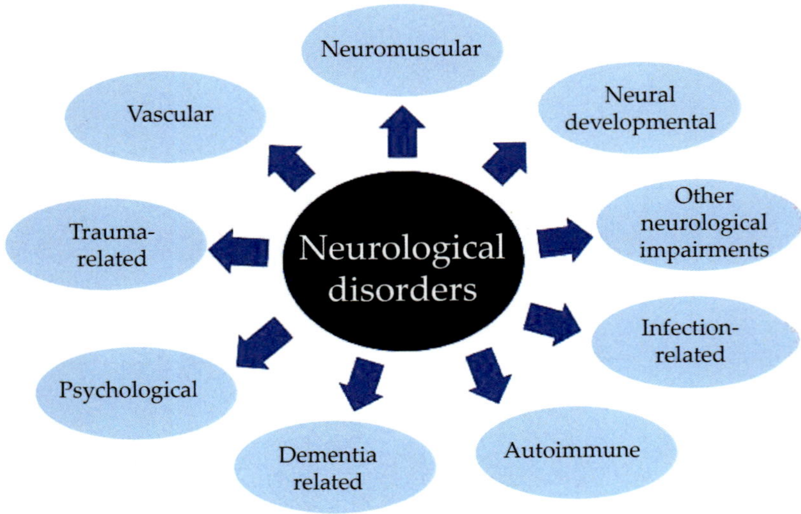

Figure 8.1. *Approaches and relationships about the neurological disorders.*

Source: https://www.intechopen.com/chapters/76045.

According to Murray et al. (2012), the prevalence of neurological diseases is projected to increase significantly in low- and middle-income countries (LMICs) over the next 10 years. Although neurological disorders have a substantial impact on patients and societies, our understanding of their epidemiology, which includes the variation in disease frequency across different locations and time periods, as well as our knowledge of associated risk factors and outcomes, is still limited, especially in LMICs. Individuals diagnosed with neurological disorders frequently necessitate substantial social and economic assistance due to the presence of physical, cognitive, and psychosocial constraints (World Health Organization, 2006). Although disability is widespread, there is a growing acknowledgment that services and resources are disproportionately limited, particularly in LMICs (WHO, 2004). Furthermore, there is a scarcity of information regarding the cost-effectiveness of interventions aimed at enhancing neurological care in these particular contexts.

These three neurological disorders, namely epilepsy, dementia, and headache disorders, are the focus of this chapter. This chapter provides an overview of the existing body of knowledge pertaining to the epidemiology, risk factors, and affordable interventions associated with these conditions. The primary emphasis is on interventions that effectively alleviate the burden on the global population, with a specific focus on their applicability to LMICs. The prevalence of neurological disorders poses a growing concern for healthcare systems on a global scale, necessitating additional research, involvement from governmental and societal entities, and enhancements in healthcare infrastructure (Figure 8.1).

Orientation and Directional Terms

Term	Definition	Illustration
Epilepsy	A neurological disorder characterized by recurrent, unprovoked seizures due to abnormal electrical activity in the brain.	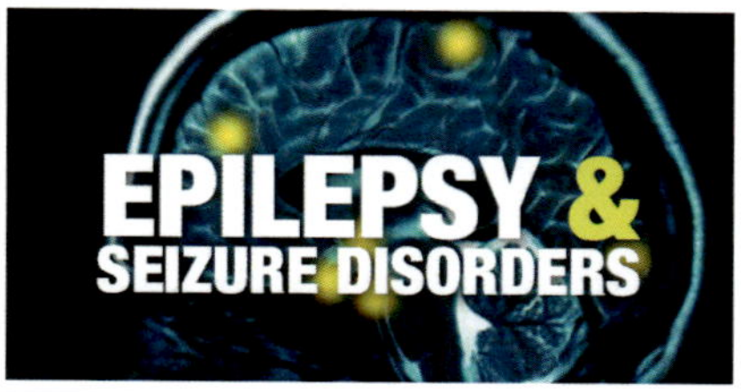
Dementia	A group of cognitive disorders marked by memory loss, impaired reasoning, and personality changes, often associated with aging.	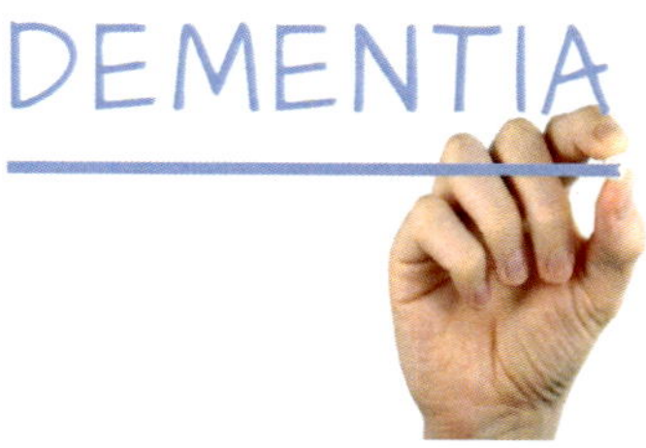
Alzheimer's Disease	A progressive neurodegenerative disease that leads to memory loss, cognitive decline, and personality changes, most common in older adults.	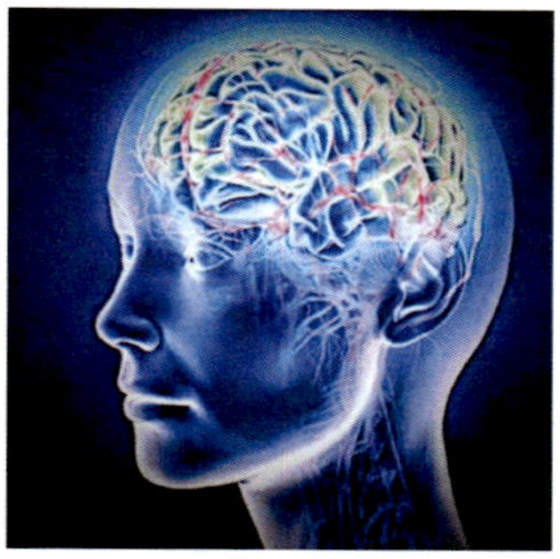
Parkinson's Disease	A degenerative disorder of the nervous system that affects movement, causing tremors, stiffness, and difficulty with balance and coordination.	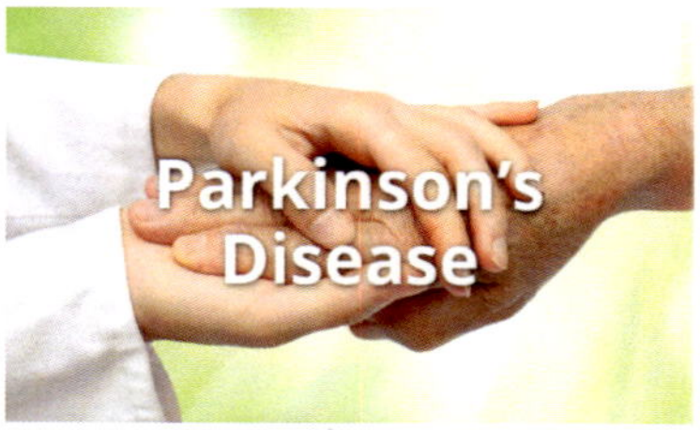
Brain Tumors	Abnormal growths of cells in the brain that can be benign or malignant, leading to various neurological symptoms depending on the tumor's size and location.	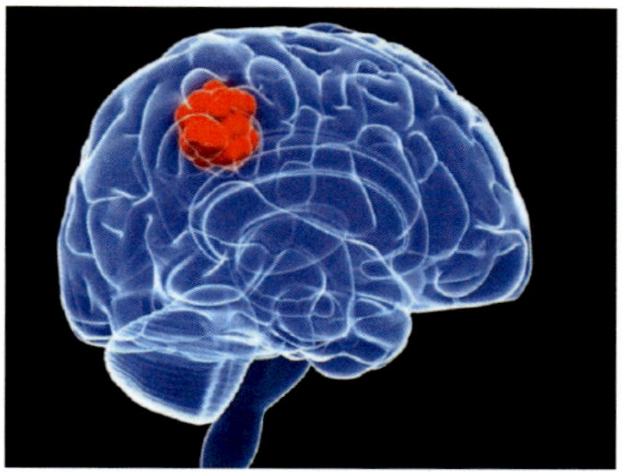

8.1. Epilepsy

8.1.1. Definition

Epilepsy is a neurological condition that is conventionally characterized by the presence of two spontaneous seizures that happen more than 24 hours apart, accompanied by a persistent tendency to produce additional seizures (Fisher et al., 2014). The enhanced definition of epilepsy was provided by the International League against Epilepsy in 2014.

Epilepsy is diagnosed when an individual satisfies any of the following criteria (Fisher et al., 2014): experiencing a minimum of two unprovoked seizures that occur more than 24 hours apart.

According to Fisher et al. (2014), epilepsy is deemed to be resolved when an individual exhibits an age-dependent syndrome that surpasses the anticipated age for this syndrome, or when the individual has maintained seizure-free status for a duration of at least 10 years and has abstained from anti-epileptic medications for a minimum of five years. Individuals who persist in experiencing seizures despite undergoing a sufficient trial of a treatment plan consisting of two well-tolerated and suitably selected anti-epileptic drugs (AEDs), whether used alone or in combination, are classified as drug resistant. Epilepsy can be categorized into three distinct classifications:

One example of epilepsy is structural or metabolic epilepsies, which can be attributed to a remote stroke.

Genetic or presumed genetic epilepsies, such as juvenile myoclonic epilepsy, are examples of epilepsy. Unidentified epilepsies (Berg et al., 2010).

Brain tumors, infectious diseases, brain injury, stroke, and hippocampal sclerosis are among the more prevalent etiologies of epilepsy. Less common etiologies encompass genetic factors, autoimmune factors, and cortical developmental malformations (Bhalla et al., 2011). Perinatal and infection-related causes frequently prevail in LMICs.

8.1.2. Epidemiology and Burden of Disease

A comprehensive global systematic review on the prevalence of the phenomenon has not been published thus far. However, existing literature has reported a range of prevalence rates in door-to-door studies, varying from 2.2 per 1,000 to 41.0 per 1,000 individuals. It is worth noting that these estimates tend to be higher in LMICs (Banerjee, Filippi, & Allen Hauser, 2009; Benamer & Grosset, 2009; Burneo, Tellez-Zenteno, & Wiebe, 2005; Forsgren et al., 2005; Mac et al., 2007). According to Ngugi et al. (2011), the median incidence per 100,000 individuals per year is greater in LMICs at 81.7 (interquartile range [IQR] 28.0–239.5) compared to high-income countries (HICs) at 45.0 (IQR 30.3–66.7).

The elevated prevalence or incidence rates observed in numerous LMICs are believed to be attributed to the presence of endemic diseases, such as malaria or neurocysticercosis, the increased occurrence of road traffic injuries and birth-related injuries, as well as disparities in medical infrastructure, the availability of preventive health programs, and the accessibility of healthcare services. The prevalence of epilepsy in HICs remains consistent until after the age of 50, at which point it begins to rise. Conversely, in LMICs, the prevalence tends to remain stable during the third and fourth decade of life, decreases in the fifth decade, and, in certain studies, reemerges after the age of 60 (Banerjee, Filippi, & Allen Hauser, 2009).

Epilepsy has been found to be correlated with premature mortality, particularly within the initial year or two following diagnosis (Neligan et al., 2010). According to Hitiris et al. (2007), the standardized mortality ratio for epilepsy is generally estimated to be around 3. The study of premature mortality is especially important in LMICs, where 85% of individuals with epilepsy survive and where the likelihood of premature death is highest (Diop et al., 2005; Jette & Trevathan, 2014; Newton & Garcia, 2012). One of the most alarming aspects is the observation that a higher percentage of fatalities in LMICs have the potential to be avoided, including incidents such as falls, drowning, burns, and status epilepticus (Diop et al., 2005; Jette & Trevathan, 2014). For instance, Ngugi et al. (2014) found that status epilepticus accounted for 38% of all deaths related to epilepsy in a large group of individuals with convulsive epilepsy in rural Kenya. According to Lowenstein et al. (2001), status epilepticus is characterized by the presence of continuous seizure activity that lasts for a duration of five minutes or longer, or the occurrence of two or more seizures without any subsequent restoration of consciousness. The provided definition holds significance due to the available evidence indicating that seizures exceeding a duration of five minutes are improbable to undergo self-termination. Acute symptomatic disorders, such as brain tumors or strokes, sudden unexpected death in individuals with epilepsy, suicide, and accidents have been identified as additional prevalent factors contributing to premature mortality (Hitiris et al., 2007).

According to the GBD 2010 report, epilepsy is the 36th most significant contributor to DALYs worldwide. Epilepsy is the 14th most significant contributor to DALYs in western Sub-Saharan Africa. Epilepsy is the 20th most common cause of young learning disabilities (YLDs) worldwide, ranking second only to migraine among brain disorders (Vos et al., 2012). Crucially, the models used in the GBD 2010 report calculate the worldwide impact of epilepsy, focusing solely on idiopathic/cryptogenic epilepsy. These models do not take into account epilepsy caused by factors like infections, stroke, or genetic syndromes, which may account for over 50% of deaths in these areas (Murray et al., 2012). Hence, the data is likely to underestimate the actual prevalence of epilepsy, particularly in LMICs.

8.1.3. Interventions

8.1.3.1. Population-Based Interventions

8.1.3.1.1. Targeting Epilepsy Risk Factors

While it is not possible to prevent genetic causes of epilepsy, public health policies can focus on primary prevention by targeting the more prevalent structural or metabolic causes. Implementing helmet usage among motorcyclists and enacting legislation against alcohol consumption while driving can effectively mitigate the likelihood of traumatic brain injury, a prevalent risk factor. Enhancing perinatal care, especially in rural regions, has the potential to decrease the occurrence and subsequent frequency of epilepsy. According to a case-control study conducted in Tanzania, 14% of children with epilepsy experienced adverse perinatal events, while none of the controls had such events (Burton et al., 2012). An association between abnormal antenatal period and active convulsive epilepsy was reported in a population-based cross-sectional and case-control study conducted in Ghana, Kenya, South Africa, Tanzania, and Uganda (Ngugi et al., 2013). While the statistical significance of abnormal delivery and home delivery was not observed, there was a noticeable association between these factors and active convulsive epilepsy. Implementing policies to manage neurocysticercosis, a prevalent risk factor in LMICs, would be a cost-effective approach to mitigate global epilepsy. In rural Salama, Honduras, a comprehensive eight-year public health and educational intervention program was initiated in 1997 with the objective of mitigating symptomatic epilepsies, specifically those resulting from perinatal insults and neurocysticercosis (Medina et al., 2011). According to Medina et al. (2011), the program encompassed various components such as educational and media campaigns, training in animal husbandry for pig farmers, implementation of water projects and appropriate sewage disposal, deworming of school students, continuous surveillance of taeniasis, and additional initiatives. According to Medina et al. (2011), there was a decrease in the prevalence of epilepsy attributed to neurocysticercosis from 36.9% in 1997 to 13.9% in 2005. The total expenditure for this study amounted to US $1.33 million, although a comprehensive economic evaluation was not undertaken to ascertain its cost-effectiveness.

A study conducted by Wohlgemut et al. (2010) investigated the effectiveness of teaching techniques in preventing epilepsy resulting from neurocysticercosis in western Kenya. The researchers observed a substantial enhancement in knowledge when employing this instructional approach. The study did not investigate whether this program decreased the occurrence of epilepsy caused by taenia solium, but the results indicate a favorable advancement. The expert consultation report on foodborne infections, specifically taeniasis/cysticercosis, suggests several strategies to guarantee the long-term prevention and management of this frequently prevalent pathogen. The aforementioned approaches are enumerated in Box 8.1; nevertheless, the report failed to provide a comprehensive assessment of the expenses associated with their implementation (WHO, 2011).

8.1.3.1.2. Anti-Stigma Interventions

Instances of civil rights violations, such as disparities in the availability of health and life insurance or the biased consideration of health insurance provisions, are frequently observed. Workplace bias and limited educational opportunities are commonplace. According to Akpan, Ikpeme, & Utuk (2013), school teachers frequently possess inadequate knowledge and hold unfavorable attitudes towards children who have seizure disorders. Stigma is commonly linked to both social and economic ramifications. Individuals afflicted with epilepsy may refrain from seeking medical intervention or communicating associated health issues to their healthcare providers, thereby exacerbating the disparity in treatment.

Enhanced understanding of epilepsy has been linked to favorable attitudes and diminished social stigma; however, the long-term viability and consequences of this relationship have yet to be ascertained (Fiest et al., 2014). Legislation and advocacy efforts are imperative in addressing stigma at the population level, necessitating a comprehensive approach. Furthermore, the dissemination of education and information to debunk misconceptions and improve seizure control among employers and teachers should empower individuals with epilepsy to pursue treatment and promote their active involvement in their communities. The formal assessment of the cost-effectiveness of interventions aimed at reducing stigma has not been conducted.

8.1.4. Legislation

The limited accessibility of anti-epileptic medications is a significant factor contributing to the disparity in epilepsy treatment in LMICs. The majority of countries do not have access to second-generation medications, and even the older anti-epileptic drugs are only occasionally available. A study conducted in Zambia examined

111 pharmacies and revealed that 49.1% of them did not stock anti-epileptic medications. Pediatric syrups commonly utilized in HICs were universally inaccessible (Chomba et al., 2010). Unfortunately, the findings from personal conversations with epilepsy care providers in other LMICs indicate that this issue may be prevalent (Chomba et al., 2010).

It is evident that the implementation of policies is necessary to ensure the continuous accessibility of cost-effective and effective anti-epileptic medications to patients on a global scale. A limited number of nations allocate a distinct budget for the provision of epilepsy services, necessitating the establishment of national funding support for epilepsy care. In 73% of low-income countries, including many countries in Africa, the Eastern Mediterranean, and South-East Asia, where the burden is highest, out-of-pocket expenses are the main means of financing epilepsy care (WHO, 2011). In numerous regions, the provision of disability benefits is lacking, resulting in patients being unable to access financial assistance.

8.1.5. Self-Management

Self-management involves enabling patients to take a more proactive role in overseeing their own healthcare. According to Fitzsimons et al. (2012), it is probable that patients will enhance their comprehension, embrace healthier lifestyles, and enhance their compliance with treatment. Self-management can assist individuals with epilepsy in effectively recognizing and controlling their seizure triggers, resulting in a decrease in seizure frequency and a reduction in the utilization of health services and healthcare expenses (Fitzsimons et al., 2012). Several studies have been conducted to investigate the efficacy of self-management education programs in both adults and children, yielding certain indications of their advantages. However, further investigation is warranted to assess the cost-effectiveness of these programs in LMICs (Bradley & Lindsay, 2008; Lindsay & Bradley, 2010).

8.1.6. Pharmacological Interventions

The determination to commence therapy with anti-epileptic medications can present difficulties. According to Kim et al. (2006), the examination of the Multicenter trial for Early Epilepsy and Single Seizures indicates limited advantages in commencing treatment for individuals who exhibit a solitary seizure, lack any identifiable neurological condition, and display normal electroencephalograms. Nevertheless, it is advisable to contemplate medical intervention for individuals who exhibit moderate to high risk, which is characterized by experiencing more than two to three seizures upon initial presentation, having underlying neurological disorders, and displaying abnormal EEGs (Kim et al., 2006). Over 60 randomized controlled trials (RCTs), primarily conducted in HICs, have investigated the effectiveness of anti-epileptic drugs. However, there remains a dearth of adequately designed RCTs that specifically assess the efficacy of these medications in patients with generalized epilepsy syndromes and in pediatric populations (Glauser et al., 2013). Although newer AEDs are generally well-tolerated and have fewer long-term side effects, their overall superiority has not been substantiated.

No studies have been conducted to compare the cost-effectiveness of anti-epileptic drugs in individuals with newly diagnosed epilepsy. The efficacy of initial monotherapy in individuals with epilepsy has been summarized in a recent systematic review. Children and adults with convulsive epilepsy should be provided with monotherapy using any of the standard anti-epileptic drugs, namely carbamazepine, phenobarbital, phenytoin, and valproic acid. Multiple studies of lower quality have provided evidence of the effectiveness of phenobarbital in treating partial onset seizures and generalized onset tonic-clonic seizures in both adults and children (Glauser et al., 2013). Considering the expenses associated with obtaining it, phenobarbital should be considered as a primary choice if its availability can be guaranteed. Carbamazepine should be provided to both children and adults experiencing partial onset seizures, if it is accessible (WHO, 2009b). The utilization of the minimum effective dosage is expected to mitigate adverse effects, enhance seizure outcomes, and reduce the duration of treatment interruption. The efficacy of valproic acid and ethosuximide in the treatment of absence seizures, particularly in pediatric patients, has been demonstrated. However, it is worth noting that valproic acid is the preferred choice due to its inclusion in the list of essential medications. Ethosuximide is offered as a supplementary pharmaceutical intervention. Nevertheless, it is advisable to refrain from using the medication in women who have the ability to bear children due to its stronger correlation with significant congenital abnormalities and inferior neurodevelopmental results. While there are newer therapeutic agents, like levetiracetam, that are not metabolized by the liver, their cost-effectiveness has not been investigated in LMICs.

Regrettably, in LMICs, the accessibility and cost-effectiveness of conventional medications are inadequate, creating obstacles to treatment. According to a study, the public sector exhibits an average availability of generic medications that is below 50% for all medications, with the exception of diazepam injection. The level of accessibility of generic oral medications in the private sector varied, with phenytoin being available at 42% and phenobarbital at 70%. The prices of generic carbamazepine and phenytoin for patients in the public sector were found to be 5 and 18 times greater than the international reference prices, respectively. Similarly, the prices for patients in the private sector were observed to be 11 and 25 times higher, respectively. The prices of both medicines from the original brand were approximately 30 times greater. According to Cameron et al. (2012), the countries with the lowest incomes exhibited the highest prices. Prioritizing the maintenance of a consistent supply at affordable prices is imperative. Around 60% of individuals in Sub-Saharan Africa lack access to automated external defibrillators (AEDs), which heightens the likelihood of seizures, seizure-related accidents, and status epilepticus. This condition is a major contributor to illness and death among individuals with epilepsy (Ba-Diop et al., 2014). Adherence to treatment and avoidance of other seizure triggers are highly effective patient-related strategies for mitigating the occurrence of status epilepticus. At a population level, the most effective approach to prevent the illness and death linked to status epilepticus is by implementing health policies that enhance the availability and accessibility of AEDs. Additionally, educating health professionals about the importance of time being crucial is crucial. According to the current operational definition of status epilepticus (Lowenstein et al., 2001), it is recommended to initiate aggressive treatment for status epilepticus after a duration of five minutes, rather than after a period of 30 minutes of ongoing seizures.

8.1.7. Management of Infectious Etiologies of Epilepsy

Neurocysticercosis frequently leads to epilepsy in LMICs. The treatment of parenchymal neurocysticercosis can be guided by recent evidence-based guidelines, as indicated by Baird et al. (2013). According to Baird et al. (2013), these guidelines indicate that using albendazole therapy, with or without corticosteroids, in combination with AEDs, is likely to be effective in enhancing outcomes. Birbeck et al. (2012) published evidence-based guidelines to provide guidance for the selection of anti-epileptic drugs in individuals with HIV/AIDS. This is due to the fact that the concurrent administration of anti-epileptic drugs and antiretroviral medications may be necessary in as many as 55% of patients. According to the guidelines, it is advisable to refrain from using enzyme-inducing antiepileptic drugs in individuals currently receiving antiretroviral regimens that incorporate protease inhibitors or nonnucleoside reverse transcriptase inhibitors. This precaution is necessary due to the potential occurrence of pharmacokinetic interactions that could lead to virologic failure. Patients may undergo pharmacokinetic assessments to ensure the effectiveness of the antiretroviral regimen if it is necessary for seizure control (Birbeck et al., 2012).

8.1.7.1. Surgical Management

The majority of cases (70% in individuals with new onset epilepsy) have a high likelihood of achieving one-year seizure freedom after attempting up to three anti-epileptic drugs. Drug resistance is observed in approximately 40% of patients in general, with a higher prevalence observed in individuals with focal epilepsy (Berg et al., 2009; Kwan & Brodie, 2000; Schiller & Najjar, 2008; Semah et al., 1998). For individuals who have not responded to three anti-epileptic medications, it is improbable that using additional anti-epileptic drugs will result in long-term freedom from seizures (Jette, Reid, & Wiebe 2014). Experts widely acknowledge that individuals who exhibit drug resistance and have not responded to two suitable antiepileptic drug trials should be deemed suitable for a surgical assessment (Jette, Reid, & Wiebe, 2014; Kwan et al., 2010; Wiebe & Jette, 2012). Children with complex syndromes, patients with stereotyped or lateralized seizures or focal findings, and children with a magnetic resonance imaging lesion amenable to surgical resection regardless of seizure frequency are among the additional patients who should be referred to a comprehensive epilepsy program for a surgical evaluation (Jette, Reid, & Wiebe, 2014; Wiebe & Jette, 2012). Various approaches have been suggested for the surgical treatment of epilepsies in settings with limited resources. Epilepsy surgery is becoming more prevalent in LMICs, yielding positive results (Asadi-Pooya & Sperling, 2008).

8.1.8. Alternative Therapies

Several alternative therapies have been suggested for the treatment of epilepsy, including dietary therapies, medical marijuana, and acupuncture. However, only dietary therapies have undergone randomized trials. According to Levy, Cooper, & Giri (2012), the ketogenic diet has the potential to enhance seizure outcomes in individuals with drug-resistant epilepsy. However, it can be challenging to tolerate, especially in adults. An observational study found that the Atkins diet was linked to enhanced seizure control. However, further research is necessary to investigate its efficacy as well as the efficacy of alternative dietary therapies, such as the modified Atkins diet and the low glycemic index diet (Levy, Cooper, & Giri, 2012). Although dietary therapies are growing in popularity, they require a significant amount of resources, are expensive, and are mainly accessible to HICs (Cross, 2013). We require cost-effective and streamlined methods for implementing these therapies in LMICs. The effectiveness of oral cannabinoids and acupuncture in the management of epilepsy is still inconclusive, as indicated by studies conducted by Cheuk & Wong (2014); and Koppel et al. (2014).

8.1.9. Strategies for Enhancing the Efficiency of Healthcare Delivery

The treatment gap refers to the unmet need for appropriate anti-epileptic treatment among individuals with active epilepsy who do not receive sufficient medical therapy. Unfortunately, individuals residing in LMICs, where the prevalence of epilepsy is widespread, are disproportionately impacted by the lack of treatment for epilepsy (Jette & Trevathan, 2014). In low-income countries, the treatment gap exceeds 75%, in many LMICs it exceeds 50%, and in most HICs it is less than 10% (Figure 8.2) (Meyer et al., 2010).

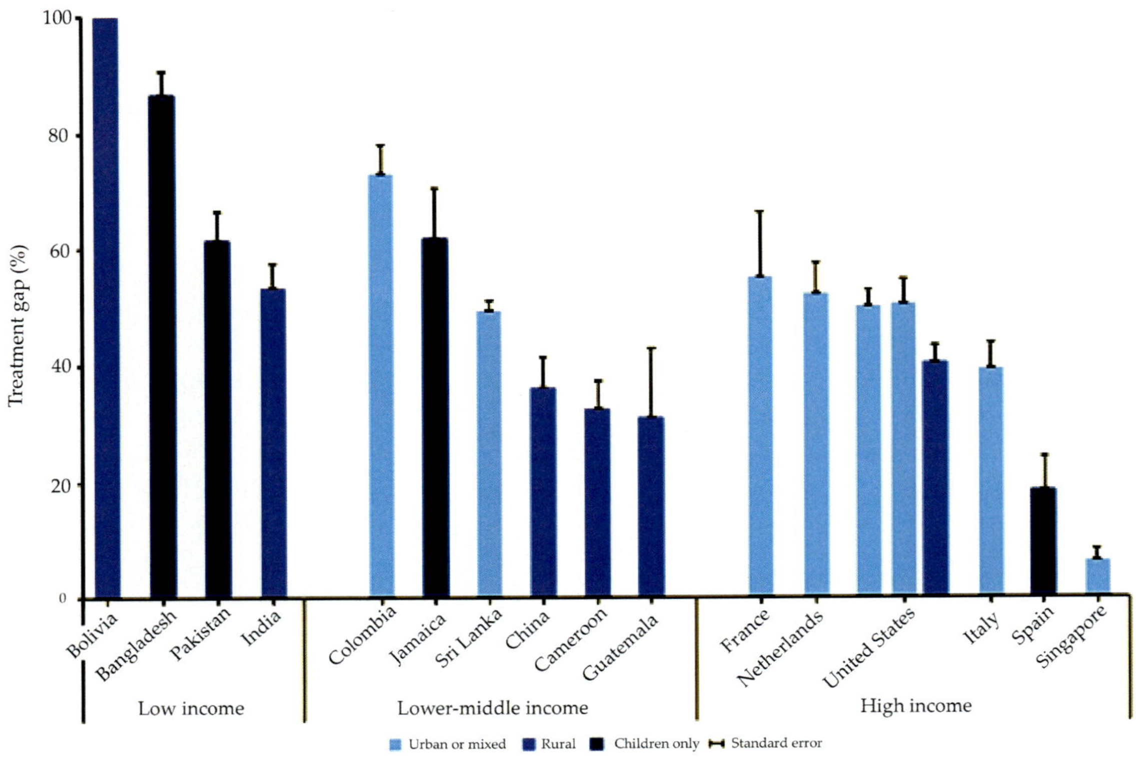

Figure 8.2. *Calculation of the treatment gap for epilepsy and the standard errors based on lifetime prevalence estimates.*

Source: Meyer et al. (2010).

The proposed mechanisms for addressing the gap in epilepsy treatment can be categorized into two main groups: healthcare system factors and patient-related factors (Cameron et al., 2012; Kale, 2002; Mbuba et al., 2008). The healthcare system is confronted with various challenges, such as limited accessibility to anti-epileptic medications, instances of missed or delayed diagnoses, incorrect prescription of treatments, failure to provide treatment options to patients, and insufficient allocation of resources and personnel (Cameron et al., 2012; Mbuba et al., 2008; Kale, 2002). The diagnosis of epilepsy primarily relies on the patient's clinical history, and primary care physicians can receive training to administer fundamental treatment. Potential patient-related factors contributing to the treatment gap encompass cultural beliefs, stigma, apprehension regarding side effects, inconvenience, and treatment expenses (Cameron et al., 2012; Kale, 2002; Mbuba et al., 2008). The various factors contributing to the disparity in epilepsy treatment should be taken into account as potential areas for assessment and intervention.

A study conducted by Cameron et al. (2012) investigated the accessibility, cost, and affordability of anti-epileptic medications across 46 nations. According to Cameron et al. (2012), the research revealed that in LMICs, the accessibility of these medications is limited, and their expenses are most elevated in regions with the most significant disparity in treatment. This study provides evidence in favor of the perspective that the accessibility and cost-effectiveness of anti-epileptic medications are significant factors in countries with limited resources.

Legislative and anti-stigma interventions are considered to be two highly influential strategies for addressing the treatment gap. Regrettably, the impact of their cost-effectiveness has not been assessed.

8.1.10. Cost-Effectiveness of Interventions

The existing body of research on cost-effectiveness primarily examines the use of medication to treat seizures. As a result, there is limited economic evidence available regarding interventions at the population and community levels, such as strategies aimed at reducing stigma. A recent study conducted in India demonstrated that providing coverage for both initial and subsequent treatment options, as well as other medical expenses, effectively reduces the financial strain caused by epilepsy. This approach is cost-efficient across all income levels and in all states of India (Megiddo et al., 2016). Chisholm & WHO-CHOICE (2005) conducted a cost-effectiveness analysis on the treatment of epilepsy in nine developing regions worldwide. Both studies have determined that the utilization of first-line medications, such as phenobarbital, is a highly efficient allocation of resources for the promotion of health (Levin & Chisholm, 2015). Research has demonstrated that surgery is a financially efficient option for suitably chosen individuals in HICs, resulting in a substantial reduction in healthcare expenses following successful surgical procedures (Jette, Reid, & Wiebe, 2014; Langfitt et al., 2007). A comprehensive examination of health economic evaluations pertaining to epilepsy surgery reveals that, on the whole, the expenses associated with each quality-adjusted life year for epilepsy surgery fall comfortably within the "very cost-effective" range as advised by the WHO (Jette & Wiebe, 2015; Langfitt, 1997). The incremental cost-effectiveness ratio in the United States was US $27,200, taking into account both direct and indirect costs. This figure is significantly lower than the country's gross domestic product per capita of US$40,000. Regrettably, there is a general absence of economic assessments regarding epilepsy surgery in children, older adults, and from LMICs. Furthermore, the majority of economic evaluations concentrate on temporal lobe surgery.

The severe ramifications of inadequately managed epilepsy encompass substantial morbidity and mortality resulting from seizures and associated injuries. The persistent social disapproval linked to seizures continues to pose a significant obstacle to the provision of clinical care in numerous areas, alongside limited availability of appropriate medications that can effectively address the needs of this demographic. To effectively address the global treatment gap of epilepsy, it is probable that legislative changes and anti-stigma interventions will emerge as the most efficacious targets. One of the necessary legislative initiatives involves advocating for improved provision of benefits for individuals with epilepsy who are functionally disabled, particularly in countries with limited resources where such support is most crucial.

8.2. Dementia

Dementia presents a distinct challenge to individuals, their families, and communities. The projected rise in the number of patients with dementia in LMICs will result in additional economic and social challenges. Dementia is frequently misunderstood as an inevitable aspect of the aging process or a condition that is incurable. Insufficient comprehension and the enduring presence of social disapproval and prejudice hinder the act of seeking assistance. As a result, the occurrence of timely diagnosis is infrequent, as the majority of individuals remain undiagnosed and face restricted availability of sufficient healthcare or social support. The treatment gap remains significant, especially in countries with persistent cultural and infrastructure barriers, due to the unavailability of pharmacotherapy and psychological and psychosocial interventions that can improve symptoms and reduce the impact on family members and caregivers.

8.2.1. Definitions

Dementia is a neuropsychiatric condition that is distinguished by the presence of cognitive deterioration, advancing behavioral and psychological symptoms (BPSD), and impairment in functioning (World Health Organization, 2012). Dementia is typically a long-lasting and moving condition. Its gradual beginning is usually marked by noticeable impairments in one or more cognitive areas, such as memory, orientation, language, and executive function. These impairments often occur in the later stages and are often accompanied by behavioral disruptions. While age is widely recognized as the primary risk factor, it is important to note that dementia is not a typical consequence of the aging process (Ganguli et al., 2000; Kukull et al., 2002; Launer et al., 1999). Dementia typically manifests as a decline in cognitive function during daily activities, and its diagnosis is typically established through a combination of physical and neurological examinations, supplemented by information gathered from informant interviews.

Dementia is a comprehensive syndrome encompassing various types of cognitive decline, such as Alzheimer's disease, vascular dementia (VaD), frontotemporal dementia, Lewy body dementia, as well as reversible causes like hypercalcemia, thyroid hormone abnormalities, deficiencies in vitamin B12 and folic acid, HIV infection, subdural hematoma, and normal pressure hydrocephalus. Alzheimer's disease constitutes approximately 50–60% of late-life dementias, while VaD represents approximately 15–20% of such cases. While there are variations in brain pathological lesions among different types of dementia, it is common for mixed forms of dementia to occur, and there is often a simultaneous presence of vascular brain damage.

8.2.2. Epidemiology and Burden of Dementia

Increasing age is the primary risk factor for dementia, with the incidence doubling every five years after the age of 65 (WHO, 2015). The process of aging in societies across all global regions is anticipated to significantly increase the number of individuals affected. Around 47 million individuals were affected by dementia in 2015, with 63% of them residing in LMICs. The projected number is expected to increase significantly, reaching 76 million by 2030 and 145 million by 2050. The majority of new cases, specifically 71%, are expected to occur in LMICs (Prince et al., 2015; WHO, 2015). These settings are anticipated to experience the most significant rise in the number of individuals with dementia due to rapid demographic shifts. Every four seconds, a new instance of dementia is identified globally, resulting in 7.7 million new cases annually. Asia accounts for approximately 50% of these new cases (WHO, 2015) (Figure 8.3).

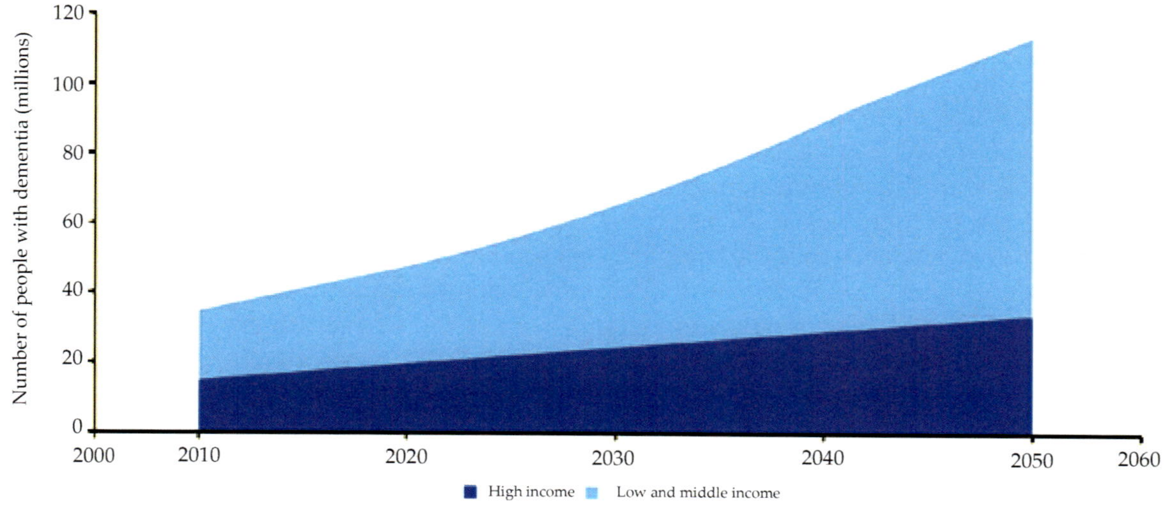

Figure 8.3. *Anticipated increase in the population of individuals affected by dementia across all income brackets from 2010 to 2050.*

Source: WHO (2012).

The prevalence of dementia in community-based samples exhibits a range of 38 to 400 cases per 100,000 individuals, with a notable upward trend observed over a span of 55 years. According to Picard et al. (2011), early-onset dementia (EOD) exhibits a higher prevalence of frontotemporal dementia (9.7%), alcohol-related dementia (9.4%), traumatic brain injury (3.8%), and Huntington's disease (3%) in comparison to late-onset dementia. While dementia is predominantly observed in older individuals, there are instances where symptoms manifest at a younger age that align with Early Onset Dementia (EOD), a condition that is not well comprehended and is often not diagnosed.

Irrespective of the age at which it begins, most patients receive care at home from their immediate family members. The necessity for individualized care commences at an early stage, escalates in intensity, and exhibits notable fluctuations over the course of the disease's natural progression. Individuals with dementia and their families may experience mood and behavioral changes, memory impairment for recent events, spatiotemporal disorientation, and problem-solving deficits in the early stages. These symptoms can lead to stressful situations even before the clinical diagnosis is made. Subsequently, the presence of mood and behavioral disorders exacerbates the overall impact of the disease.

According to Kales et al. (2014), the subsequent phases are distinguished by widespread engagement with psychological and behavioral manifestations, such as repetitive actions, hallucinations, aggression, and wandering. These symptoms exhibit a strong correlation with institutionalization, as opposed to cognitive deficits (Richardson et al., 2013). The provision of care for individuals with dementia is correlated with heightened levels of physical and emotional stress. Research indicates that caregivers frequently experience emotions of seclusion, unease, and despondency, which diminish their overall well-being and potentially influence the standard of care they deliver (Reitz, Brayne, & Mayeux, 2011). The collective anguish experienced by caregivers is a fundamental element of the burden associated with dementia (Donaldson & Burns, 1999).

8.2.3. Worldwide Impact of Dementia

Dementia has emerged as a substantial economic burden on a global scale (*see* Figure 8.4). Dementia is the primary cause of dependence among older adults worldwide, with up to 50% of those requiring care being affected by the disease. As per the 2010 GBD report, the DALYs caused by Alzheimer's disease and other forms of dementia have increased twofold over the last two decades. Dementia is considered the primary cause of DALYs in older age compared to other chronic diseases due to its significant correlation with death and reliance. In LMICs, where life expectancy is rising and resources for providing healthcare for older adults are limited or unavailable, the DALYs associated with dementia may continue to rise.

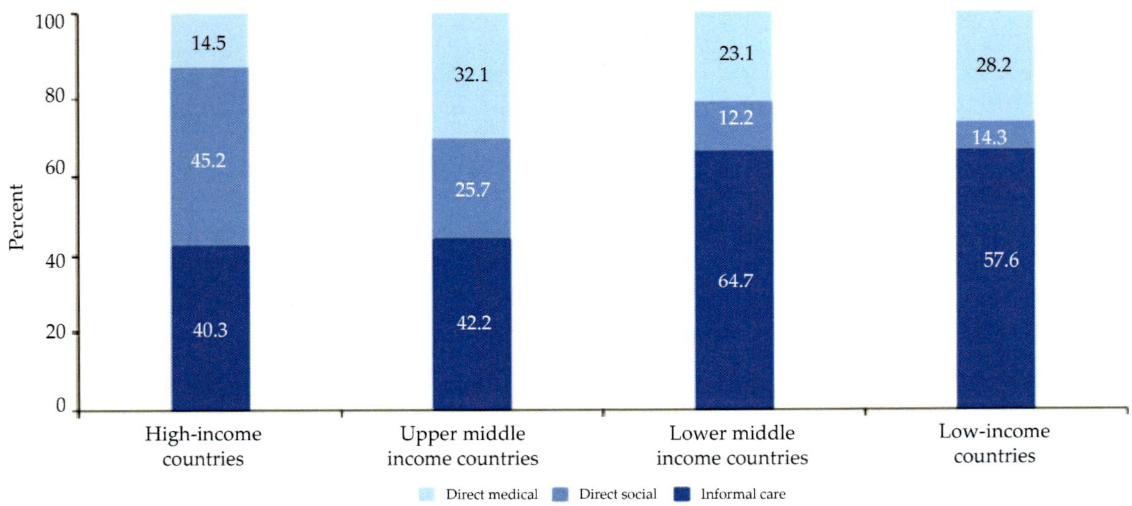

Figure 8.4. *Allocation of the overall societal expenses associated with dementia care, categorized by World Bank income levels.*

Source: WHO (2012).

The primary determinant of institutionalization among older adults in HICs is the extent of care required. In LMICs, the likelihood of institutionalization is low. Individuals with dementia typically remain in their own homes until the disease reaches its advanced stages. They receive care from informal caregivers, who are typically close relatives and women.

The direct costs encompass the utilization of health services, healthcare expenses, and the need for institutionalization. The indirect costs pertain to the reduction in work hours to provide care. Both of these factors impose substantial economic challenges on individuals, families, and societies.

The year 2013 witnessed a worldwide economic expenditure of US $604 billion, which accounted for roughly 1% of the global gross domestic product (WHO, 2015). In HICs, there is a proportional increase in both direct and indirect costs. Furthermore, the allocation of expenses among medical, societal, and informal care exhibits significant disparities among different regions and health system entities. According to Leibson et al. (2015), hospital inpatient expenses accounted for 70% of the direct costs associated with common dementia, primarily due to psychiatric treatment. The indirect expenses associated with informal care are likely to extend well beyond the loss of income. Caring for individuals with dementia can have harmful consequences on families and social relationships, especially in environments where there are misconceptions about the causes and progression of the condition.

8.2.4. Interventions

Interventions must target four crucial domains:

- Timely diagnosis;
- The evaluation and upkeep of one's physical well-being;
- Assessment and treatment of BPSD: focusing on cognition, activity, and well-being;
- Assistance for individuals providing care;
- The identification and assessment of dementia.

Currently, there is insufficient evidence to justify the implementation of dementia screening in the general population. Screening tools are commonly employed in primary health services to assess individuals who express initial apprehensions regarding their cognitive abilities. The Mini-Mental State Examination (Folstein, Folstein, & McHugh, 1973) has been developed in concise formats, with a time commitment of no more than five minutes. However, in contrast to the Mini-Mental State Examination, which has undergone validation in various settings and languages, none of the abbreviated versions have undergone validation in LMICs. Consequently, their utilization is currently not advised.

Diagnosis necessitates a comprehensive clinical and informant interview, as well as a thorough mechanical examination. Population-based studies, such as the 10/66 culture-fair diagnostic algorithm (Prince et al., 2003), provide evidence indicating that diagnosis can be accomplished through the utilization of meticulously designed interviews and examinations administered by proficient community health workers. Modifications for implementation in clinical settings are necessary, however, the practicality and cost-efficiency of laboratory tests employed in HICs to rule out treatable types of dementia may restrict their application in LMICs. Evidence from HICs suggests that the practice of revealing the dementia diagnosis can enhance planning and potentially reduce distress. However, there is a lack of evidence from LMICs.

The design of programs and activities should be influenced by the local culture, language, and beliefs, and should involve stakeholders, policy makers, the media, and local healthcare services. It is imperative to augment health and social services in order to effectively address the anticipated surge in service demand.

8.2.5. Assessment of Physical and Care Needs

When evaluating BPSD and its severity, it is important to take into account information regarding care arrangements and available resources. Conducting a thorough physical examination is of utmost significance in order to effectively monitor potential manifestations of hearing and visual impairment, pain, constipation, urinary tract infections, and bedsores, which could potentially contribute to the worsening of psychological symptoms. The extent to which physical assessment enhances the prognosis of dementia, specifically in relation to the progression of cognitive impairment, remains largely unexplored. It is imperative to diligently monitor the nutritional status throughout the duration of the disease. Weight loss is a prevalent occurrence that can commence prior to receiving a diagnosis. The reduction in body weight has the potential to elevate rates of illness and death. However, caregivers can be provided with guidance on basic strategies and methods to address issues associated with indifference and unpleasant feeding behaviors. Additionally, they can receive nutritional education to enhance the caloric and nutritional value of meals. It is imperative to promote the monitoring and efficient management of vascular risk factors, such as hypertension, hypercholesterolemia, tobacco use, obesity, and diabetes, in order to enhance the secondary prevention of cerebrovascular events. Furthermore, a substantial body of compelling evidence derived from mechanistic and meticulously designed prospective cohort studies supports the notion that mitigating the prevalence of high blood pressure and hypertension during middle age, as well as diabetes during middle and later stages of life, alongside reducing tobacco consumption and enhancing educational attainment, can significantly diminish the risk of dementia among populations (Prince et al., 2014).

8.2.6. Pharmacological Interventions

Pharmacological treatment targets encompass cognitive impairment, behavioral symptoms such as agitation and aggression, and psychological symptoms including depression, anxiety, and psychosis. The Institute for Quality and Efficiency in Healthcare (2014) has provided a substantial amount of evidence supporting the effectiveness of cholinesterase inhibitors (ChEIs), including donepezil, rivastigmine, and galantamine, in managing mild to moderate Alzheimer's disease. Each of these medications is linked to similar and temporary enhancements in cognitive function, overall clinical condition, and daily activities. Nevertheless, the available evidence for ChEIs in LMICs is restricted. Furthermore, the effectiveness of this category of medications in treating severe dementia remains uncertain, although galantamine has been found to improve behavioral symptoms (Institute for Quality and Efficiency in Healthcare, 2014). Memantine, a fourth pharmaceutical agent utilized in the management of cognitive impairment, exhibits a distinct mechanism of action and is generally well-tolerated. However, the available evidence regarding its effectiveness is constrained to individuals presenting with moderate to severe dementia. ChEIs and memantine exhibit lower efficacy in the treatment of VaD compared to alternative forms. Their effectiveness in treating behavioral disturbances has not been confirmed; trials sponsored by the manufacturer and subsequent analysis suggest minor enhancements.

The utilization of haloperidol and atypical antipsychotic medications in the management of agitation and behavioral symptoms in individuals with Borderline Personality Spectrum Disorder (BPSD) demonstrates modest therapeutic outcomes, particularly in relation to aggression. However, it is crucial to consider the potential mortality risk associated with these interventions (Kales et al., 2012). The utilization of atypical antipsychotic medications for the treatment of psychosis in individuals with dementia has been extensively documented. However, a comprehensive analysis of their effectiveness revealed that solely aripiprazole and risperidone exhibited a statistically and clinically significant impact on psychiatric symptoms (Tan et al., 2015). A crucial consideration regarding the utilization of these medications in dementia is the correlated heightened susceptibility to mortality and cerebrovascular adverse events. According to Banerjee, Filippi, & Allen Hauser (2009), the existing body of literature on antipsychotic treatment in older individuals with dementia indicates that while there was only a slight improvement in behavioral disturbance after a period of 6–12 weeks, there was a notable rise in the absolute mortality risk by approximately 1%. According to the literature, if antipsychotics are prescribed for dementia for more than 6–12 weeks, it is likely that there will be significant harm associated with continued antipsychotic treatment in dementia. Consequently, a considerable number of experts advocate for the utilization of nonpharmacological interventions, such as psychological and training approaches, as a means to mitigate BPSD, as opposed to the administration of antipsychotic medications (Deudon et al., 2009).

The efficacy of antidepressants in individuals with dementia was found to be inconclusive in a meta-analysis conducted by Leong in 2014. The utilization of antidepressants for the management of BPSD has been suggested, yielding promising outcomes (Henry, Williamson, & Tampi, 2011).

8.2.7. Nonpharmacological Interventions

A meticulously executed randomized controlled trial (RCT) in the United Kingdom, involving cognitive stimulation techniques such as reality orientation, games, and information processing-based discussions, as well as a small pilot trial conducted in Brazil, indicate that the cognitive advantages derived from this intervention are comparable to those observed in cognitive enhancement interventions (ChEIs) (Aguirre et al., 2013). Additional targeted cognitive training yielded no advantages. Cognitive rehabilitation, a personalized treatment aimed at improving remaining cognitive abilities and the capacity to manage impairments, demonstrated potential in uncontrolled case studies conducted in HICs. The findings of a meta-analysis encompassing four trials investigating the efficacy of reminiscence therapy, which involves the exploration of past activities, events, and experiences, indicate that this therapeutic approach yields positive outcomes in terms of cognition, mood, and caregiver strain within a short timeframe. However, it is important to note that the quality of these trials was suboptimal (Bahar-Fuchs, Clare, & Woods, 2013; Woods et al., 2005, 2012).

8.2.8. Interventions for Caregivers

There exists a substantial body of literature that supports the advantages of caregiver interventions. The aforementioned interventions encompass psycho-educational approaches, frequently involving caregiver training, psychological therapies like cognitive behavioral therapy and counseling, caregiver support, and respite care. Numerous interventions integrate multiple elements of this nature. The examined results encompass caregiver stress, depression, and subjective welfare; behavioral disruption and mood in the recipient of care; and institutionalization.

Numerous caregiver-focused interventions have been found to effectively mitigate strain and alleviate depression. Among these interventions, cognitive behavioral therapy has been identified as particularly influential in addressing depression (Aboulafia-Brakha et al., 2014; Martín-Carrasco et al., 2009; Selwood et al., 2007; Van Mierlo et al., 2012). The development of caregiver training models for dementia care has been observed, exemplified by the Maximizing Independence at Home project (Tanner et al., 2015). To achieve effectiveness, psycho-educational interventions necessitate the active involvement of the caregiver. Carer support resulted in enhanced well-being, but did not yield any other outcomes.

Methodologically flawed RCTs for respite care did not demonstrate any positive effects on any outcome (Grant et al., 2003; Maayan, Soares-Weiser, & Lee, 2014). However, according to nonrandomized studies conducted by Ornstein et al. (2014), it has been found that respite care has a significant impact on reducing caregiver strain and psychological morbidity. Interventions aimed at the caregiver may yield modest yet noteworthy positive impacts on the behavior of individuals with dementia. A comprehensive analysis of 10 RCTs revealed a significant decrease of 40% in the combined likelihood of institutionalization. The successful interventions were characterized by their structured, intensive, and multicomponent nature, providing a range of services and supports for participants to choose from (Tam-Tham et al., 2013). Two small-scale trials conducted in India and Russia demonstrated significantly greater treatment effects on caregiver psychological morbidity and strain compared to interventions typically observed in HICs (Gavrilova et al., 2009; Dias et al., 2008).

8.2.9. Interventions to Optimize Healthcare Delivery

8.2.9.1. Interventions to Increase Demand for Services

The act of increasing public, caregiver, and health worker awareness has the potential to result in heightened demands for services. Awareness-raising among children and young adults can serve as a means to foster intergenerational solidarity. In numerous LMICs, a significant number of individuals with dementia reside in multigenerational households alongside young children, who serve as the primary caregivers and are more inclined to seek assistance. The implementation of disability pensions and caregiver benefits in LMICs is expected to result in a rise in the demand for diagnostic assessments. Crucially, endeavors to enhance awareness must be accompanied by reforms in the health system and services, ensuring that seeking help is met with a provision of better equipped and more prompt services.

8.2.9.2. Interventions to Improve the Capacity of Healthcare Teams

Primary healthcare services in LMICs frequently prove inadequate for older individuals due to their clinic-based nature, emphasis on basic curative interventions, and the burden of heavy workloads. Due to the vulnerability of elderly individuals with dementia, it is necessary to conduct outreach efforts to evaluate and handle patients in their own residences. Incorporating dementia care into any chronic disease care strategy is imperative. The primary emphasis in the training of nonspecialist health professionals should be on the identification of cases and effectively communicating the diagnosis to patients and caregivers, along with providing relevant information, conducting needs assessments, and offering training and support. Training programs can encompass service-based approaches, as well as modifications to curricula in medical and nursing schools, public health institutions, and rural health programs. The planning and coordination of medical and community care services are imperative to effectively address the growing demand for support as the disease advances.

8.2.9.3. Community-Based Initiatives for Implementing Efficacious Interventions

Community health workers or experienced caregivers can deliver programs to support caregivers either individually or in groups. The presence of strain, potentially linked to BPSD, should prompt the implementation of more comprehensive interventions such as psychological evaluation and depression therapy for the caregiver, respite care, and education and training for the caregiver. Horizontally constructed, community-based programs that cater to the general needs of frail, dependent, older individuals and their caregivers, regardless of whether these needs stem from cognitive, mental, or physical disorders, have the potential to integrate such interventions. Recent research has shown that delivering caregiver interventions through the Internet is effective (Czaja & Rubert, 2002; Marziali & Garcia, 2011).

8.2.10. The Cost-Effectiveness of Interventions for Dementia

According to Prince et al. (2015), the global societal expenditure associated with dementia surpassed a sum of US $818 billion in the year 2015. The direct costs encompass the utilization of health services and the process of institutionalization, while the indirect costs pertain to the inability to engage in employment and the provision of care for caregivers. Both categories of expenses place substantial economic strains on individuals, families, and societies. The costs of informal care are significantly higher in LMICs, whereas the direct costs for social care make up more than half of the costs in HICs (Prince et al., 2015). Multiple studies, primarily conducted in HICs, have assessed the cost-effectiveness of interventions for dementia. Specific difficulties encountered in these studies include the variability in the causes of dementia and the assessment of cost-effectiveness in individuals with less severe cognitive impairment.

8.2.11. Screening

In the Republic of Korea, a comprehensive early detection program for dementia was conducted, revealing that the financial implications per quality-adjusted life year derived from early screening varied between US $24,150 and US $35,661, contingent upon the specific age cohort. The likelihood of screening being economically efficient was greatest among individuals aged 75 years and above, across a broad spectrum of willingness to pay (Yu et al., 2015). Disease modifying therapies have demonstrated the highest cost-effectiveness in treating moderate to severe dementia (Plosker & Lyseng-Williamson, 2005).

8.2.12. Pharmacotherapy

Memantine is a cost-effective treatment, as supported by pharmacoeconomic data from Europe and the United States. Two cost-effectiveness studies have been carried out in Finland and the United Kingdom to evaluate the effectiveness of memantine in treating moderate-to-severe Alzheimer's disease. The study simulated patient progression by considering factors such as dependency, residential setting, and cognitive function (Francois et al., 2004; Jones et al., 2004). According to Wimo et al. (2003), a resource utilization and cost analysis conducted in conjunction with a pivotal trial in patients with moderate-to-severe Alzheimer's disease in the United States revealed that memantine resulted in a reduction of total societal costs by US$1,090 per patient per month over a period of 28 weeks. This comparison was made in comparison to the absence of pharmacological treatment. The findings were predominantly influenced by decreases in overall caregiver expenses, encompassing the foregone time dedicated to caregiving responsibilities, as well as direct nonmedical costs, which encompassed the expenses associated with providing care in a nursing home or comparable establishment.

A study conducted in Canada revealed that the administration of rivastigmine resulted in cost savings in the direct expenses associated with the care of individuals diagnosed with Alzheimer's disease, surpassing the initial cost of the medication after a period of two years of treatment (Hauber et al., 2000). The sensitivity analysis conducted on a 20-year Markov cohort model of disease modifying treatment in Alzheimer's disease, using a Swedish population, found that disease modifying therapy did not result in any cost savings. However, the majority of options demonstrated cost effectiveness compared to the chosen willingness to pay (Skoldunger et al., 2013). In a separate investigation examining the efficacy of cholinesterase inhibitors or memantine in the management of mild to moderate VaD, it was determined that the administration of donepezil at a dosage of 10 mg orally per day yielded the highest cost-effectiveness (Wong et al., 2009).

8.2.13. Alternative Therapies

Cognitive stimulation therapy has demonstrated cost-effectiveness for individuals with mild-to-moderate dementia when administered biweekly for a duration of 7 weeks. However, its effects were found to be modest when continued for an extended period in conjunction with the use of acetylcholinesterase inhibitors (D'Amico et al., 2015). The study revealed that an exercise intervention exhibited the capacity to be economically efficient in relation to behavioral and psychological symptoms. However, it did not demonstrate cost-effectiveness when evaluating quality-adjusted life year gains. According to Livingston et al. (2014), the START (STrAtegies for RelaTives) study was conducted as a randomized controlled trial to assess the clinical effectiveness and cost-effectiveness of a manual-based coping strategy program in enhancing the mental well-being of carers of individuals with dementia. The study determined that the intervention was cost-effective in terms of both caregiver and patient outcomes, as well as meeting the thresholds set by the National Institute for Health and Care Excellence. According to Dahlrup et al. (2014), a health economic analysis was conducted to examine the resource costs and costs associated with formal care in relation to a psychosocial intervention for family caregivers of individuals with dementia. The findings revealed that participants in the intervention group reported a higher quality of life when their spouse resided at home.

Conducting research on early diagnosis is crucial considering the potential for more effective treatments in the initial phases of the disease, when diagnosis is more challenging. Currently, the field of dementia lacks disease-modifying pharmacological interventions, and the effectiveness of medications aimed at alleviating symptoms seems to be limited (Birks, 2006; McShane, Areosa Sastre, & Minakaran, 2006). The announcement made by world political leaders during the G8 meeting in London in 2013 regarding the ambitious objective of finding a cure for Alzheimer's disease by 2025 highlights the acknowledgment of dementia as a significant global health concern and a top priority. Nevertheless, the pursuit of a remedy should not deplete resources from the investigation of alterable risk factors, which continues to be vital for prevention, with the potential to postpone the onset of symptoms or decelerate the progression of the disease. The inaugural WHO Ministerial Conference on Global Action Against Dementia took place in March 2015 with the aim of raising awareness about the public health and economic difficulties caused by dementia. It also sought to enhance comprehension of the duties and obligations of Member States and stakeholders. As a result, conference participants endorsed a Call for Action. Undoubtedly, it is crucial to adopt a comprehensive public health strategy to tackle the intricate issues associated with dementia.

8.3. Headache Disorders

Migraine, TTH, and MOH are three headache disorders that hold significant public health importance. In aggregate, these three factors constitute the third most prevalent contributor to disability among global populations (Murray et al., 2012; Steiner et al., 2015; Stovner et al., 2007; Vos et al., 2012).

According to the WHO (2011), headache disorders are the leading reason for seeking medical attention in primary care and neurology settings. This condition often leads to visits to various healthcare professionals, including internists, ear, nose, and throat specialists, ophthalmologists, dentists, psychologists, and advocates of complementary and alternative medical practices. The occurrence of headache is a frequently observed symptom in emergency departments. The ramifications of chronic migraine encompass various adverse effects such as pain, disability, reduced productivity, financial setbacks, and compromised quality of life. Hence, while headaches typically do not indicate significant underlying medical conditions, their causal relationship with individual experiences of pain, disability, and reduced quality of life renders them a substantial factor in the development of poor health.

8.3.1. Definitions

8.3.1.1. Migraine

The onset of migraine is frequently observed during adolescence and frequently persists throughout an individual's lifespan. The frequency of episodic attacks typically occurs once or twice a month, although it can vary significantly depending on lifestyle and environmental factors. In females, the occurrence is greater due to a hormonally-influenced correlation with menstruation.

The most distinctive manifestations of an attack include headache, nausea, and photophobia. Approximately 10% of all migraine attacks, and only one-third of individuals with migraine, experience headaches that are preceded by aura symptoms, predominantly visual in nature. The duration of the headache spans from several hours to a period of two to three days. It is commonly characterized by its moderate or severe nature, unilateral onset, pulsating nature, and exacerbation by regular physical exertion (International Headache Society, 2013). Chronic migraine, characterized by headache episodes occurring on 15 or more days per month and/or the absence of episodic episodes, is a highly debilitating manifestation (Natoli et al., 2010).

8.3.1.2. Tension-Type Headache

TTH is a disorder characterized by significant variability, typically emerging during adolescence, and reaching its highest levels in individuals in their 30s. Migraine is characterized by the absence of distinct features and accompanying symptoms, as headaches are typically mild or moderate in intensity, widespread in nature, and characterized by sensations of pressure or tightness (International Headache Society, 2013).

8.3.1.3. Headache Caused by Excessive Use of Medication

MOH is being acknowledged as a disorder of significant public health significance due to three factors: it is a characteristic of migraine or (less frequently) TTH; it is extremely debilitating at the individual level; and it is caused by medical intervention and can be prevented. The prevalence of MOH in the general population is estimated to be approximately 1 to 2% (Westergaard et al., 2014). In the chronic headache population, it is reported to affect up to 67% of individuals, while in specialized headache centers, it is estimated to affect 30–50% of patients (Evers, Jensen, and European Federation of Neurological Societies, 2011). The underlying factor is the persistent and excessive utilization of medications initially prescribed for the treatment of sporadic headaches (Diener & Limmroth, 2004). The excessive utilization of all these medications is linked to this issue, although the process by which it arises undoubtedly differs among different categories of drugs (Steiner et al., 2007).

8.3.2. Epidemiology and Burden of Disease

Estimating the worldwide impact of headache disorders is a difficult undertaking due to the lack of data for many LMICs, differences in the methods used in epidemiological studies, and variations in cultural attitudes towards reporting complaints. A significant portion of the global population resides in nations where the prevalence and impact of headaches are not fully understood (Stovner et al., 2007). However, previous studies have provided estimates indicating that the worldwide prevalence of migraine within a one-year period is 14.7%, while the prevalence of TTH among adults aged 18–65 is 20.8% (Murray et al., 2012). The incidence of all forms of headache, including chronic migraine, chronic TTH, and MOH, occurring on 15 or more days per month, is 3% (Stovner et al., 2007). While Asia has a lower prevalence of migraine compared to Africa, a study conducted in Zambia has revealed a high one-year prevalence of migraine (22.9%). Additionally, there is a significant occurrence of headache on 15 or more days a month (11.5%) and probable mental health disorders (7.1%), which have a substantial economic impact (Mbewe et al., 2015).

8.3.3. Interventions

Globally, a minimum of 50% of headaches are treated by individuals themselves, including in HICs (WHO, 2011). According to the WHO (2011), it is recommended that primary care settings offer professional healthcare for the majority of cases. Additionally, Steiner et al. (2007) have provided guidelines for the management of headache disorders in these settings. It is important for historical analysis and examination to carefully consider warning signs that may indicate the presence of an underlying condition (Steiner et al., 2007).

It is possible to use various tools, such as the HALT questionnaire, to evaluate the impact of headache symptoms on individual patients. According to Steiner & Martelletti (2007), practical objectives of management involve recognizing that primary headaches are not curable but can be effectively controlled. Our subsequent treatment deliberations will be centered on the topic of migraine.

8.3.4. Self-Management

Migraine is frequently associated with stress as a predisposing factor. Enhancing coping mechanisms represents an alternative therapeutic strategy; however, the efficacy of psychological therapies in the management of migraines remains uncertain. The majority of research has primarily concentrated on the advanced and intensive treatment of specific instances of incapacitating and untreatable headache, which has limited applicability to the field of public health. However, there is a possibility of providing group behavioral training at a low cost, and there is even some minimal evidence of its benefits (Mérelle et al., 2008). This approach could be further investigated in LMICs.

Obesity has been identified as a significant risk factor for migraine, particularly in cases of frequent migraine (Evans et al., 2012). Engaging in regular physical activity and maintaining physical fitness can yield advantageous outcomes. According to a study conducted by Evans et al. (2012), there was a notable enhancement in headache symptoms among obese adolescents with migraine who engaged in a 12-month weight-loss intervention.

8.3.5. Pharmacological Treatments

According to Steiner et al. (2007), it is recommended to adopt a stepped-care approach that begins with acute treatment utilizing basic analgesics, such as aspirin or various other nonsteroidal anti-inflammatory drugs. There is substantial evidence supporting the effectiveness and tolerability of aspirin (Kirthi, Derry, & Moore, 2013), ibuprofen (Rabbie, Derry, & Moore, 2013), and diclofenac potassium (Derry, Rabbie, & Moore, 2013). The optimal result of acute treatment is the attainment of complete pain relief within a two-hour timeframe, without any reoccurrence or requirement for additional medication, and without any adverse events. This phenomenon is infrequently observed when relying solely on basic analgesics. The outcome commonly known as sustained headache relief (SHR) is characterized by the reduction of pain to a level no worse than mild within a two-hour period following treatment, without any recurrence or requirement for additional medication. It is assumed that mild pain is not linked to disability, and SHR indicates complete functional recovery when there was initial functional impairment. According to Kirthi, Derry, & Moore (2013), aspirin alone provides SHR in approximately 39% of users. This effect is considered modest as it leaves 61% without this benefit. However, it is worth noting that aspirin is one of the most cost-effective interventions for improving public health, as stated by Linde, Steiner, & Chisholm (2015). Aspirin possesses the benefits of being widely accessible and included in the World Health Organization's essential medicines list (WHO, 2013). Ibuprofen is associated with a slightly higher proportion of users (45%) who experience SHR, although the cost may vary and not always be higher (Rabbie, Derry, & Moore, 2013). According to Derry, Rabbie, & Moore (2013), Diclofenac exhibits a higher cost-effectiveness ratio compared to other medications. There is a contention that the anti-inflammatory impact holds significance in the management of acute migraines, leading to the assertion that paracetamol is comparatively less efficacious than aspirin (at equivalent expense) or alternative nonsteroidal anti-inflammatory medications (Derry & Moore, 2013; Steiner et al., 2007).

The utilization of antiemetics in acute treatment should not be limited solely to patients experiencing vomiting or having a high likelihood of vomiting. Nausea is a highly unpleasant and incapacitating symptom of a migraine episode and should be managed effectively (Silberstein et al., 2012). Migraine is characterized by gastric stasis, which can be improved by using prokinetic antiemetics like domperidone or metoclopramide. These medications enhance the emptying of the stomach and increase the effectiveness of oral analgesics in treating migraines.

The typical subsequent phase in the management process involves acute treatment, wherein specific anti-migraine therapy is either substituted or added (Steiner et al., 2007). Ergotamine tartrate continues to be utilized in numerous countries (World Health Organization, 2011); however, its bioavailability is limited, its efficacy is suboptimal, and it carries potential adverse effects. There are seven specific anti-migraine medications, known as triptan agents, that are available in many countries. They exhibit slight variations in their pharmacokinetics and efficacy, but the disparities are negligible compared to the significant price disparities of up to 10 times between sumatriptan (available in generic forms) and the other six medications. There are four formulations of Sumatriptan, namely oral, intranasal, rectal, and subcutaneous. According to Derry, Derry, & Moore (2012), the administration of Sumatriptan 50 mg orally results in SHR in approximately 35% of individuals, similar to aspirin. However, Sumatriptan exhibits a distinct mechanism of action, and the responses to each medication are not interdependent. According to Linde, Steiner, & Chisholm (2015), the cost-effectiveness of sumatriptan is significantly lower compared to aspirin when used alone. Consequently, it is typically reserved as a secondary treatment option for individuals who do not respond to initial treatments (Steiner et al., 2007). Regular and frequent use of acute medications, exceeding two days per week, poses a risk for the development of MOH in both adults and children.

Prophylactic medications are employed during the third step of treatment to mitigate the occurrence of attacks in cases where acute therapy proves insufficient (Steiner et al., 2007). Propranolol (Linde et al., 2013b), amitriptyline (Dodick et al., 2009), valproate (specifically sodium valproate or valproic acid) (Linde et al., 2013b), and topiramate (Diener et al., 2004; Linde et al., 2013a) have been supported by sufficient or strong evidence regarding their effectiveness and tolerability. In order to evaluate the effectiveness of migraine attacks prevented, it is necessary to compare the outcome with an untreated baseline. This baseline is applicable to both propranolol (28%) and amitriptyline (44%) (Linde, Steiner, & Chisholm, 2015). The effectiveness of divalproex sodium, sodium valproate, topiramate, metoprolol, propranolol, and timolol in preventing migraines was demonstrated in a review conducted by the American Academy of Neurology (Silberstein et al., 2012). Propranolol and amitriptyline have similar and low costs, while topiramate is significantly more expensive. Amitriptyline may be the preferred prophylactic drug when conserving resources is the primary concern (Linde, Steiner, & Chisholm, 2015). Nevertheless, the specific mechanism by which these medications work in treating migraines remains unclear, and the lack of response to one medication does not necessarily indicate the lack of response to others (Steiner et al., 2007). These alternative medications may be considered when amitriptyline proves to be ineffective and resources allow.

8.3.6. Alternative Therapies

Acupuncture and physical therapies, such as spinal manipulation, necessitate direct therapist-patient interaction and are resource-intensive. However, their effectiveness is questionable, as evidenced by studies conducted by Bronfort et al. (2004); and Linde et al. (2009), which raises doubts about their recommendation. The potential advantages observed in clinical trials may not be reproducible in practical settings, where therapists work within time limitations.

8.3.7. Programs for Public Education

The implementation of public education programs has the potential to enhance migraine outcomes. Lifestyle factors can increase an individual's susceptibility to or exacerbate migraine. While there is limited evidence supporting the effectiveness of lifestyle modifications in controlling migraines, it is a logical approach to avoid trigger factors (Steiner et al., 2007).

Public education regarding the escalating susceptibility to migraines in individuals with obesity (Bronfort et al., 2004) may yield certain advantages, as headaches are currently experienced, unlike numerous other adverse health outcomes associated with obesity. Public education has been identified as a highly effective strategy for managing a potential epidemic of mental health disorders (MOH) resulting from mistreated migraines. According to recent findings from the Global Campaign against Headache (Mbewe et al., 2015), it has been indicated that this issue may be particularly prevalent in LMICs, where the cost and accessibility of medications are comparatively higher than those of healthcare services. The initial efficacy of basic analgesics promotes their continued utilization, which is not problematic when used infrequently. As the frequency increases, there is a greater dependence and a higher risk of MOH. After the establishment of MOH, there is a high probability that medication overuse will increase.

Adding educational programs to the use of over-the-counter and prescription medications in LMICs seems to result in additional health benefits that can be achieved at reasonable additional costs (Linde, Steiner, & Chisholm, 2015). Pharmacists can serve as a crucial resource for the public regarding headache disorders, treatments, and the risks associated with excessive medication usage. However, this can only be achieved if their role is explicitly acknowledged in their reimbursement and if their advice is actively sought. Moreover, the cost-effectiveness of treatments could potentially be enhanced through the implementation of public education programs aimed at enhancing treatment adherence (Linde, Steiner, & Chisholm, 2015).

8.3.8. Strategies for Enhancing the Efficiency of Healthcare Delivery

According to a worldwide survey, 33% of the countries surveyed suggested enhancing the structure and provision of healthcare for headaches in order to ensure efficient and fair care (WHO, 2011). Organizing services to accomplish this objective is undeniably a formidable task, and no singular solution may be suitable in every context. According to Steiner et al. (2007), the majority of patients do not need specialized knowledge or specific tests. Additionally, the Global Campaign against Headache for Europe's three-tier service model, developed by Steiner et al. (2011), is extremely flexible. In China (Yu et al., 2014), and in Sverdlovsk Oblast, Russia (Lebedeva et al., 2013), this model has been employed in demonstration projects to establish headache services. According to the model, approximately 90% of patients receive primary care, typically administered by physicians, while the remaining 1% necessitate specialized care that is exclusively provided within a hospital setting. The remaining 9% of individuals do not necessitate specialized medical attention, but they may encounter challenges in diagnosis or treatment that would be enhanced by receiving care at a higher level. The delivery of this standard of care is contingent upon available resources and the presence of local health service organizations. In order for the model to function effectively, each level must uphold a gatekeeper function towards higher levels. Paradoxically, nations that have made investments in headache services have predominantly done so through the establishment of specialized headache clinics. Globally, specialists treat 10% of headache patients, as reported by the WHO in 2011. This suggests that there is significant potential for reallocating resources to benefit a larger number of patients if the resources available at lower levels were more effectively utilized. The formal integration of pharmacists into healthcare systems is imperative.

8.3.8.1. The Education and Development of Healthcare Providers

The efficacy of primary healthcare services relies on the providers, such as physicians, clinical officers, or nurses, possessing the fundamental knowledge necessary. The evidence unequivocally demonstrates shortcomings, and improved professional education emerged as the most prominent recommendation for improvement in the global survey conducted by the WHO in 2011. According to Linde, Steiner, & Chisholm (2015), providing training to primary care physicians in the management of migraines has the potential to enhance patient outcomes and enhance the cost-effectiveness of prescription medications. In addition, this training could potentially decrease waste by reducing the excessive number of unnecessary investigations conducted to support diagnoses (WHO, 2011).

8.3.9. Cost-Effectiveness of Interventions

The current state of resource allocation decisions for headache disorders in LMICs is characterized by a dearth of nationally conducted cost-effectiveness studies. A recent study conducted a cost-effectiveness modeling analysis on the treatment of migraines in four countries: China (an upper-middle-income country), India (a lower-middle-income country), Russia (a high-income country), and Zambia (a lower-middle-income country). According to Linde, Steiner, & Chisholm (2015), the analysis determined that the administration of aspirin as an acute treatment resulted in a year of healthy life at a cost of less than US$100. This finding positions as one of the most effective interventions for enhancing population health. Paracetamol was not subjected to a cost-effectiveness analysis because the only evidence of SHR was obtained from 42 patient cases in the United States who were highly atypical (Linde, Steiner, & Chisholm, 2015). According to Steiner et al. (2007), the cost-effectiveness of sumatriptan as a standalone treatment for acute migraine is significantly lower compared to aspirin, with a difference of at least two orders of magnitude. This suggests that sumatriptan is typically reserved as a secondary treatment option for individuals who do not respond to initial treatments.

According to Linde, Steiner, & Chisholm (2015), the cost-effectiveness of prophylactic medications is comparatively lower than that of acute therapy involving simple analgesics. However, it is significantly more cost-effective than acute therapy involving the combination of analgesics and triptans, if necessary. However, it is important to note that this observation may only hold true if prophylactics are exclusively prescribed to individuals experiencing three or more attacks per month. Implementing educational initiatives, such as posters and leaflets in pharmacies, to promote the use of both over-the-counter and prescription medications seems to enhance overall population health outcomes at a reasonable additional expense. Similarly, providing training to healthcare providers has been found to have a positive impact (Linde, Steiner, & Chisholm, 2015).

The implementation of structured headache services, which are rooted in primary care and complemented by educational initiatives targeting professionals and the general public, appears to be the most viable approach for the majority of nations. These services necessitate the redistribution of resources, which can be readily justified from an economic standpoint. Significantly, the provision of services for migraine would concurrently address the prevalence of other prevalent and incapacitating headache disorders. The potential improvements in population health that can be attained through the implementation of efficient headache management strategies are significant and not contingent upon the reduction of indirect expenses associated with these conditions. The economic burden on society due to reduced productivity caused by migraines is substantial: exceeding €100 billion (US $100 billion) annually in the European Union (Linde et al., 2012), surpassing the healthcare expenses associated with headaches in any country (WHO, 2011). Investing more in the effective treatment of migraines through well-structured health services, coupled with education, could potentially result in cost savings in the long run (WHO, 2011).

8.4. Aging and Neurological Disorders

Existing research suggests that the process of aging initiates with subclinical alterations occurring at the molecular level. The factors contributing to genomic instability encompass the accumulation of mutations, telomere attrition, and epigenetic alterations. These defects increase rapidly over time, causing a "snowball effect" and ultimately resulting in the deterioration of the brain's structure and function. This includes the gradual loss of neurons, decreased levels of neurotransmitters, excessive inflammation, and damaged blood vessels, which can lead to infarction and small bleeding. Moreover, the diminishing efficacy of DNA repair mechanisms heightens the vulnerability to reactive oxygen species (ROS) and spontaneous mutagenesis, leading to the development of age-related neoplasia. Furthermore, the prevalent malnutrition and malabsorption observed in older individuals can result in a deficiency of vitamin B12 and folic acid, which are essential for the metabolism of homocysteine, ultimately leading to vascular harm. Collectively, these factors contribute to the occurrence of cerebral impairment during advanced stages of life and significantly augment the susceptibility to the onset of central nervous system (CNS) disorders, including stroke, epilepsy, Parkinson's disease, Alzheimer's disease, and various forms of dementia.

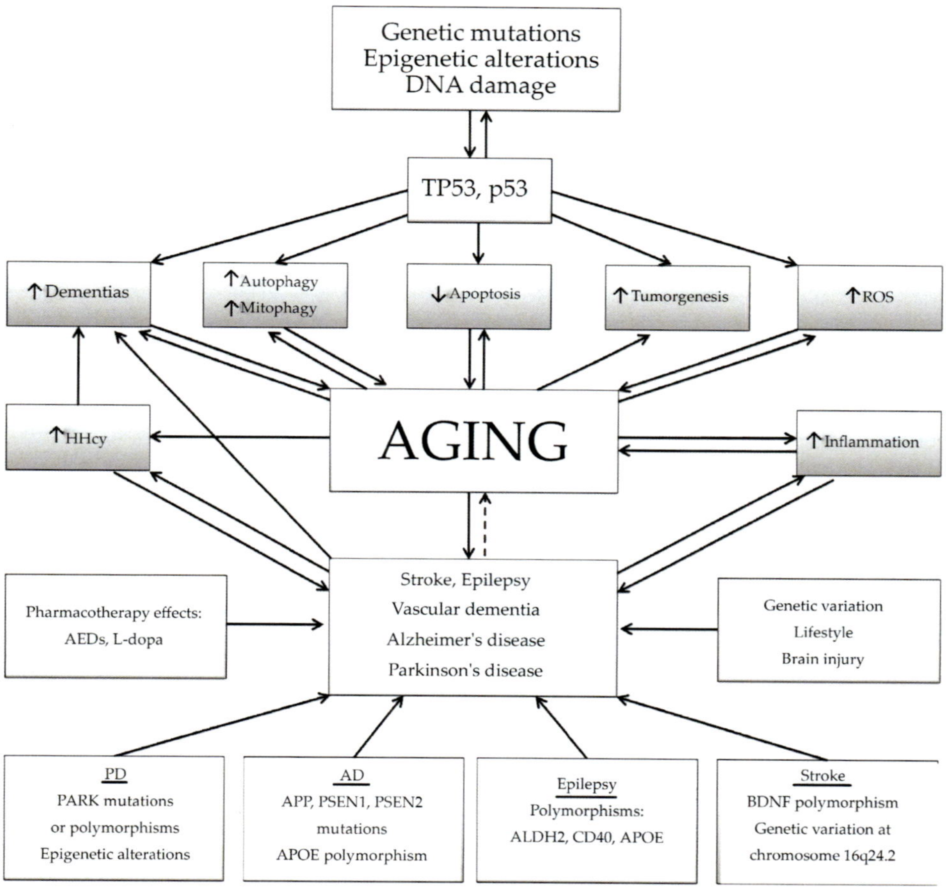

Figure 8.5. *The molecular determinants linked to the process of aging and the development of age-related neurological disorders. The molecular-level pathological changes initiate oxidative stress and disrupt the cell cycle, resulting in cellular deterioration and systemic decline in the aging organism. Genetic variation has the potential to contribute to the development of age-related neurological disorders. The acronyms ROS, HHcy, AEDs, AD, and PD refer to reactive oxygen species, hyperhomocysteinemia, antiepileptic drugs, Alzheimer's disease, and Parkinson's disease, respectively.*

Source: https://www.intechopen.com/chapters/55869.

Physiological aging commences subsequent to the age of 60. Alterations in the function of central cholinergic neurons are observed in both animal models and humans during the process of senescence. The observed alterations primarily encompass diminished quantities of cholinergic receptors, diminished production and secretion of acetylcholine, and a significant decline in the quantity of muscarinic cholinergic neurons. These changes are potentially associated with the age-related cognitive impairments commonly observed in individuals diagnosed with Alzheimer's disease. Furthermore, individuals with Parkinson's disease commonly experience a reduction in dopaminergic neurons by 40–50% in the substantia nigra and a decrease in dopamine (DA) levels in the striatum by the end of their sixth decade of life. These changes are characteristic of the condition.

The extended lifespan observed in many developed countries seems to have resulted in an elevated occurrence of strokes. In addition to the phenomenon of an aging population, the escalating prevalence of hypertension, diabetes, obesity, and cardiovascular disorders exerts a substantial influence on the rise in stroke occurrences. These diseases exhibit a higher incidence as individuals grow older.

Vascular changes in the brain (approximately 5%) and degenerative diseases of the CNS (10–20%) are the primary causes of epilepsy in the elderly. Patients with Alzheimer's disease, demyelinating diseases (such as MS), metabolic disorders, toxic and hormonal disorders, or individuals with a history of brain injuries or CNS infection may also experience seizures.

The complete understanding of the mechanisms underlying the onset of neurological disorders in older individuals remains incomplete. The regulation of cell death in the aging brain lacks known mechanisms. The impact of cell age on apoptosis and other neuronal death mechanisms, as well as the factors influencing the vulnerability to developing neurological diseases in old age, remains uncertain. Gaining insight into the factors contributing to the rising prevalence of neurological disorders among older individuals can aid in their prevention and enhance their overall well-being during old age (Figure 8.5).

8.4.1. The Molecular Mechanisms of Aging

Aging is caused by molecular mechanisms such as genome instability resulting from the buildup of gene mutations, telomere attrition, and epigenetic changes. Curiously, instability is more prevalent in certain regions of the genome compared to others. The correlation and interplay among the aforementioned mechanisms result in the deterioration of functionality in aging organisms.

8.4.1.1. The Process of Aging Resulting From DNA Damage

The theory of aging posits that somatic mutations occur in a stochastic manner throughout an organism's lifespan, and their gradual accumulation ultimately impacts crucial processes such as DNA synthesis, degradation, and repair, thereby leading to the occurrence of the "error catastrophe." Genetic harm manifests in both nuclear DNA (nDNA) and mitochondrial DNA (mtDNA). Nevertheless, mitochondria possess an oxidative milieu as a consequence of numerous redox reactions occurring within the electron transport chain. Additionally, their DNA repair mechanism exhibits lower efficiency, leading to a greater accumulation of damaged mDNA compared to nDNA. The decline in autophagy and mitophagy activity could potentially contribute to the buildup of mtDNA mutations and mitochondrial dysfunction in the context of aging.

Exogenous factors, such as physical, chemical, or biological agents, as well as endogenous factors, including DNA replication errors and ROS, can both disrupt the integrity and stability of DNA. The replication process is responsible for the majority of DNA damage, which is primarily repaired by an intricate network of DNA repair mechanisms. The MMR system ensures the accuracy and reliability of replication. Unrepaired damage triggers the activation of the checkpoint response, resulting in cell senescence or death. This process can also disrupt tissue and disrupt the body's homeostasis. The depletion of crucial MMR proteins has been documented in the process of aging. The inquiry arises as to whether this decline is a causal factor or a consequence of senescence.

Tumor protein 53 (p53), encoded by the *TP53* gene, plays a crucial role in regulating various cellular processes, including reversible and irreversible cell cycle arrest and senescence. The protein undergoes activation in response to diverse stress factors, leading to the initiation of apoptosis or autophagic cell death, contingent upon the specific cell category. The process of cellular aging is initiated with the purpose of inhibiting the proliferation of impaired cells and the development of tumors. P53 is activated by two primary categories of signals: DNA damage and oncogenic stress. Research has shown that senescent cells experience a decline in p53 function, as 50% of human neoplasms have a mutated version of the TP53 gene. Furthermore, the presence of TP53 mutations has been documented in age-related dementias, including Alzheimer's disease, in both human subjects and its murine model (Figure 8.5).

8.4.1.2. The Role of Telomeres

Telomere attrition represents an additional molecular mechanism that contributes to the process of senescence. Telomeres are located at the terminus of each chromatid and serve as a structural element of chromosomes. They are composed of DNA and proteins that bind to telomeres. The telomere DNA consists of the repetitive sequence 5 -TTAGGG-3 , which is repeated between 150 and 2,000 times. Telomeres primarily serve to safeguard against genetic information loss during replication and to prevent abnormal recombination, chromosome fusion, or chromosomal degradation caused by exonucleases. During cellular division, the telomere sequence undergoes a reduction in length ranging from 50 to 200 base pairs (bp), resulting in alterations to the structure of telomeres. The biological clock is widely regarded as a primary mechanism for determining the potential number of cell divisions. Hayflick's observations pertaining to somatic cells delineated the upper limit of divisions beyond which cells cease to undergo division while retaining metabolic activity. The Hayflick limit, which is subject to variation depending on the tissue type and organism, represents the uppermost limit. It is widely acknowledged that a decrease in the quantity of divisions serves as a deterrent against the accumulation of mutations.

8.4.1.3. Epigenetics of Aging

Epigenetic modifications, such as DNA methylation and histone modifications, are additional molecular mechanisms implicated in the process of aging. As individuals age, there is a deregulation of the epigenome. The decline in global DNA methylation levels is observed as individuals age, and alterations in the methylation profile have the potential to contribute to age-related immune deficiencies. The process of chemically modifying histones encompasses various modifications such as acetylation, methylation, phosphorylation, ubiquitination, deamination, citrullination, sumoylation, ADP ribosylation, and proline isomerization. These modifications result in alterations in the interactions between histones and DNA, as well as between histones themselves. Both alterations in the DNA methylation pattern and histone modifications have the ability to directly impact the arrangement of chromatin, leading to the exposure of distinct regions of the DNA to transcriptional factors and subsequently influencing the expression of various genes. Epigenetic investigations have provided evidence of gradual alterations at the transcriptomic level that are linked to the process of aging. The period between 49 and 56 years of age in humans appears to play a crucial role in the process of transcriptional senescence. Gene expression changes, whether they increase or decrease, occur over time and are subject to change (Figure 8.5).

8.4.1.4. Aging of the Brain

Moreover, senescence encompasses the process of aging in the cerebral white matter and gray matter, which involves the gradual loss of neurons, reduced levels of neurotransmitters, heightened inflammation, compromised structural integrity, the formation of lesions, infarction, and microbleeds. The aging process has an impact on various cell types, including neurons, glial cells (such as astrocytes, oligodendrocytes, and microglia), vascular cells, and the basal lamina matrix. This aging process disrupts their ability to maintain metabolic and ion homeostasis in the CNS, regulate cerebral blood flow, conduct impulses, and perform phagocytosis. As individuals age, the decrease in white matter volume is nearly three times greater, resulting in a loss of 28% of neurons, compared to the decrease in gray matter volume, which affects 10% of neurons. Hence, alterations in working memory can lead to a deterioration in both behavior and cognition among older individuals. Moreover, it has been observed that older individuals exhibit a diminished capacity for working memory repair. White matter alterations are evident in diseases such as stroke, Parkinson's disease, and Alzheimer's disease.

Ageing is characterized by a multitude of molecular alterations, which collectively establish an extensive network of interconnections. The determination of whether age-related diseases are attributed to a snowball effect of senescence or if they are instead a consequence of individual variability is rendered exceedingly challenging. Both hypotheses appear to hold validity, as aging is a significant risk factor for various diseases including stroke, epilepsy, Parkinson's disease, Alzheimer's disease, and brain tumors. However, it is not a definitive causal factor, as depicted in Figure 8.5.

8.4.2. Aging and Dementia

Dementia, which is a type of cognitive decline, is closely linked to advanced age. Approximately 10% of individuals aged 65 and above experience some form of memory impairment. Alzheimer's disease and VaD are the primary etiologies of dementia. The incidence of dementia exhibits a positive correlation with advancing age, impacting approximately half of individuals aged 85 years and above. Dementia is a degenerative condition that ultimately results in profound impairment and total reliance on caregivers.

8.4.2.1. Vascular Dementia

VaD was initially conceptualized as a progressive consequence of recurrent cerebral lesions. The advancement of brain imaging techniques unveiled the prevalence of silent ischemic lesions, which subsequently emerged as a prominent factor contributing to dementia. Epidemiological research has demonstrated that vascular dysfunction is responsible for approximately 10–20% of dementia cases. In the general population, the prevalence of VaD ranges from 1.2% to 4.2% among individuals aged 65 years and above, contingent upon the chosen methodological approach. There exists a significant correlation between the occurrence of VaD and age. The findings of a study conducted in Canada indicate a notable rise in the prevalence of vascular cognitive impairment, with rates increasing from 2.0% among individuals aged 65 to 74 years to 13.7% among those aged 85 years and above. The trend of increasing incidence of vasculosis (VaD) in senescence was confirmed by a meta-analysis conducted in 1998, which synthesized the results of 23 studies conducted globally. The significance and impact of vascular-related memory deficits have been amplified due to the growing longevity observed in numerous populations. The findings of a comprehensive longitudinal study revealed a twofold increase in the prevalence of post-stroke dementia from 1984 to 2001.

Numerous studies have examined the risk factors associated with CNS vascular lesions, apart from age. Hypertension, heart disease, diabetes with insulin resistance, and dyslipidemia have been identified as factors associated with an elevated susceptibility to the development of vascular disease (VaD). It is crucial to acknowledge that the findings obtained by various authors sometimes conflict with one another. VaD has been found to be associated with a cluster of cardiovascular risk factors known as "metabolic syndrome," which encompasses dyslipidemia, obesity, hypertension, and insulin resistance. Furthermore, it was observed that individuals exhibiting complete symptomatic metabolic syndrome achieved lower scores in neuropsychological assessments. Furthermore, it has been demonstrated that HHcy, which has previously been linked to VaD and stroke, is also associated with VaD.

Numerous studies have also provided evidence indicating that a symptomatic stroke event, predominantly observed in the elderly population, can result in memory impairments in a range of 6 to 32% of patients, contingent upon the duration of the follow-up period spanning from 3 months to 20 years. Pre-existing mild cognitive impairment before a stroke raises the likelihood of developing dementia after the stroke, and the decline in memory appears to occur more quickly in subsequent stroke episodes. In a similar vein, it was observed that individuals who experienced multiple strokes exhibited more significant cognitive impairment in comparison to those who had only experienced a single vascular incident (Figure 8.5).

8.4.3. Alzheimer's Disease

In older adults, Alzheimer's disease is the prevailing type of dementia. Alzheimer's disease is a degenerative neurodegenerative disorder that worsens over time, with aging being the main contributing factor. Alzheimer's disease can be classified into two primary clinical subtypes: familial Alzheimer's disease, which is distinguished by its early onset (prior to the age of 65) and often involves mutations in the APP, PSEN1, and PSEN2 genes. The genetic triad under consideration accounts for approximately 50% of the observed cases of FAD. Nevertheless, the occurrence of mutations in these genes is exceedingly infrequent within the human population. Following this, a significant proportion (90%) of cases of Alzheimer's disease are classified as sporadic (SAD) and primarily affect individuals aged 65 years and above. The complex nature of the disease poses significant challenges in identifying a definitive causative factor for Seasonal Affective Disorder (SAD). As of the present time, approximately 700 genes have been linked to Alzheimer's disease, with the E4 allele of the APOE gene being the most extensively studied risk factor for seasonal affective disorder (SAD).

The diagnosis of probable Alzheimer's disease relies on clinical criteria. However, the disease can only be definitively diagnosed after death through histopathologic examination of the brain, which reveals distinctive lesions such as Aβ plaques and neurofibrillary tangles formed by hyperphosphorylated protein tau. An amyloid precursor protein (APP), which is encoded by the *APP* gene, undergoes pathological cleavage through the action of β- and γ-secretases, which are encoded by the BACE and PSEN genes, respectively. One potential factor contributing to neurodegeneration in Alzheimer's disease brains is the presence of Aβ plaques and neurofibrillary tangles. These presences are associated with the morphological and functional decline of neurons and synapses, as well as the occurrence of excessive neuroinflammatory processes. Martin et al. demonstrated that the activation of receptors on microglia and monocyte-derived macrophages may be similar in both aging and Aβ pathology. In addition, individuals who possess the APOE E4 allele and rare variants in other genes, including HLA-DRB5/DRB1, INPP5D, MEF2C, CR1, CLU, and TREM2, may demonstrate a heightened level of microglial activation compared to those who do not carry these alleles. This elucidates the increased susceptibility of elderly individuals with unfavorable genetic variants to heightened neuroinflammatory reactions, resulting in neuronal degeneration and the onset of dementia.

The neurons that are primarily impacted by Alzheimer's disease are those that express acetylcholine (ACh) receptors, commonly referred to as "cholinergic neurons" (AChN). The gradual loss and degeneration of these specific cells is a characteristic feature of dementia, which manifests over time as individuals age and the disease progresses. Age-related apoptosis of acetylcholinesterase (AChN) results in a decline in ACh levels in the brain. ACh has been demonstrated to be the neurotransmitter that exhibits the greatest reduction in the majority of patients with Alzheimer's disease. Genetic factors, such as the presence of the pathogenic APOE E4 allele, appear to exert a substantial influence on the synthesis and secretion of ACh. Figure 8.5 demonstrates that the age-related decline in ACh levels released by the hippocampus was more pronounced in mice with human APOE E4/E4 compared to mice with APOE E3/E3 variants, as observed in the study on transgenic mice expressing human APOE. The primary cholinergic component of the brain is the basal forebrain, which undergoes neurodegeneration in both advanced aging and the early stages of Alzheimer's disease and other forms of dementia. The degeneration of basal forebrain is attributed to a decline in cholinergic neurotransmission and a decrease in the quantity of ACh within synaptic clefts. This is subsequently followed by the loss of cholinergic receptors, ultimately leading to the death of acetylcholine neurons. According to the "cholinergic deficit hypothesis," this particular process leads to the manifestation of behavioral and cognitive impairment, particularly in the form of learning difficulties, which tend to progress at an accelerated pace as individuals age.

It is important to mention that in Alzheimer's disease, like in VaD and stroke, there may be an elevation in the concentration of Hcy. This can result in harm to the blood vessels, leading to reduced blood flow and ineffective delivery of nutrients to neurons. As a result, the withered cells become more susceptible to ROS and apoptosis. HHcy is additionally linked to a reduction in the glutathione reservoir, which leads to the degradation of defense mechanisms against free radicals, thereby exacerbating neuronal loss and neurodegeneration.

8.4.4. Parkinson's Disease and Aging

Parkinson's disease is a neurodegenerative condition that occurs with age and is characterized by experiencing resting tremor, rigidity, and bradykinesia. The prevalence of Parkinson's disease patients is on the rise over time as a result of population aging. The precise pathomechanism underlying Parkinson's disease remains uncertain; however, it is established that the degenerative process initiates several years prior to the manifestation of clinical symptoms. The defining characteristic of Parkinson's disease is the demise of dopaminergic neurons in the substantia nigra (SN), a consequence of the formation of Lewy bodies (LBs) caused by dysfunction in the ubiquitin-proteasome system and disruptions in the proteins alpha-synuclein (ASN) and Parkin. The molecular features of Parkinson's disease encompass heightened production of ROS resulting from impaired mitochondrial function, juxtaposed with diminished mitophagy, neuroinflammation, and depletion of neurotrophic factors. Additionally, Parkinson's disease is associated with exposure to 1-methyl-4-phenyl-1, 2,3,6-tetrahydropyridine (MPTP) or paraquat, trichloroethylene or polychlorinated biphenyls, iron (the concentration of which rises in the supraoptic region with advancing age), copper, manganese, or mutations in PARK genes. Mitochondrial dysfunction is linked to the merging of ASN, apoptosis, the buildup of impaired mitochondria, and alterations in the functioning of complex 1. The aging process is associated with a decrease in mitochondrial function, as well as inflammation and alterations in DA metabolism.

The most significant risk factor for developing PD is increasing age. Parkinson's disease has a prevalence rate of approximately 1% among individuals aged 60 and above, and 5% among those aged 85 and above. The progression of DA neuron loss with aging has been observed since 1987, albeit at a slower rate compared to Parkinson's disease. Furthermore, LB can be found in elderly individuals who do not have Parkinson's disease. The aging brain exhibits an increased susceptibility to stressor stimuli and the production of ROS, leading to the impairment and eventual demise of sympathetic neurons. Conversely, a reduction or complete absence of ROS scavengers, such as neuromelanin, in the brain affected by Parkinson's disease may be the initial cause of damage to DA neurons, rather than a consequence of this damage.

Numerous epigenetic mechanisms, including alterations in DNA methylation patterns and histone modifications, exert a significant influence on the aging process and contribute to the development of Parkinson's disease. Measuring the DNA methylation pattern is sufficient to characterize the epigenetic clock. Notably, individuals with Parkinson's disease exhibit a higher rate of aging acceleration in comparison to adults of the same age. Hypomethylation of the SNCA gene, which encodes ASN, results in an upregulation of ASN expression and has been detected in the SN of patients with Parkinson's disease. ASN can also impact histone acetylation, which is a characteristic of genes that are active during transcription, and increase the formation of ASN fibrils.

The functional decline of the blood-brain barrier (BBB) during the process of normal aging can lead to neuroinflammation and the subsequent onset of neurodegenerative disorders. The occurrence of disruptions in BBB permeability during the senescence process could potentially contribute to the development of WM lesions, thereby impacting the effectiveness of treatment. During the process of ASN aggregation in PD, the production of ROS and the levels of proinflammatory cytokines or toxic agents may worsen the disruptions of the BBB.

The presence of HHcy in Parkinson's disease may play a role in the development of the disease, but the specific mechanism of interaction has not yet been identified. HHcy and age are both risk factors for the development of dementia in patients with Parkinson's disease. L-dopa treatment may be the cause of HHcy in individuals with Parkinson's disease. Hcy is generated through the process of methylation of L-dopa in patients, facilitated by the enzyme catechol-O-methyltransferase (COMT). Additional molecular-level side effects of L-dopa encompass heightened oxidative stress, along with modified levels of catecholamines and apoptotic proteins. Elevated Hcy levels may exacerbate the damage of DA neurons caused by oxidative stress (Figure 8.5). A mouse study has demonstrated that increased Hcy levels enhance the susceptibility to MPTP and the development of Parkinson's disease-like dysfunction.

8.4.5. Brain Tumors in the Elderly

Brain tumors, which are classified into four grades according to WHO criteria, are a type of CNS disease that primarily affects the elderly. Grade IV is considered the most malignant grade. Malignant glioma (MGs) is the most common form of primary brain tumor in adults, with the highest occurrence occurring between the ages of 40 and 65. Most MGs occur randomly, with ionizing radiation being the sole identified risk factor. Glioblastoma multiforme (GBM) is the prevailing form of glioma, classified as a grade IV astrocytic tumor by the WHO. It accounts for approximately 50% of all gliomas, with the highest prevalence observed in individuals aged 70 to 90 years. The prognosis of GBM is negatively influenced by advanced age. One notable attribute of GBM is its escalating incidence in correlation with advancing age. Consequently, as the median life expectancy continues to rise, it is anticipated that the patient population will expand in the forthcoming decades. Primary CNS lymphomas and meningiomas are additional forms of brain tumors that frequently occur in the elderly population.

GBM is a diverse group of tumors, consisting of two main types: primary glioblastomas making up 85–90% of cases, and secondary GBMs originating from low-grade astrocytomas, accounting for 10–15% of cases. While both types may not be distinguishable under a microscope, they exhibit genetic differences. Primary GBMs are characterized by genetic abnormalities, including the amplification and mutation of the EGFR gene, absence of heterozygosity on chromosome 10q, inactivation of the PTEN homolog gene, and infrequent occurrences of mutations in the IDH and TP53 genes. In contrast, the genetic basis of secondary GBM is distinguished by genetic mutations occurring in the IDH and/or TP53 genes, alongside the activation of platelet-derived growth factor receptors. In 2010, The Cancer Genome Atlas (TCGA) Research Network established a classification system for GBM based on gene expression. Four subtypes of GBM were identified by the authors. The distinguishing features of the subtypes are as follows: proneural GBM exhibits changes in the PDGFRA gene and point mutations in IDH1, classical GBM displays abnormalities in EGFR, and mesenchymal GBM shows abnormalities in NF1. Neural GBM, as the fourth subtype, is distinguished by the presence of neuron markers including NEFL, GABRA1, SYT1, and SLC12A5. The sensitivity of each subtype of GBM to radiotherapy and chemotherapy varies. Therefore, the identification of the genetic type of a surgically excised or biopsied lesion could serve as a safeguard for patients, preventing the administration of unnecessary and ineffective treatment.

Regrettably, GBMs commonly prove to be untreatable in the elderly population, as the majority of these patients have a survival rate of less than 6 months. The identification of primary brain tumors in elderly individuals can present additional complexities and delays as a result of nonspecific symptoms that may be concealed by physiological and cognitive alterations commonly associated with the natural aging phenomenon. Furthermore, there is a lack of adequate representation of elderly patients in numerous clinical trials. The available literature suggests that, towards the end of the 20th century, there was a decline in the likelihood of receiving medical interventions, such as surgery and/or radiotherapy, as patients advanced in age. Treatment was administered to 82% of patients under the age of 65, while only 47% of individuals over the age of 65 and only 25% of patients over the age of 75 received any form of therapy. Furthermore, it was observed that individuals who underwent radiotherapy and/or surgery exhibited a notably diminished rate of survival upon reaching the age threshold of 60 years.

While the pathological processes may vary across different subtypes of glioma, there exists a shared set of molecular events. The activation of ERK or Akt pathways is induced by growth factor receptor tyrosine kinases, leading to downstream signaling. The absence of p53 activation is subsequently accompanied by the inability to initiate DNA repair mechanisms and the induction of cell death through apoptosis. Another detrimental feature observed in GBM is the induction of vascular endothelial growth factor (VEGF) secretion by the cells, which plays a crucial role in the process of angiogenesis. GBM secretes VEGF, which leads to the formation of blood vessels in the tumor, increased permeability of the BBB, and the development of swelling outside the cells. Ultimately, the advancement of tumor invasion occurs as a result of the expansion of vasculature.

While brain tumors can be highly invasive, it is worth mentioning that in elderly patients, they can be effectively treated using maximally safe surgical resection, radiotherapy, and/or chemotherapy with Temozolomide. Temozolomide is particularly recommended as the first-line treatment for patients with the MGMT promoter, depending on the specific subtype of the tumor. Bevacizumab (BV, Avastin®) is currently under investigation as a potential treatment for brain tumors, alongside radiotherapy and/or Temozolomide. The humanized IgG1 monoclonal antibody Bevacizumab exhibits a strong affinity for VEGF and effectively deactivates the growth factor. Therefore, BV facilitates the regression of tumors and reduces the likelihood of cerebral edema. Remarkably, research has shown that while advanced age is a detrimental prognostic factor, BV exhibited greater efficacy in older patients (...55 years of age). Those who received BV treatment maintained better health for a longer duration and required lower doses of steroids. The results were consistent with the research conducted by Nghiemphu et al., which showed that the expression of VEGF was 1.4 times greater in older patients compared to younger individuals. Therefore, inhibiting VEGF could potentially lead to a more favorable outcome in these patients.

One potential explanation for the higher prevalence of brain tumors among older individuals could be attributed to a decline in the efficacy of repair mechanisms. The deactivation of genes responsible for DNA repair, such as TP53 and MGMT mentioned earlier, may progress as individuals age. The potential consequence of this phenomenon is the heightened buildup of DNA damage, which subsequently triggers the activation of proto-oncogenes and the suppression of tumor suppressor genes. These alterations, caused by either mutation or epigenetic modifications, can lead to further disruption of cellular repair mechanisms, making cells more vulnerable to ROS and spontaneous mutagenesis. This, in turn, initiates the positive feedback loop of neoplasia (Figure 8.6).

In brief, the process of senescence initiates at the molecular level and progressively results in the deterioration of brain cell morphology and functional impairment. Ultimately, these factors contribute to the decline of the CNS and an elevated susceptibility to the onset of neurological disorders.

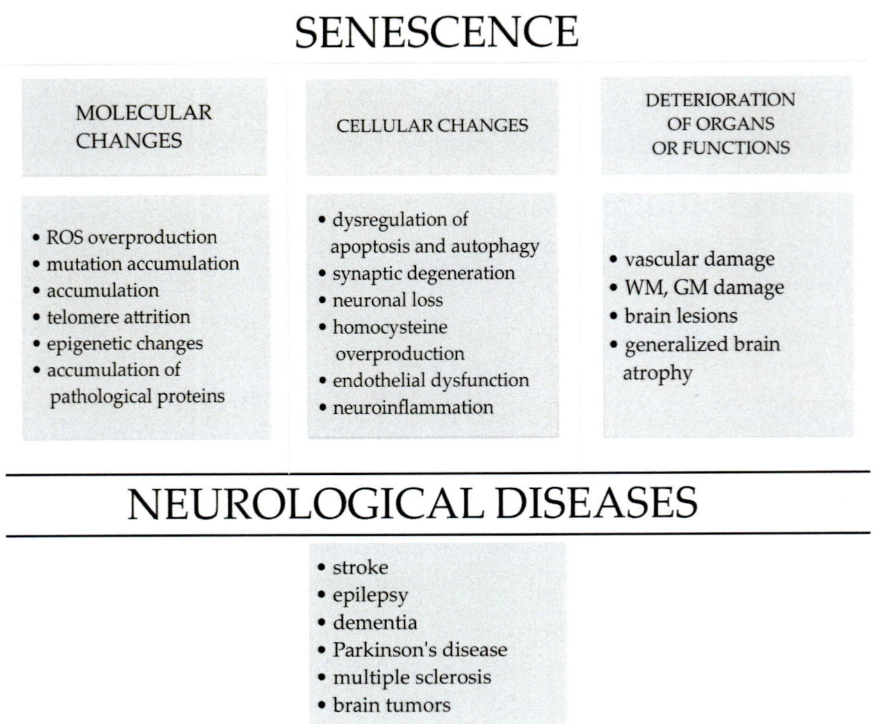

Figure 8.6. *Neurological diseases may be linked to alterations that occur during the senescence process. The molecular-level pathological changes impact the cells of the aging organism, resulting in systemic deterioration and the development of age-related neurological diseases. Reactive oxygen species, white matter (WM), and gray matter (GM) are three distinct components of the brain.*

Source: https://www.intechopen.com/chapters/55869.

8.5. Summary

- Aging is intrinsically linked to an increased risk of neurological disorders, reflecting a significant area of concern in the medical and scientific communities. As individuals age, the brain and nervous system undergo various changes that can predispose them to conditions such as Alzheimer's disease, Parkinson's disease, stroke, and other forms of dementia.
- These disorders are characterized by a progressive decline in cognitive and motor functions, severely impacting the quality of life of affected individuals and presenting substantial challenges for caregivers and healthcare systems.
- Research in this field focuses on understanding the mechanisms behind the aging process and how it contributes to the development of neurological diseases.
- Factors such as genetic predispositions, lifestyle choices, and environmental influences are under investigation to determine their roles in the onset and progression of these conditions.

- Advances in neuroimaging, biomarker identification, and molecular biology are facilitating early diagnosis and the development of targeted therapies, aiming to slow disease progression and improve patient outcomes.
- Despite these efforts, aging-related neurological disorders remain a leading cause of disability and mortality worldwide, underscoring the importance of continued research, prevention strategies, and support for those affected.

A Closer Look

Parkinson's Disease

Parkinson's disease (PD) is a neurodegenerative disorder that primarily affects movement due to the gradual loss of dopamine-producing neurons in a part of the brain known as the substantia nigra. As dopamine levels decline, individuals with PD experience motor symptoms like tremors, bradykinesia (slowness of movement), rigidity, and postural instability. Parkinson's disease is progressive, meaning symptoms worsen over time, leading to significant challenges in daily functioning. The exact cause of PD remains unclear, but a combination of genetic and environmental factors is believed to contribute to the disease.

The diagnosis of Parkinson's disease is primarily clinical, relying on patient history and neurological examination. There is no definitive test to diagnose PD, which can complicate early detection. Imaging techniques like dopamine transporter scans (DaTscans) may assist in diagnosis by showing reduced dopamine levels in the brain, but these are used selectively. Early symptoms of PD are often subtle, including a slight tremor in one hand or stiffness in the body. Over time, these symptoms intensify, affecting coordination, balance, and eventually leading to more severe physical disability.

Pharmacotherapy is central to managing PD symptoms, with Levodopa being the most commonly prescribed medication. Levodopa is converted into dopamine in the brain, temporarily alleviating motor symptoms. However, as the disease progresses, the effectiveness of Levodopa may diminish, and patients may experience "on-off" fluctuations where symptoms unpredictably worsen or improve. Other medications, such as dopamine agonists and MAO-B inhibitors, are also used to enhance dopamine activity or inhibit its breakdown, providing symptom relief. However, long-term use of these drugs can lead to side effects, including dyskinesias (involuntary movements) and hallucinations. Beyond pharmacotherapy, lifestyle modifications and supportive therapies play an essential role in managing PD. Physical therapy helps patients maintain mobility and improve balance, while occupational therapy aids in adapting daily activities to the limitations imposed by the disease. Additionally, deep brain stimulation (DBS), a surgical procedure, has been used for patients with advanced PD who do not respond well to medication. DBS involves implanting electrodes in specific brain areas to regulate abnormal electrical signals, improving motor function and reducing tremors.

Research in Parkinson's disease is actively exploring various fronts, including neuroprotective treatments that might slow disease progression and gene therapies aimed at restoring dopamine levels. Stem cell therapy is another promising area under investigation, as it holds the potential to replace damaged neurons and restore dopamine production. Genetic research has also identified several mutations linked to PD, offering insights into its mechanisms and potential therapeutic targets. While there is currently no cure for Parkinson's disease, these advancements provide hope for future therapies that may not only alleviate symptoms but also modify the disease course, improving quality of life for millions worldwide.

References

1. Aboulafia-Brakha, T., Suchecki, D., Gouveia-Paulino, F., Nitrini, R., & Ptak, R., (2014). "Cognitive-Behavioural Group Therapy Improves a Psychophysiological Marker of Stress in Caregivers of Patients with Alzheimer's Disease." *Aging Mental Health. 18*(6), 801–808.
2. Aguirre, E., Woods, R. T., Spector, A., & Orrell, M., (2013). "Cognitive Stimulation for Dementia: A Systematic Review of the Evidence of Effectiveness from Randomized Controlled Trials." *Ageing Research Reviews. 12*(1), 253–262.
3. Akpan, M. U., Ikpeme, E. E., & Utuk, E. O., (2013). "Teachers' Knowledge and Attitudes towards Seizure Disorder: A Comparative Study of Urban and Rural School Teachers in Akwa Ibom State, Nigeria." *Nigerian Journal of Clinical Practice. 16*(3), 365–370.
4. Asadi-Pooya, A. A., & Sperling, M. R., (2008). "Strategies for Surgical Treatment of Epilepsies in Developing Countries." *Epilepsia. 49*(3), 381–385.
5. Ba-Diop, A., Marin, B., Druet-Cabanac, M., Ngougou, E. B., Newton, C. R., & Preux, P. M., (2014). "Epidemiology, Causes, and Treatment of Epilepsy in Sub-Saharan Africa." The Lancet Neurology. *13*(10), 1029–1044. doi:10.1016/S1474-4422(14)70114-0.
6. Bahar-Fuchs, A., Clare, L., & Woods, B., (2013). "Cognitive Training and Cognitive Rehabilitation for Mild to Moderate Alzheimer's Disease and Vascular Dementia." *Cochrane Database of Systematic Reviews, 6*, CD003260. PubMed PMID:23740535.
7. Baird, R. A., Wiebe, S., Zunt, J. R., Halperin, J. J., Gronseth, G., et al., (2013). "Evidence-Based Guideline: Treatment of Parenchymal Neurocysticercosis: Report of the Guideline Development Subcommittee of the American Academy of Neurology." *Neurology. 80*(15), 1424–29. doi:10.1212/WNL.0b013e31828c2f3e.
8. Banerjee, P. N., Filippi, D., Hauser W Allen. (2009). "The Descriptive Epidemiology of Epilepsy—A Review." *Epilepsy Research. 85*(1), 31–45. doi:10.1016/j.eplepsyres.2009.03.003.
9. Benamer, H. T., & Grosset, D. G., (2009). "A Systematic Review of the Epidemiology of Epilepsy in Arab Countries." *Epilepsia. 50*(10), 2301–04. doi:10.1111/j.1528-1167.2009.02058.x.
10. Berg, A. T., Berkovic, S. F., Brodie, M. J., Buchhalter, J., Cross J H., et al., (2010). "Revised Terminology and Concepts for Organization of Seizures and Epilepsies: Report of the ILAE Commission on Classification and Terminology, 2005–2009." *Epilepsia. 51*(4), 676–685. doi:EPI2522 [pii].10.1111/j.1528-1167.2010.02522.x.
11. Berg, A. T., Levy, S. R., Testa, F. M., D'Souza, R., (2009). "Remission of Epilepsy after Two Drug Failures in Children: A Prospective Study." *Annals of Neurology. 65*(5), 510–519. doi:10.1002/ana.21642.
12. Bhalla, D., Godet, B., Druet-Cabanac, M., & Preux, P. M., (2011). "Etiologies of Epilepsy: A Comprehensive Review." *Expert Review of Neurotherapeutics. 11*(6), 861–876. doi:10.1586/ern.11.51.
13. Birbeck, G. L., French, J. A., Perucca, E., Simpson, D. M., Fraimow, H., et al., (2012). "Evidence-Based Guideline: Antiepileptic Drug Selection for People with HIV/AIDS: Report of the Quality Standards Subcommittee of the American Academy of Neurology and the Ad Hoc Task Force of the Commission on Therapeutic Strategies of the International League Against Epilepsy." *Neurology. 78*(2), 139–145. doi:10.1212/WNL.0b013e31823efcf8.

14. Birks, J., (2006). "Cholinesterase Inhibitors for Alzheimer's Disease." *Cochrane Database Systematic Reviews. 25*(1), CD005593.

15. Bradley, P. M., & Lindsay, B., (2008). "Care Delivery and Self-Management Strategies for Adults with Epilepsy." *Cochrane Database of Systematic Reviews, 1*, CD006244. doi:10.1002/14651858.CD006244.pub2.

16. Bronfort, G., Nilsson, N., Haas, M., Evans, R., Goldsmith C H., et al., (2004). "Non-Invasive Physical Treatments for Chronic/Recurrent Headache." *Cochrane Database of Systematic Reviews, 3*, CD001878.

17. Burneo, J. G., Tellez-Zenteno, J., & Wiebe, S., (2005). "Understanding the Burden of Epilepsy in Latin America: A Systematic Review of Its Prevalence and Incidence." *Epilepsy Research. 66*(1–3), 63–74. doi:S0920-1211(05)00138-5 [pii]10.1016/j.eplepsyres.2005.07.002.

18. Burton, K. J., Rogathe, J., Whittaker, R., Mankad, K., Hunter, E., et al., (2012). "Epilepsy in Tanzanian Children: Association with Perinatal Events and Other Risk Factors." *Epilepsia. 53*(4), 752–760. doi:10.1111/j.1528-1167.2011.03395.x.

19. Cameron, A., Bansal, A., Dua, T., Hill, S. R., Moshe S L., et al., (2012). "Mapping the Availability, Price, and Affordability of Antiepileptic Drugs in 46 Countries." *Epilepsia. 53*(6), 962–969. doi:10.1111/j.1528-1167.2012.03446.x.

20. Cheuk, D. K., & Wong, V., (2014). "Acupuncture for Epilepsy." *Cochrane Database of Systematic Reviews, 5*, CD005062. doi:10.1002/14651858.CD005062.pub4.

21. Chisholm, D., & WHO-CHOICE. (2005). "Cost-Effectiveness of First-Line Antiepileptic Drug Treatments in the Developing World: A Population-Level Analysis." *Epilepsia. 46*(5), 751–759.

22. Chomba, E. N., Haworth, A., Mbewe, E., Atadzhanov, M., Ndubani, P., et al., (2010). "The Current Availability of Antiepileptic Drugs in Zambia: Implications for the ILAE/WHO 'Out of the Shadows' Campaign." *American Journal of Tropical Medicine and Hygiene. 83*(3), 571–574. doi:10.4269/ajtmh.2010.10-0100.

23. Cross, J. H., (2013). "New Research with Diets and Epilepsy." *Journal of Child Neurology. 28*(8), 970–974. doi:10.1177/0883073813487593.

24. Czaja, S. J., & Rubert, M. P., (2002). "Telecommunications Technology as an Aid to Family Caregivers of Persons with Dementia." *Psychosomatic Medicine. 64*(3), 469–476.

25. Dahlrup, B., Nordell, E., Steen Carlsson, K., & Elmståhl, S., (2014). "Health Economic Analysis on a Psychosocial Intervention for Family Caregivers of Persons with Dementia." *Dementia and Geriatric Cognitive Disorders. 37*(3–4), 181–195.

26. Derry, C. J., Derry, S., & Moore, R. A., (2012). "Sumatriptan (Oral Route of Administration) for Acute Migraine Attacks in Adults." *Cochrane Database of Systematic Reviews, 2,* Article No. CD008615. doi:10.1002/14651858.CD008615.pub2.

27. Derry, S., & Moore, R. A., (2013). "Paracetamol (Acetaminophen) with or without an Antiemetic for Acute Migraine Headaches in Adults." *Cochrane Database of Systematic Reviews, 4*, CD008040. doi:10.1002/14651858.CD008040.pub3.

28. Derry, S., Rabbie, R., & Moore, R. A., (2013). "Diclofenac with or without an Antiemetic for Acute Migraine Headaches in Adults." *Cochrane Database Systematic Reviews, 4*, CD008783.

29. Deudon, A., Maubourguet, N., Gervais, X., Leone, E., Brocker, P., et al., (2009). "Non-Pharmacological Management of Behavioural Symptoms in Nursing Homes." *International Journal of Geriatric Psychiatry, 12*, 1386–95. doi:10.1002/gps.2275.

30. Dias, A., Dewey, M. E., D'Souza, J., Dhume, R., Motghare, D. D., Shaji K S., et al., (2008). "The Effectiveness of a Home Care Program for Supporting Caregivers of Persons with Dementia in Developing Countries: A Randomised Controlled Trial from Goa, India." *PLoS One. 3*(6), e2333. doi:10.1371/journal.pone.0002333.

31. Diener, H. C., & Limmroth, V., (2004). "Medication-Overuse Headache: A Worldwide Problem." *The Lancet Neurology.* 3(8), 475–483.

32. Diener, H. C., Tfelt-Hansen, P., Dahlof, C., Lainez, M. J., Sandrini, G., Wang, S. J., Neto, W., Vijapurkar, U., Doyle, A., Jacobs, D., & Group, M. S., (2004). "Topiramate in Migraine Prophylaxis: Results from a Placebo-Controlled Trial with Propranolol as an Active Control." *Journal of Neurology. 251*(8), 943–950. doi:10.1007/s00415-004-0464-6.

33. Diop, A. G., Hesdorffer, D. C., Logroscino, G., & Hauser, W. A., (2005). "Epilepsy and Mortality in Africa: A Review of the Literature." *Epilepsia. 46*(Suppl. 11), 33–35. doi:10.1111/j.1528-1167.2005.00405.x.

34. Dodick, D. W., Freitag, F., Banks, J., Saper, J., Xiang, J., et al., (2009). "Topiramate versus Amitriptyline in Migraine Prevention: A 26-Week, Multicenter, Randomized, Double-Blind, Double-Dummy, Parallel-Group Noninferiority Trial in Adult Migraineurs." *Clinical Therapeutics. 31*(3), 542–559. doi:10.1016/j.clinthera.2009.03.020.

35. Donaldson, C., & Burns, A., (1999). "Burden of Alzheimer's Disease: Helping the Patient and Caregiver." *Journal of Geriatric Psychiatry Neurology. 12*(1), 21–28.

36. Evans, R. W., Williams, M. A., Rapoport, A. M., & Peterlin, B. L., (2012). "The Association of Obesity with Episodic and Chronic Migraine." *Headache. 52*(4), 663–671. doi:10.1111/j.1526-4610.2012.02114.x.

37. Evers, S., Jensen, R., and European Federation of Neurological Societies. (2011). "Treatment of Medication Overuse Headache—Guideline of the EFNS Headache Panel." *European Journal of Neurology. 18*(9), 1115–21. doi:10.1111/j.1468-1331.2011.03497.x.

38. Fiest, K. M., Birbeck, G. L., Jacoby, A., & Jette, N., (2014). "Stigma in Epilepsy." *Current Neurology and Neuroscience Reports. 14*(5), 444. doi:10.1007/s11910-014-0444-x.

39. Fisher, R. S., Acevedo, C., Arzimanoglou, A., Bogacz, A., Cross J H., et al., (2014). "ILAE Official Report: A Practical Clinical Definition of Epilepsy." *Epilepsia. 55*(4), 475–482. doi:10.1111/epi.12550.

40. Fitzsimons, M., Normand, C., Varley, J., & Delanty, N., (2012). "Evidence-Based Models of Care for People with Epilepsy." *Epilepsy & Behavior. 23*(1), 1–6. doi:10.1016/j.yebeh.2011.10.019.

41. Folstein, M., Folstein, S., & McHugh, P. R., (1973). "Clinical Predictors of Improvement after Electroconvulsive Therapy of Patients with Schizophrenia, Neurotic Reactions, and Affective Disorders." *Biological Psychiatry. 7*(2), 147–152.

42. Forsgren, L., Beghi, E., Oun, A., & Sillanpaa, M., (2005). "The Epidemiology of Epilepsy in Europe—A Systematic Review." *European Journal of Neurology. 12*(4), 245–253. doi:10.1111/j.1468-1331.2004.00992.x.

43. Francois, C., Sintonen, H., Sulkava, R., & Riva, B., (2004). "Cost Effectiveness of Memantine

in Moderately Severe to Severe Alzheimer's Disease: A Markov Model in Finland." *Clinical Drug Investigations. 24*(7), 373–384.

44. Ganguli, M., Chandra, V., Kamboh, M. I., Johnston, J. M., Dodge H H., et al., (2000). "Apolipoprotein E Polymorphism and Alzheimer Disease: The Indo-US Cross-National Dementia Study." *Arch Neurology. 57*(6), 824–830.

45. Gavrilova, S. I., Cerri, C. P., Mikhaylova, N., Sokolova, O., Banerjee, S., et al., (2009). "Helping Carers to Care—The 10/66 Dementia Research Group's Randomized Control Trial of a Caregiver Intervention in Russia." *International Journal of Geriatric Psychiatry. 24*(4), 347–354.

46. Glauser, T., Ben-Menachem, E., Bourgeois, B., Cnaan, A., Guerreiro, C., et al., (2013). "Updated ILAE Evidence Review of Antiepileptic Drug Efficacy and Effectiveness as Initial Monotherapy for Epileptic Seizures and Syndromes." *Epilepsia. 54*(3), 551–563. doi:10.1111/epi.12074.

47. Grant, I., McKibbin, C. L., Taylor, M. J., Mills, P., Dimsdale, J., Ziegler, M., & Patterson, T. L., (2003). "In-Home Respite Intervention Reduces Plasma Epinephrine in Stressed Alzheimer Caregivers." *American Journal of Geriatric Psychiatry. 11*(1), 62–72.

48. Hauber, A. B., Gnanasakthy, A., & Mauskopf, J. A., (2000). "Savings in the Cost of Caring for Patients with Alzheimer's Disease in Canada: An Analysis of Treatment with Rivastigmine." *Clinical Therapeutics, 4*, 439–451.

49. Henry, G., Williamson, D., & Tampi, R. R., (2011). "Efficacy and Tolerability of Antidepressants in the Treatment of Behavioral and Psychological Symptoms of Dementia, a Literature Review of Evidence." *American Journal of Alzheimer's Disease and Other Dementias. 26*(3), 169–183.

50. Hitiris, N., Mohanraj, R., Norrie, J., & Brodie, M. J., (2007). "Mortality in Epilepsy." *Epilepsy and Behavior. 10*(3), 363–376.

51. Institute for Quality and Efficiency in Health Care. (2014). https://www.iqwig.de/en/home.2724.html.

52. International Headache Society. (2013). "The International Classification of Headache Disorders, 3rd edition (beta version)." *Cephalalgia. 33*(9), 629–808. doi:10.1177/0333102413485658.

53. Jette, N., Reid, A. Y., & Wiebe, S., (2014). "Surgical Management of Epilepsy." *Canadian Medical Association Journal* [Journal de l'Association medicale canadienne]. doi:10.1503/cmaj.121291.

54. Jette, N., & Trevathan, E., (2014). "Saving Lives by Treating Epilepsy in Developing Countries." *Neurology. 82*(7), 552–553. doi:10.1212/WNL.0000000000000133.

55. Jette, N., & Wiebe, S. S., (2015). "Health Economics Issues." In *Long-Term Outcomes of Epilepsy Surgery in Adults and Children*, first edition, edited by Malmgren, K., Baxendale, S., Cross, H., editors. Springer.

56. Jones, R. W., McCrone, P., & Guilhaume, C., (2004). "Cost Effectiveness of Memantine in Alzheimer's Disease: An Analysis Based on a Probabilistic Markov Model From a UK Perspective." *Aging. 21*(9), 607–620.

57. Kale, R., (2002). "Global Campaign against Epilepsy: The Treatment Gap." *Epilepsia. 43*(Suppl. 6), 31–33.

58. Kales, H. C., Gitlin, L. N., Lyketsos C. G., & Detroit Expert Panel on Assessment and Management of Neuropsychiatric Symptoms of Dementia. (2014). "Management of Neuropsychiatric Symptoms of Dementia in Clinical Settings: Recommendations from a Multidisciplinary Expert Panel." *Journal of the American Geriatrics Society. 62*(4), 762–769. doi:10.1111/jgs.12730.

59. Kales, H. C., Kim, H. M., Zivin, K., Valenstein, M., Seyfried L S., et al., (2012). "Risk of Mortality among Individual Antipsychotics in Patients with Dementia." *The American Journal of Psychiatry. 169*(1), 71–79. doi:10.1176/appi.ajp.2011.11030347.

60. Kim, L. G., Johnson, T. L., Marson, A. G., & Chadwick, D. W., (2006). "Prediction of Risk of Seizure Recurrence after a Single Seizure and Early Epilepsy: Further Results from the MESS Trial." *The Lancet Neurology. 5*(4), 317–322. doi:10.1016/S1474-4422(06)70383-0.

61. Kirthi, V., Derry, S., & Moore, R. A., (2013). "Aspirin with or without an Antiemetic for Acute Migraine Headaches in Adults." *Cochrane Database Systematic Reviews, 4*, CD008041. doi:10.1002/14651858.CD008041.pub3.

62. Koppel, B. S., Brust, J. C., Fife, T., Bronstein, J., Youssof, S., et al., (2014). "Systematic Review: Efficacy and Safety of Medical Marijuana in Selected Neurologic Disorders: Report of the Guideline Development Subcommittee of the American Academy of Neurology." *Neurology. 82*(17), 1556–63. doi:10.1212/WNL.0000000000000363.

63. Kukull, W. A., Higdon, R., Bowen, J. D., McCormick, W. C., Teri, L., et al., (2002). "Dementia and Alzheimer Disease Incidence: A Prospective Cohort Study." *Archives of Neurology. 59*(11), 1737–46.

64. Kwan, P., Arzimanoglou, A., Berg, A. T., Brodie, M. J., Allen H W., et al., (2010). "Definition of Drug Resistant Epilepsy: Consensus Proposal by the Ad Hoc Task Force of the ILAE Commission on Therapeutic Strategies." *Epilepsia. 51*(6), 1069–77.

65. Kwan, P., & Brodie, M. J., (2000). "Early Identification of Refractory Epilepsy." *The New England Journal of Medicine. 342*(5), 314–319.

66. Langfitt, J. T., Holloway, R. G., McDermott, M. P., Messing, S., Sarosky, K., et al., (2007). "Health Care Costs Decline after Successful Epilepsy Surgery." *Neurology. 68*(16), 1290–98.

67. Langfitt, J. T., (1997). "Cost-Effectiveness of Anterotemporal Lobectomy in Medically Intractable Complex Partial Epilepsy." *Epilepsia. 38*(2), 154–163.

68. Launer, L. J., Andersen, K., Dewey, M. E., Letenneur, L., Ott, A., et al., (1999). "Rates and Risk Factors for Dementia and Alzheimer's Disease: Results from EURODEM Pooled Analyses. EURODEM Incidence Research Group and Work Groups. European Studies of Dementia." *Neurology. 52*(1), 78–84.

69. Lebedeva, E. R., Olesen, J., Osipova, V. V., Volkova, L. I., Tabeeva G R., et al., (2013). "The Yekaterinburg Headache Initiative: An Interventional Project, within the Global Campaign against Headache, to Reduce the Burden of Headache in Russia." *Journal of Headache and Pain. 14*(1), 101. doi:10.1186/1129-2377-14-101.

70. Leibson, C. L., Long, K. H., Ransom, J. E., Roberts, R. O., Hass S L., et al., (2015). "Direct Medical Costs and Source of Cost Differences across the Spectrum of Cognitive Decline: A Population-Based Study." *Alzheimer's Dement. 11*(8), 917–932. doi:10.1016/j.jalz.2015.01.007.

71. Leong, C., (2014). "Antidepressants for Depression in Patients with Dementia: A Review of the Literature." *Consultant Pharmacist. 29*(4), 254–263. doi:10.4140/TCP.n.2014.254.

72. Levin, C., & Chisholm, D., (2015). "Cost-Effectiveness and Affordability of Interventions, Policies, and Platforms for the Prevention and Treatment of Mental, Neurological, and Substance Use Disorders." In *Disease Control Priorities* (third edition), Volume 4, Mental, Neurological, and Substance Use Disorders, edited by Patel, V., Chisholm, D., Dua, T., Laxminarayan, R., Medina-Mora, M. E., editors. Washington, DC: World Bank.

73. Levy, R. G., Cooper, P. N., & Giri, P., (2012). "Ketogenic Diet and Other Dietary Treatments for Epilepsy." *Cochrane Database of Systematic Reviews, 3*, CD001903. doi:10.1002/14651858.CD001903.pub2.

74. Linde, K., Allais, G., Brinkhaus, B., Manheimer, E., Vickers, A., & White, A. R., (2009). "Acupuncture for Migraine Prophylaxis." *Cochrane Database of Systematic Reviews, 1*, CD001218. doi:10.1002/14651858.CD001218.pub2.

75. Linde, K., & Rossnagel, K., (2004). "Propranolol for Migraine Prophylaxis." *Cochrane Database of Systematic Reviews, 2*, CD003225.

76. Linde, M., Gustavsson, A., Stovner, L. J., Steiner, T. J., Barré, J., et al., (2012). "The Cost of Headache Disorders in Europe: The Eurolight Project." *European Journal of Neurology. 19*(5), 703–711. doi:10.1111/j.1468-1331.2011.03612.x.Epub 2011 Dec 5.

77. Linde, M., Mulleners, W. M., Chronicle, E. P., & McCrory, D. C., (2013a). "Topiramate for the Prophylaxis of Episodic Migraine in Adults." *Cochrane Database of Systematic Reviews, 6*, CD010611. doi:10.1002/14651858.

78. Linde, M., Mulleners, W. M., Chronicle, E. P., & McCrory, D. C., (2013b). "Valproate (Valproic Acid or Sodium Valproate or a Combination of the Two) for the Prophylaxis of Episodic Migraine in Adults." *Cochrane Database of Systematic Reviews, 6,* CD010611. doi:10.1002/14651858.

79. Linde, M., Steiner, T. J., & Chisholm, D., (2015). "Cost-Effectiveness Analysis of Interventions for Migraine in Four Low- and Middle-Income Countries." *Journal of Headache Pain. 18*(16), 15. doi:10.1186/s10194-015-0496-6.

80. Lindsay, B., & Bradley, P. M., (2010). "Care Delivery and Self-Management Strategies for Children with Epilepsy." *Cochrane Database of Systematic Reviews, 12*, CD006245. doi:10.1002/14651858.CD006245.pub2.

81. Livingston, G., Barber, J., Rapaport, P., Knapp, M., Griffin, M., et al., (2014). "Long-Term Clinical and Cost-Effectiveness of Psychological Intervention for Family Carers of People with Dementia: A Single-Blind, Randomised, Controlled Trial." *Lancet Psychiatry, 7*, 539–548. doi:10.1016/S2215-0366(14)00073-X. Epub (2014). Dec 3.

82. Lowenstein, D. H., Alldredge, B. K., Allen, F., Neuhaus, J., Corry, M., et al., (2001). "The Prehospital Treatment of Status Epilepticus (PHTSE) Study: Design and Methodology." *Controlled Clinical Trials, 22*, 290–309.

83. Maayan, N., Soares-Weiser, K., & Lee, H., (2014). "Respite Care for People with Dementia and their Carers." *Cochrane Database of Systematic Reviews; 1*, CD004396. doi:10.1002/14651858.CD004396.pub3.

84. Mac, T. L., Tran, D. S., Quet, F., Odermatt, P., Preux P M., et al., (2007). "Epidemiology, Aetiology, and Clinical Management of Epilepsy in Asia: A Systematic Review." *The Lancet Neurology. 6*(6), 533–543.

85. Martín-Carrasco, M., Martín, M. F., Valero, C. P., Millán, P. R., García C I., et al., (2009). "Effectiveness of a Psychoeducational Intervention Program in the Reduction of Caregiver Burden in Alzheimer's Disease Patients' Caregivers." *International Journal of Geriatric Psychiatry. 24*(5), 489–499.

86. Marziali, E., & Garcia, L. J., (2011). "Dementia Caregivers' Responses to 2 Internet-Based Intervention Programs." *American Journal of Alzheimer's Diseases and Other Dementias. 26*(1), 36–43.

87. Mbewe, E., Zairemthiama, P., Paul, R., Birbeck, G. L., & Steiner, T. J., (2015). "The Burden of Primary Headache Disorders in Zambia: National Estimates from a Population-Based Door-to-Door Survey." *Journal of Headache Pain, 16*, 513.

88. Mbuba, C. K., Ngugi, A. K., Newton, C. R., & Carter, J. A., (2008). "The Epilepsy Treatment Gap in Developing Countries: A Systematic Review of the Magnitude, Causes, and Intervention Strategies." *Epilepsia. 49*(9), 1491–503. doi:10.1111/j.1528-1167.2008.01693.x.

89. McShane, R., Sastre A Areosa, Minakaran, N., (2006). "Memantine for Dementia." *Cochrane Database of Systematic Reviews, 2*, CD003154.

90. Medina, M. T., Aguilar-Estrada, R. L., Alvarez, A., Duron, R. M., Martinez, L., et al., (2011). "Reduction in Rate of Epilepsy from Neurocysticercosis by Community Interventions: The Salama, Honduras Study." *Epilepsia. 52*(6), 1177–85. doi:10.1111/j.1528-1167.2010.02945.x.

91. Megiddo, I., Colson, A., Chisholm, D., Dua, T., Nandi, A., et al., (2016). "Health and Economic Benefits of Public Financing of Epilepsy Treatment in India: An Agent-Based Simulation Model." *Epilepsia.* (2016). Epub. doi:10.1111/epi.13294.

92. Mérelle, S. Y., Sorbi, M. J., van Doornen, L. J., & Passchier, J., (2008). "Lay Trainers with Migraine for a Home-based Behavioral Training: A 6-Month Follow-Up Study." *Headache. 48*(9), 1311–25.

93. Meyer, A. C., Dua, T., Ma, J., Saxena, S., & Birbeck, G., (2010). "Global Disparities in the Epilepsy Treatment Gap: A Systematic Review." *Bulletin of the World Health Organization. 88*(4), 260–266. doi:10.2471/BLT.09.064147.

94. Murray, C. J., Vos, T., Lozano, R., Naghavi, M., Flaxman A D., et al., (2012). "Disability-Adjusted Life Years (DALYs) for 291 Diseases and Injuries in 21 Regions, 1990–2010: A Systematic Analysis for the Global Burden of Disease Study (2010). " *The Lancet. 380*(9859), 2197–223. doi:10.1016/S0140-6736(12)61689-4.

95. Natoli, J. L., Manack, A., Dean, B., Butler, Q., Turkel C C., et al., (2010). "Global Prevalence of Chronic Migraine: A Systematic Review." *Cephalalgia. 30*(5), 599–609. doi:10.1111/j.1468-2982.2009.01941.x.

96. Neligan, A., Bell, G. S., Shorvon, S. D., & Sander, J. W., (2010). "Temporal Trends in the Mortality of People with Epilepsy: A Review." *Epilepsia. 51*(11), 2241–2246. doi:10.1111/j.1528-1167.2010.02711.x.

97. Newton, C. R., & Garcia, H. H., (2012). "Epilepsy in Poor Regions of the World." *The Lancet. 380*(9848), 1193–201. doi:10.1016/S0140-6736(12)61381-6.

98. Ngugi, A. K., Bottomley, C., Fegan, G., Chengo, E., Odhiambo, R., et al., (2014). "Premature Mortality in Active Convulsive Epilepsy in Rural Kenya: Causes and Associated Factors." *Neurology. 82*(7), 582–589. doi:10.1212/WNL.0000000000000123.

99. Ngugi, A. K., Bottomley, C., Kleinschmidt, I., Wagner, R. G., Kakooza-Mwesige, A., et al., (2013). "Prevalence of Active Convulsive Epilepsy in Sub-Saharan Africa and Associated Risk Factors: Cross-Sectional and Case-Control Studies." *The Lancet Neurology. 12*(3), 253–263. doi:10.1016/S1474-4422(13)70003-6.

100. Ngugi, A. K., Kariuki, S. M., Bottomley, C., Kleinschmidt, I., Sander J W., et al., (2011). "Incidence of Epilepsy: A Systematic Review and Meta-Analysis." *Neurology. 77*(10), 1005–12. doi:10.1212/WNL.0b013e31822cfc90.

101. Ornstein, K., Gaugler, J. E., Zahodne, L., & Stern, Y., (2014). "The Heterogeneous Course of Depressive Symptoms for the Dementia Caregiver." *International Journal of Aging and Human Development. 78*(2), 133–148.

102. Picard, C., Pasquier, F., Martinaud, O., Hannequin, D., & Godefroy, O., (2011). "Early Onset Dementia: Characteristics in a Large Cohort from Academic Memory Clinics." *Alzheimer Disease and Associated Disorders. 25*(3), 203–205. doi:10.1097/WAD.0b013e3182056be7.

103. Prince, M. J., Wu, F., Guo, Y., Robledo L M Gutierrez, O'Donnell, M., et al., (2015). "The Burden of Disease in Older People and Implications for Health Policy and Practice." *The Lancet. 385*(9967), 549–562. doi:10.1016/S0140-6736(14)61347-7.

104. Prince, M., Acosta, D., Chiu, H., Scazufca, M., Varghese, M., et al., (2003). "Dementia Diagnosis in Developing Countries: A Cross-Cultural Validation Study." *The Lancet. 361*(9361), 909–917.

105. Prince, M., Albanese, E., Guerchet, M., & Prina, M., (2014). World Alzheimer's Report (2014). Dementia *and Risk Reduction: An Analysis of Protective and Modifiable Factors.* London: Alzheimer's Disease International.

106. Rabbie, R., Derry, S., & Moore, R. A., (2013). "Ibuprofen with or without an Antiemetic for Acute Migraine Headaches in Adults." *Cochrane Database of Systematic Reviews, 4,* CD008039. doi:10.1002/14651858.CD008039.pub3.

107. Reitz, C., Brayne, C., & Mayeux, R., (2011). "Epidemiology of Alzheimer Disease." Nature Reviews *Neurology. 7*(3), 137–152. doi:10.1038/nrneurol.2011.2.

108. Richardson, T. J., Lee, S. J., Berg-Weger, M., & Grossberg, G. T., (2013). "Caregiver Health: Health of Caregivers of Alzheimer's and Other Dementia Patients." *Current Psychiatry Reports. 15*(7), 367. doi:10.1007/s11920-013-0367-2.

109. Schiller, Y., & Najjar, Y., (2008). "Quantifying the Response to Antiepileptic Drugs: Effect of Past Treatment History." *Neurology. 70*(1), 54–65. doi:10.1212/01.wnl.0000286959.22040.6e.

110. Selwood, A., Johnston, K., Katona, C., Lyketsos, C., & Livingston, G., (2007). "Systematic Review of the Effect of Psychological Interventions on Family Caregivers of People with Dementia. *Journal of Affective Disorders. 101*(1–3), 75–89.

111. Semah, F., Picot, M. C., Adam, C., Broglin, D., Arzimanoglou, A., et al., (1998). "Is the Underlying Cause of Epilepsy a Major Prognostic Factor for Recurrence?" *Neurology. 51*(5), 1256–62.

112. Silberstein, S. D., Holland, S., Freitag, F., Dodick, D. W., Argoff, C., & Ashman, E., (2012). "Quality Standards Subcommittee of the American Academy of Neurology and the American Headache Society. Evidence-Based Guideline Update: Pharmacologic Treatment for Episodic Migraine Prevention in Adults: Report of the Quality Standards Subcommittee of the American Academy of Neurology and the American Headache Society." *Neurology. 78*(17), 1337–45. doi:10.1212/WNL.0b013e3182535d20.

113. Sköldunger, A., Johnell, K., Winblad, B., & Wimo, A., (2013). "Mortality and Treatment Costs Have a Great Impact on the Cost-Effectiveness of Disease Modifying Treatment in Alzheimer's Disease: A Simulation Study." *Current Alzheimer Research. 10*(2), 207–216.

114. Steiner, T. J., Antonaci, F., Jensen, R., Lainez M J A, Lanteri-Minet, M., et al., (2011). "Recommendations for Headache Service Organisation and Delivery in Europe." *Journal of Headache Pain. 12*(4), 419–426.

115. Steiner, T. J., Birbeck, G. L., Jensen, R. H., Katsarava, Z., Stovner, L. J., & Martelletti, P., (2015). "Headache Disorders Are Third Cause of Disability Worldwide." *Journal of Headache Pain 6*, 58. doi:10.1186/s10194-015-0544-2.

116. Steiner, T. J., & Martelletti, P., (2007). "Aids for Management of Common Headache Disorders in Primary Care." *Journal of Headache Pain* (Suppl. 1), S2.

117. Steiner, T. J., Paemeleire, K., Jensen, R., Valade, D., Savi, L., et al., (2007). "European Principles of Management of Common Headache Disorders in Primary Care." *Journal of Headache Pain. 8*(Suppl. 1), S3–47.

118. Stovner, L., Hagen, K., Jensen, R., Katsarava, Z., Lipton, R., et al., (2007). "The Global Burden of Headache: A Documentation of Headache Prevalence and Disability Worldwide." *Cephalalgia. 27*(3), 193–210.

119. Tam-Tham, H., Cepoiu-Martin, M., Ronksley, P. E., Maxwell, C. J., & Hemmelgarn, B. R., (2013). "Dementia Case Management and Risk of Long-Term Care Placement: A Systematic Review and Meta-Analysis." *International Journal of Geriatric Psychiatry. 28*(9), 889–902.

120. Tan, L., Tan, L., Wang, H. F., Wang, J., Tan C C., et al., (2015). "Efficacy and Safety of Atypical Antipsychotic Drug Treatment for Dementia: A Systematic Review and Meta-Analysis." *Alzheimer's Research and Therapy. 7*(1), 20. doi:10.1186/s13195-015-0102-9.

121. Tanner, J. A., Black, B. S., Johnston, D., Hess, E., Leoutsakos J M., et al., (2015). "A Randomized Controlled Trial of a Community-Based Dementia Care Coordination Intervention: Effects of MIND at Home on Caregiver Outcomes." *American Journal of Geriatric Psychiatry. 23*(4), 391–402. doi:10.1016/j.jagp.2014.08.00.

122. Van Mierlo, L. D., Meiland, F. J., Roest H G Van der, Droes, R. M., (2012). "Personalised Caregiver Support: Effectiveness of Psychosocial Interventions in Subgroups of Caregivers of People with Dementia." *International Journal of Psychiatry. 27*(1), 1–14. doi:10.1002/gps.2694. Epub (2011).

123. Vos, T., Flaxman, A. D., Naghavi, M., Lozano, R., Michaud, C., et al., (2012). "Years Lived with Disability (YLDs) for 1160 Sequelae of 289 Diseases and Injuries 1990–2010: A Systematic Analysis for the Global Burden of Disease Study (2010). " *The Lancet. 380*(9859), 2163–2196. doi:10.1016/S0140-6736(12)61729-2.

124. Westergaard, M. L., Hansen, E. H., Glümer, C., Olessen, J., & Jensen, R. H., (2014). "Definitions of Medication-Overuse Headache in Healthy Lifestyle Behaviour and Stress in Chronic Headache: Results from a Population-Based Studies and Their Implications in Prevalence Estimates: A Systematic Review." *Cephalalgia 34*, 409–425.

125. WHO (World Health Organization). (2004). *Atlas: Country Resources for Neurological Disorders.* Geneva: WHO.

126. WHO (World Health Organization). (2006). *Neurological Disorders: Public Health Challenges.* Geneva: WHO.

127. WHO (World Health Organization). (2009a). *Report of the WHO Expert Consultation on Foodborne Trematode Infections and Taeniasis/Cysticercosis.* Geneva: WHO.

128. WHO (World Health Organization). (2009b). *mhGAP Intervention Guide for Mental, Neurological, and Substance Use Disorders in Non-Specialized Health Settings.* Geneva: WHO.

129. WHO (World Health Organization). (2011). *Lifting the Burden: The Global Campaign to Reduce the Burden of Headache*. Geneva: WHO.

130. WHO (World Health Organization). (2012). *Dementia-A Public Health Priority*. Geneva: WHO.

131. WHO (World Health Organization). (2015). *First WHO Ministerial Conference on Global Action Against Dementia.* Geneva: WHO.

132. Wiebe, S., & Jette, N., (2012). "Pharmacoresistance and the Role of Surgery in Difficult to Treat Epilepsy." *Nature Reviews. Neurology. 8*(12), 669–677. doi:10.1038/nrneurol.2012.181.

133. Wimo, A., Winblad, B., Stoffler, A., Wirth, Y., & Mobius, H. J., (2003). "Resource Utilisation and Cost Analysis of Memantine in Patients with Moderate to Severe Alzheimer's Disease." *Pharmacoeconomics. 21*(5), 327–350.

134. Wohlgemut, J., Dewey, C., Levy, M., & Mutua, F., (2010). "Evaluating the Efficacy of Teaching Methods Regarding Prevention of Human Epilepsy Caused by Taenia Solium Neurocysticercosis in Western Kenya." *American Journal of Tropical Medicine and Hygiene. 82*(4), 634–642. doi:10.4269/ajtmh.2010.09-0404.

135. Wong, C. L., Bansback, N., Lee, P. E., & Anis, A. H., (2009). "Cost-Effectiveness: Cholinesterase Inhibitors and Memantine in Vascular Dementia." *Canadian Journal of Neurological Sciences. 36*(6), 735–739.

136. Woods, B., Aguirre, E., Spector, A. E., & Orrell, M., (2012). "Cognitive Stimulation to Improve Cognitive Functioning in People with Dementia." *Cochrane Database of Systematic Reviews 2*, CD005562. PubMed PMID: 22336813.

137. Woods, B., Spector, A., Jones, C., Orrell, M., & Davies, S., (2005). "Reminiscence Therapy for Dementia." *Cochrane Database of Systematic Reviews, 2*, CD001120.

138. Yu, S. Y., Lee, T. J., Jang, S. H., Han, J. W., Kim, T. H., & Kim, K. W., (2015). "Cost-Effectiveness of Nationwide Opportunistic Screening Program for Dementia in South Korea." *Journal of Alzheimer's Disease. 44*(1), 195–204. doi:10.3233/JAD-141632.

139. Yu, S., Zhang, M., Zhou, J., Liu, R., Wan, Q., & Li, Y., (2014). "Headache Care in China." *Headache 54,* 601–609.

INDEX

A

B

C

D

E

F

G

H

I

J

K

L

M

N

O

P

FSC
www.fsc.org
MIX
Papier | Fördert
gute Waldnutzung
FSC® C083411

Kolibri 360 GmbH
Ferdinand-Jühlke-Straße 7
99095 Erfurt, Deutschland
produktsicherheit@kolibri360.de